THE MANY FACES OF HEALTH, COMPETENCE AND WELL-BEING IN OLD AGE

The Many Faces of Health, Competence and Well-Being in Old Age

Integrating Epidemiological, Psychological and Social Perspectives

Edited by

HANS-WERNER WAHL
German Centre for Research on Ageing, University of Heidelberg, Germany

HERMANN BRENNER
German Centre for Research on Ageing, University of Heidelberg, Germany

HEIDRUN MOLLENKOPF
German Centre for Research on Ageing, University of Heidelberg, Germany

DIETRICH ROTHENBACHER
German Centre for Research on Ageing, University of Heidelberg, Germany

and

CHRISTOPH ROTT
German Centre for Research on Ageing, University of Heidelberg, Germany

Springer

A C.I.P. Catalogue record for this book is available from the Library of Congress.

ISBN-10 1-4020-4137-3 (HB)
ISBN-13 978-1-4020-4137-2 (HB)
ISBN-10 1-4020-4138-1 (e-book)
ISBN-13 978-1-4020-4138-9 (e-book)

Published by Springer,
P.O. Box 17, 3300 AA Dordrecht, The Netherlands.

www.springer.com

Printed on acid-free paper

Printed in the Netherlands.

CONTENTS

INTRODUCTION

Hans-Werner Wahl, Hermann Brenner, Heidrun Mollenkopf,
Dietrich Rothenbacher and Christoph Rott

Ageing research has been identified as a prototypical field of inquiry deserving the full exploitation of single discipline approaches and interdisciplinary synergies amongst these single perspectives. Although this is a generally accepted insight, there still is a strong need to provide models of how this global and most fundamental challenge can be dealt with. It seems in any case necessary to narrow down the wide scope of ageing research issues to sets of key constructs most promising in terms of interdisciplinary cross-fertilisation. Against this, the major aim of the book is to provide a comprehensive treatment of one well-selected set of key issues of recent ageing research, i.e. health, competence and well-being. In addition, the book's ambition is to identify priorities for future ageing research and to further new avenues for interdisciplinary approaches and social policy applications.

The substance of the book is based on an international conference which took place on June 18 and 19, 2004 in Heidelberg, Germany. Framed within the array of health, competence and well-being perspectives in ageing research, the idea of the conference was to provide an integrated presentation of findings generated in the German Centre for Research on Ageing at the University of Heidelberg (Deutsches Zentrum für Alternsforschung, DZFA). The centre's three departments, i.e. the Department of Epidemiology, the Department of Social and Environmental Gerontology and the Department of Adult Development, are particularly prone to contribute significantly to the issues of health, competence and well-being. In addition, a substantial number of world-known ageing researchers was asked to comment on the centre's contributions.

In this book, the major conference contributions have been compiled to address the attention of a wide scholarly audience in gerontology and life-span research. More specifically, the book aims to treat the key constructs—health, competence and well-being—on converging research streams which seldom have come to a joint venture in the ageing research literature. First, social-ecological research starts from the insight that major processes and outcomes of ageing such as day-to-day competence are shaped by social and physical-spatial environments. Second, geropsychology research is mainly driven by a life-span developmental conception of ageing and deals with core issues such as personality and the ageing mind. Third, epidemiology offers by its descriptive and analytic approach fundamental disease, function and prevention related data able to underfeed and complement the "normal ageing" perspective, which strongly informs social and behavioural ageing research.

Each of the three major research directions is outlined by a short introduction. Then, three contributions treating in an empirical manner key research questions related to each of these constructs are presented followed by respective commentary papers written by international experts. Besides, two papers revealing still more directly the potential synergies of combing the three research approaches and a respective discussion paper build a major section of the book. In the final part of the book, still another level of reflection on the book's contents is purposefully introduced based on the input of two outstanding policy-oriented ageing researchers, who are raising issues critical for the application of future ageing research in societal and political (specifically European) contexts.

Finally, in the appendix, the abstracts of the rich set of posters, which also have been presented during the conference by young scholars, have been included.

We hope that this book will convey the spirit of interdisciplinarity in ageing research, which was lively present and further developed during the conference, to a wide scholarly audience of researchers who were unable to attend, and that the book may further stimulate interdisciplinarity in a research field that is rapidly growing in importance in all parts of the world.

This book could not have been completed without the help and contribution of many helpful minds and hands. While it is not possible to specifically name all of them here, we would like to express, at the very least, our special thanks to the speakers and many discussants from the large and distinguished audience for their stimulating contributions to the conference, Ursula Kloé, Marion DeMille and Andreas Sokoll for ensuring the smooth running of the conference, Ursula König for professional compilation and Jan Cargile for proofreading of the papers, Welmoed Spahr and Marianna Pascale for their support from Springer Verlag, and last but not least, The German Federal Ministry for Family, Senior Citizens, Women and Youth for generous financial support.

PART I

FOCUSING ON SOCIAL-ECOLOGICAL RESEARCH—CONTRIBUTIONS TO HEALTH, COMPETENCE, AND WELL-BEING IN OLD AGE

HANS-WERNER WAHL

INTRODUCTION: THE PERSON–ENVIRONMENT PERSPECTIVE IN AGEING RESEARCH

The person–environment perspective in ageing research, frequently coined environmental gerontology, draws upon the idea that old age is a period of adult development profoundly influenced and shaped by the environment. Because age-related losses in vision, mobility, and cognitive capacity have a direct impact on the relationship between the organism and the environment, the older person is particularly vulnerable to environmental demands. In other words, this research paradigm views contextual factors as crucial determinants of everyday behaviour and well-being in later life.

From its inception, environmental gerontology has placed strong emphasis on enhancing the theoretical understanding of person–environment relations as people age (see Scheidt & Windley, 1998; Wahl, 2001; Wahl, Scheidt, & Windley, 2004; Wahl & Weisman, 2003). This is important because there was (and still is) a tendency in the gerontology scholarly work to "de-contexualise" human ageing from the environment, that is, from those day-to-day surroundings in which a person's ageing actually takes place. Also, environmental gerontology has focussed in particular on the physical and spatial component of the context of ageing, while concurrently acknowledging the close links between physical, social, and cultural environments.

The "Gestalt switch" from ageing persons to ageing person–environment systems has come in historical terms by no means accidentally; it has taken not only one, but a diversity of theoretical avenues, and yet a clear need to develop and refine existing conceptualisations remains. A rising interest in environmental gerontology and its related theories emerged from the Chicago School of Urban Sociology during the 1920s and 1930s (e.g. Park, Burgess, & McKenzie, 1925). Man-made environments such as run-down urban districts were regarded explicitly and for the first time as detrimental to man's existence, health, and welfare. In the 1930s and 1940s, the theoretical writings of the German psychologist Lewin (e.g. Lewin, 1951 for an overview) promoted the insight that behaviour should be regarded as a function of both the person and the environment, while greatly influencing the development of contextual thinking in the behavioural and social sciences. During the same historical period, Murray (1938), the American personality researcher, introduced the term "press" as an indication that external forces impact both the objectively and subjectively perceived levels of personal growth.

A more proximal influence on the development of environmental perspectives in gerontology was provided by the fast growing role of social science impulses within gerontology by the end of the 1940s, setting the stage for the new field of social gerontology (Tibbitts, 1960). In addition to the traditionally strong consideration of biology and medical conditions, factors such as economic circumstances, family and

H. W. Wahl et al. (eds.), The Many Faces of Health, Competence and Well-Being in Old Age, 3–6.

social surroundings, housing and neighborhood quality (to name just a few such social influences) were each acknowledged as able to shape ageing, in many respects, similarly to changing bodily functions. Finally, the emergence of environmental psychology in the 1960s and 1970s provided yet another set of proximal roots for environmental gerontology. Because of the assumed vulnerability of the ageing organism for environmental demand, as well as the existence of specially designed environments for ageing people (such as long-term care institutions), old age has been an attractive area for environmental psychology since its inception (e.g. Pastalan & Carson, 1970). This provided another major cue toward the development of environmental gerontology by the end of the 1960s.

Main theoretical approaches still actively used in environmental gerontology are as follows: In the *press–competence model* suggested by Lawton and Nahemow (1973) with direct referral to Murray (1938) and Lewin (1951), a major assumption is that it is the lowered competence of the older person in conjunction with high "environmental press" which negatively impacts behaviour and well-being. In still earlier conceptual and empirical work (Lawton & Simon, 1968), the term *Environmental Docility Hypothesis* has been coined to address this basic mechanism in person–environment relations as people age. For example, early empirical research (Lawton & Simon, 1968) revealed to what degree social interaction patterns of elders in institutional settings depend on physical distances; longer distances were found to more strongly undermine social relations, thus pointing to the "environmental docility" of the older organism. The press–competence model purposely takes a more a general approach, thus allowing both "environmental press" and "competence" to be filled with various content such as sensory loss, loss in physical mobility, or cognitive decline (competence), as well as low housing standard, bad neighbourhood conditions, or underdeveloped public transport, among other out-of-home mobility concerns (environmental press). Also, behaviour can mean basic functioning in day-to-day life (such as dressing or washing) or leisure involvement; well-being echoes positive and negative affect as well as cognitive evaluations such as satisfaction with life.

The *person–environment fit model* has strongly underlined the role of motivation within person–environment processes as people age. The basic assumption is that misfits between given needs and given environmental options to fulfil these needs are linked to lowered behavioural functioning and well-being. Empirical support for this assumption has been reported from studies conducted specifically in institutional settings (Kahana, 1982). Carp and Carp (1984), which suggested a greater differentiation of the person–environment fit model in distinguishing between older persons' basic and higher-order needs in their relation to both the potential and the limits of a given environment. While person–environment misfit in the basic need domain will predominantly result in reduced behavioural autonomy, misfit in the higher-order realm will predominantly undermine emotional well-being and mental health.

In contrast to the foregoing approaches that point mostly to the role of the objective environment, *place attachment concepts* address the gamut of processes operating when ageing individuals form affective, cognitive, and behavioural ties to their physical–spatial surroundings (Oswald & Wahl, 2003; Rubinstein & Parmelee, 1992). Place attachment-related concepts may be reflected in the strength of such bonding, as well as in different meaning facets associated with places, such as home environments or specific landscapes. One approach suggested by Rowles (1983) has focussed on the many faces of insideness of places in old age. Whereas *social insideness* arises from everyday social exchange over long periods of time, *physical insideness* is characterised by familiarities and routines within given settings such as the home environment. A third element of PA is labelled as *autobiographical insideness*. In the words of Rowles (1983): "Place becomes a landscape of memories, providing a sense of identity." (p. 114).

Besides these classic environmental gerontology approaches, person–environment perspectives in ageing research also deserve a broader view, drawing particularly from *social science and ageing conceptual thinking*; ageing is seen as depending on societal conditions, providing person–environment constellations of equality as well as inequality. In addition, person–environment constellations echoed in housing and outdoor mobility options, for example, also reflect social indicator shaping processes and outcomes of ageing.

The three contributions of the book that address person–environment perspectives are each anchored in the conceptual network as described in this introduction. Further, all three papers strive to strengthen the empirical basis of these theoretical perspectives based on the re-consideration and reframing of classic research themes of environmental gerontology, new research paradigms and methodological avenues. The paper by Oswald et al. focuses on the issue of housing in old and very old age, driven mainly by a behavioural science perspective on ageing. Special emphasis is put on the conceptual and empirical argument that assessment tools that address both objective and subjective person–environment relations are needed in order to better understand the basic dynamics and variations in "ageing in place" processes. The Mollenkopf et al. paper adds to this by broadening the scope of person–environment relations to out-of-home mobility issues from a European perspective. The impetus of this work comes from a sociology of ageing perspective and is thus a more meso to macro view on person–environment interchange. Finally, the paper of Wahl et al. uses the research paradigm of age-related vision loss as a means to examine environmental vulnerabilities as people age.

AFFILIATION

German Centre for Research on Ageing at the University of Heidelberg

REFERENCES

Carp, F. M., & Carp, A. (1984). A complementary/congruence model of well-being or mental health for the community elderly. In I. Altman, M. P. Lawton, & J. F. Wohlwill (Eds.), *Human behavior and environment: Vol. 7. Elderly people and the environment* (pp. 279–336). New York: Plenum Press.

Kahana, E. (1982). A congruence model of person–environment interaction. In M. P. Lawton, P. G. Windley, & T. O. Byerts (Eds.), *Aging and the environment: Theoretical approaches* (pp. 97–121). New York: Springer.

Lawton, M. P., & Nahemow, L. (1973). Ecology and the aging process. In C. Eisdorfer & M. P. Lawton (Eds.), *The psychology of adult development and aging* (pp. 619–674). Washington, DC: American Psychological Association.

Lawton, M. P., & Simon, B. B. (1968). The ecology of social relationships in housing for the elderly. *The Gerontologist, 8,* 108–115.

Lewin, K. (1951). *Field theory in social science.* New York: Harper.

Murray, H. A. (1938). *Explorations in personality: A clinical and experimental study of fifty men of college age.* Oxford: Oxford University Press.

Oswald, F., & Wahl, H.-W. (2003). Place attachment across the life span. In J. R. Miller, R. M. Lerner, L. B. Schiamberg, & P. M. Anderson (Eds.), *Human ecology: An encyclopedia of children, families, communities, and environments* (Vol. 2, pp. 568–572). Santa Barbara, CA: ABC-Clio Press.

Park, R. E., Burgess, E. W., & McKenzie, R. D. (1925). *The city.* Chicago: Chicago University Press.

Pastalan, L. A., & Carson, D. H. (Eds.). (1970). *Spatial behavior of older people.* The University of Michigan: Institute of Gerontology.

Rowles, G. D. (1983). Geographical dimensions of social support in rural Appalachia. In G. D. Rowles & R. J. Ohta (Eds.), *Aging and milieu: Environmental perspectives on growing old* (pp. 111–130). New York: Academic Press.

Rubinstein, R. L., & Parmelee, P. A. (1992). Attachment to place and representation of life course by the elderly. In I. Altman & S. M. Low (Eds.), *Human behavior and environment: Vol. 12. Place attachment* (pp. 139–163). New York: Plenum Press.

Scheidt, R. J., & Windley, P. G. (Eds.). (1998). *Environment and aging theory: A focus on housing.* Westport, CT: Greenwood Press.

Tibbitts, C. (Ed.). (1960). *Handbook of social gerontology: Societal aspects of aging.* Chicago: University of Chicago Press.

Wahl, H.-W. (2001). Environmental influences on aging and behavior. In J. E. Birren & K. W. Schaie (Eds.), *Handbook of the psychology of aging* (5th ed., pp. 215–237). San Diego: Academic Press.

Wahl, H.-W., Scheidt, R., & Windley, P. G. (Eds.). (2004). *Aging in context: Socio-physical environments* (Annual Review of Gerontology and Geriatrics, 2003). New York: Springer.

Wahl, H.-W., & Weisman, J. (2003). Environmental gerontology at the beginning of the new millennium: Reflections on its historical, empirical, and theoretical development. *The Gerontologist, 43*, 616–627.

FRANK OSWALD, HANS-WERNER WAHL, DÖRTE NAUMANN, HEIDRUN MOLLENKOPF and ANNETTE HIEBER

THE ROLE OF THE HOME ENVIRONMENT IN MIDDLE AND LATE ADULTHOOD

1. AGEING AND THE HOME ENVIRONMENT: TOWARDS AN INTEGRATIVE THEORETICAL FRAMEWORK

Human development over the life span is characterised by person–environment (p–e) exchange processes (Bronfenbrenner, 1999), covering subjective experiences as well as objective behaviour. In order to address the complexity of ageing in place from a predominantly psychological point of view, a conceptual framework that emphasises two processes of p–e exchange in later life is suggested, and integrates many of the theoretical approaches offered in the field in the last decades. These processes are labelled "belonging" and "agency" (Oswald & Wahl, 2004; Wahl & Lang, 2003; Wahl & Oswald, 2004, in press) (Figure 1). Processes of belonging account for the full range of subjective experiences, while processes of agency emphasise the full range of objective behaviours. Having experienced life-long bonding to certain places in later life, processes of belonging are based on the increasing amount of environmental experience, leading to subjective evaluation and interpretation of places, allocation of meaning, as well as to cognitive and emotional representation and place attachment. Processes of agency, in contrast, deal with behaviour in relation to passive and active use, compensation, adaptation, retrofitting and creation of places, which are especially important in old age because of the decrease in functional capacity and behavioural flexibility. Both processes are considered to be particularly important for p–e exchange in the immediate home environment. The home becomes more relevant to people as they age, due to the increased time older people spend at home, as well as the many activities that take place at home (Baltes, Maas, Wilms, & Borchelt, 1999).

Thus, the research programme underlying this work is driven by the basic assumption that processes of housing-related belonging and processes of housing-related agency are two fundamental processes of ageing in place. However, both types of processes are not considered independent from each other in everyday life. Furthermore, we would argue that processes of p–e exchange are related to housing-related outcome variables. Two types of outcomes are introduced by way of dichotomisation into housing-related identity and housing-related autonomy. As far as the ageing self at home is concerned, a major goal in later life is to maintain identity and personality—as far as the ageing body is concerned, a major goal is to remain independent at home for as long as possible. To reach both aims, processes of housing-related agency and belonging are assumed to be instrumental. Finally, we argue that both outcomes are

H. W. Wahl et al. (eds.), The Many Faces of Health, Competence and Well-Being in Old Age, 7–24.

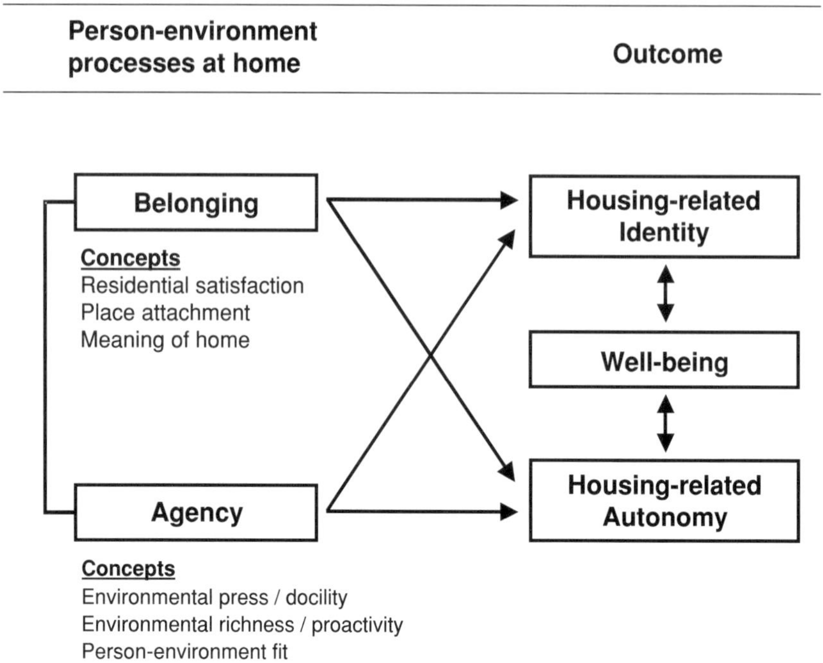

Figure 1. A conceptual framework on housing in later life.

related to subjective well-being and healthy ageing at large. Based on concepts from developmental psychology and environmental gerontology, both types of p–e processes and outcomes are introduced next.

1.1. Processes of Housing-Related Belonging

Processes of belonging are based on concepts and theories on *residential satisfaction* (Aragonés, Francescato, & Gärling, 2002; Galster, 1987; Pinquart & Burmedi, 2004; Weideman & Anderson, 1985), addressing, for instance, varieties in subjective global evaluations of the home due to age or geographic location, as well as the relation of residential satisfaction and life satisfaction. Often, residential satisfaction is assessed by single-item self-evaluations (Oswald, Wahl, Mollenkopf, & Schilling, 2003). Theories on *place attachment* and identity (Altman & Low, 1992; Hidalgo & Hernadez, 2001; Neisser, 1988; Proshansky, Fabian, & Kaminoff, 1983; Stedman, 2002) emphasise domains of belonging in a more differentiated way. Other than residential satisfaction evaluations, place attachment is not only related to attitudinal components of the home, but to aspects of physical, social and personal bonding on behavioural, cognitive and emotional levels, which are often assessed by global attachment evaluations, e.g. on indoor versus outdoor place attachment (Oswald, Hieber, Wahl, & Mollenkopf, 2005).

Furthermore, concepts of the individual *meaning of home* deal with the outcomes of place attachment processes in great detail. Since older adults have often lived a long period of time in the same residence, cognitive and emotional aspects of the meaning of home are often strongly linked to biography, but independent from housing satisfaction or objective housing conditions. Such links may become manifest through processes of reflecting on the past, symbolically represented in certain places and cherished objects within the home. Thus, one characteristic of belonging is to address non-goal-oriented cognitive and emotional bonding. It also covers behavioural bonding at home, where familiarity and routines have been developed over time. This insight is based on many (mostly qualitative) empirical studies (Feldman, 1990, 1996; Lalli, 1992; Proshansky et al., 1983; Relph, 1976; Rowles, 1983; Rubinstein, 1989; Rubinstein & Parmelee, 1992; Sixsmith, 1986; Sixsmith & Sixsmith, 1991; Tuan, 1980; Zingmark, Norberg, & Sandman, 1995), leading to a categorization of domains of meaning, covering physical, behavioural, cognitive, emotional and social aspects (Oswald & Wahl, in press). Further processes of belonging are related to specific psychological mechanisms, such as housing-related internal and external control belief strategies (Oswald, Wahl, Martin, & Mollenkopf, 2003) or perceived usability of areas of the home environment (Fänge & Iwarsson, 2003).

One major assumption drawn from the literature with regard to these non-goal-directed processes of housing-related belonging in old age is that belonging mainly contributes to housing-related identity (Born, 2002; Neisser, 1988). As social geographer Rowles has put it: processes of place attachment and allocation of meaning (of home) reflect different patterns of physical, autobiographical and social "insideness" as a result of the long duration of living in the same place (Rowles, 1983). "Place becomes a landscape of memories, providing a sense of identity (. . .)" (Rowles, 1983, p. 114; see also Rowles & Watkins, 2003). For instance, people often perceive the risk of losing their homes (especially in very old age or when suffering from competence loss) as closely related to the risk of losing crucial parts of their selves, characterized by their way of ageing in place. However, we would argue that although the focus is on non-goal-oriented cognitive and emotional bonding, processes of belonging are also instrumental in daily life as the home is cognitively represented "inside" the person. For instance, perceiving oneself as active and judging housing-related behaviour as important can trigger one's everyday routines, activities and organisation, and thus, be a resource for housing-related autonomy (Rowles, Oswald, & Hunter, 2004).

1.2. Processes of Housing-Related Agency

As people age, it is argued that the home serves to compensate for the reduced functional capacity of the ageing individual, especially when suffering from competence loss or of functional capacities. To maintain independence and to avoid institutionalisation, either environmental changes (e.g. moving) or purposeful behavioural adaptations (e.g. retrofitting) must occur (e.g. Lawton, 1977; Scheidt & Windley, 1985; Wahl, 2001). Processes of agency are based on concepts and theories, derive from "*environmental docility hypothesis*" and the "ecological theory of ageing" (ETA) (Lawton, 1982,

1987; Lawton & Nahemow, 1973; Nahemow, 2000). The main assumption, that as people age their capacity to behaviourally adapt to existing environmental press decreases overall, is due to an increasing number of functional limitations. Thus, older people in general need to react to environmental press in order to remain independent (Lawton & Nahemow, 1973). The related "ETA" describes behaviour and affect as a function of the level of personal competence and environmental press (Lawton, 1982, 1989, 1998; Nahemow, 2000). Behavioural adaptation in that sense is reduced to docile reactions on existing circumstances. In extension of this model, "*environmental proactivity hypothesis*" assumes that older adults are not simply pawns in their environment, but can proactively change housing conditions according to their own wishes and needs in order to maintain independence, allowing older adults to cope with environmental press and to profit from environmental richness (Lawton, 1985, 1989).

One facet of environmental behaviour in regard to both environmental docility and proactivity is to optimise environmental control at home by ways of "environmental centralisation" (Rubinstein & Parmelee, 1992). Observational data have shown a recurring tendency for environmental centralisation, especially around the most favoured places at home and especially when people suffer from competence loss. People arrange essential things as well as subjectively important objects around them, which enables them to reach everything from one place. Further characteristics of the favoured place are a good view into different directions (window, entrance) and remote controls for several functions (door opener, TV). This offers adaptive potential in maintaining and enhancing competence in the immediate environment and thus, through a process of miniaturisation, establishing "control centres" or "living centres" (Lawton, 1985; Oswald & Wahl, 2005; Rubinstein & Parmelee, 1992).

As opposed to small-scale indoor environmental centralisation, one of the most radical types of housing-related agency is relocation, for instance, moving from one home to another. Addressing the underlying motivation to move in a differentiated way may serve to detect the extent to which older people move in order to cope with increasing environmental press or to proactively benefit from environmental richness (Oswald & Rowles, in press). Further theoretical concepts address the level of individual congruence or incongruence on several domains of p–e exchange, e.g. in the "congruence model of p–e fit" (Kahana, 1982) and the "complementary/congruence model" (Carp & Carp, 1984). A critical message inherent in "*p–e fit*" concepts is that the level of behavioural competence in a certain domain corresponds with the given level of environmental press (e.g. barriers at home), leading to adaptation (fit) versus maladaptation (misfit). It is argued that the equilibrium between individual competence and environmental press is especially unstable in very old age, as adaptation capacities decrease. One example of p–e fit in this regard is the correspondence of housing-related subjective needs and objective circumstances leading to p–e fit indices on different domains of housing (Oswald et al., 2005). Another example is the correspondence of functional limitations with environmental barriers at home leading to certain degrees of housing accessibility as an indicator for p–e fit (Iwarsson & Slaug, 2001).

One major assumption to be drawn from the literature with regard to these goal-directed processes of housing-related agency in old age is that processes of agency mainly contribute to housing-related autonomy, for instance, by compensating with barriers at home when faced with functional limitations by means of environmental adaptation or centralisation (Lawton, 1985; Nahemow, 2000) or by relocation. However, we would argue that although the focus is to maintain autonomy, processes of agency also address aspects of the ageing self at home, for instance, by establishing meaningful "living centres" instead of exclusive "control centres" (Rubinstein & Parmelee, 1992), or by moving to a new home based on higher-order needs, i.e. to fulfil personal wishes, and thus contribute to housing-related identity.

The overarching conceptual framework (Figure 1) has been instrumental in conducting a series of qualitative and quantitative studies, in which some portions of these omnibus concepts and relationships were the targets of analysis. However, from a broader perspective, environmental gerontology deals with concepts like adaptation as an example for a mixture of both p–e exchange processes (belonging and agency). Older people living at home and suffering from competence loss can adapt to environmental problems in terms of behavioural, cognitive and emotional adaptation (Wahl, Oswald, & Zimprich, 1999). They may objectively reduce their action range *and* subjectively re-evaluate their interior spaces as more valuable in contrast to the outdoor environment which is no longer accessible to them. Thus, adaptation to the home environment in later life does not just refer to the behaviour, but is symbolic in nature (Rubinstein & De Medeiros, 2004).

1.3. Basic Research Questions

Against the background of the conceptual framework, four major questions are addressed within the research program on housing in middle and late adulthood. In the first step, we want to further shed light on the processes of housing-related belonging by exploring residential satisfaction, place attachment and meaning of home. On a global level, we ask for residential satisfaction distribution among elders of different ages and in different geographic locations as well as for the relation of residential satisfaction and life satisfaction. Next, we ask for global indoor versus outdoor place attachment evaluations in middle and late adulthood in different urban settings. Finally, we ask for patterns of meaning of home in relation to functional competence. In the second step, processes of agency take centre stage. Emphasising the most important parts of the indoor environment, we ask for processes of environmental centralisation in relation to functional capacities at home. Next, on the opposite side of the scale of agency, we ask for the relation of moving from home to home and its underlying motivation. Finally, two examples of p–e fit are presented by asking for the correspondence of housing needs and housing conditions as well as for patterns of housing accessibility in different age groups and settings. In the third step, we ask for the relationship between processes of housing-related agency and belonging. And fourth, the question is, how are p–e processes of housing-related agency and belonging related to outcomes of housing-related identity and autonomy and well-being at large.

2. MAJOR FINDINGS OF OWN RESEARCH PROGRAM

First, selected findings from our own studies on processes of housing-related belonging are presented, followed second by processes of housing-related agency. Third, findings on the relationship of belonging and agency are presented. Fourth, results from studies on the relationship of housing-related agency/belonging and identity/autonomy are provided.

2.1. On the Variability of Processes of Housing-Related Belonging

2.1.1. Variety of Residential Satisfaction in Relation to Age and Living in Different Settings

As part of the Interdisciplinary Longitudinal Study on Adult Development ("ILSE"), external global expert ratings on residential satisfaction versus residential stress, based on a broad range of housing-related information, were assessed in semi-structured explorations (Oswald, Schmitt, Wahl, & Lang, 2004). A total of 898 individuals from East and West Germany (born 1950–1952 and 1930–1932, respectively) who participated at two measurement points (T1–T2: 4.1 years) were examined. One goal was to assess the variety of residential satisfaction evaluations among different age groups living in different settings (i.e. East versus West Germany after reunification). Another goal was to examine the role of home experience in relation to well-being in later life from a longitudinal perspective. Findings revealed higher residential satisfaction scores in the older age group compared to the younger cohort in both settings. As predicted, both the extent of residential satisfaction (level) and the amount of (mainly positive) changes in residential satisfaction over a period of 4 years (slope) had an impact on life satisfaction in middle and late adulthood in East and West Germany, whereas the number of objective environmental changes (e.g. retrofitting, relocation) had not (Oswald et al., 2004). The findings underpin the need to consider processes of belonging in ageing studies concerning those already in middle adulthood and inspire further investigation of belonging beyond satisfaction ratings.

2.1.2. Variety of Place Attachment in Relation to Age and Different Urban Settings

Processes of belonging in terms of global single-item self-evaluations on indoor versus outdoor place attachment were assessed in the study "Heidelberg 2002", with 365 older adults, aged 51–80 years, living in three different urban neighbourhoods. The concept of place attachment was introduced by means of explanation and a set of examples on different types of cognitive, emotional and behavioural bonding to the indoor and outdoor environment (Oswald et al., 2005). Whereas indoor place attachment ratings were comparable among participants of different age groups and from different neighbourhoods, outdoor place attachment differed due to age and urban setting. The older the participants, the stronger was outdoor place attachment, eventually reflecting an increase of belonging that was parallel to a decrease of alternative options, e.g. to move away. In other words, if you cannot move away you may prefer to stay in a neighbourhood that is considered a valuable place to live. Thus, high place attachment scores in very old age may contribute to a stable housing-related identity. However, there were also district differences in outdoor place attachment. Highest scores were reported in the rich and most scenic neighbourhood, whereas lowest scores were found in the poor and partially run-down district. In sum, the findings strengthen the link between housing-related belonging and identity and open the floor to further assess processes of belonging in a more detailed way, e.g. by assessing facets of meaning of home.

2.1.3. Variety of Meaning of Home in Relation to Functional Limitations in Old Age
The focus here was to identify domains of meaning of home and to examine meaning patterns among elders with different types of competence loss. It was assumed that the effect of environment-related competence losses in old age leads the individual to develop idiosyncratic meanings of home patterns. Data from the qualitative–quantitative study "PASA" with 126 healthy and severely impaired older adults between the ages of 61 and 92 revealed that individuals report different meaning patterns due to their health (Oswald & Wahl, 2001, 2005). One-third of the participants were in good health, one-third suffered from severe mobility impairment, and one-third were blind. Data are based on in-depth interviews that were tape-recorded, transcribed and categorised into five global categories (Oswald, 1996, 2003). The identified meaning of home categories were: (1) "physical", focusing on the experience of housing conditions such as experience of the residential area, access and furnishing; (2) "behavioural", related to the everyday behaviour of the person at home and to proactive ways of manipulating or rearranging items in the home; (3) "cognitive", representing statements of cognition, especially biographical bonding to the home, such as the experience of familiarity and insideness; (4) "emotional", expressing emotional bonding including the experience of privacy, safety, pleasure and stimulation; and (5) "social", consisting of statements that express relationships with fellow-lodgers, neighbours or visitors. Many of the non-goal-directed aspects of physical, autobiographical and social insideness were found within the meaning patterns of all participants, indicating a strong link between processes of belonging and housing-related identity. However, behavioural aspects of meaning, for instance, do not reflect observed behaviour in terms of agency at home but address the importance of the experience of agency, which is part of the process of housing-related belonging. Furthermore, there was a diversity of meanings in all groups of these community-dwelling participants, although these differences may be a consequence of individual health issues (Figure 2).

Concerning group differences, healthy participants were more appreciative of the physical location, access and amenity aspects of the home. Impaired participants emphasised the cognitive and biographical significance of the home. Concerning behavioural and social aspects, blind participants concentrated more on their social and cognitive sphere and less on behavioural and physical aspects of the home, while the meaning patterns of the mobility-impaired participants include behavioural aspects to a greater extent. About the same share of statements were made with regard to emotional themes in all three groups. In sum, cognitive and emotional aspects of home are important "non-observable" characteristics of belonging, particularly when suffering

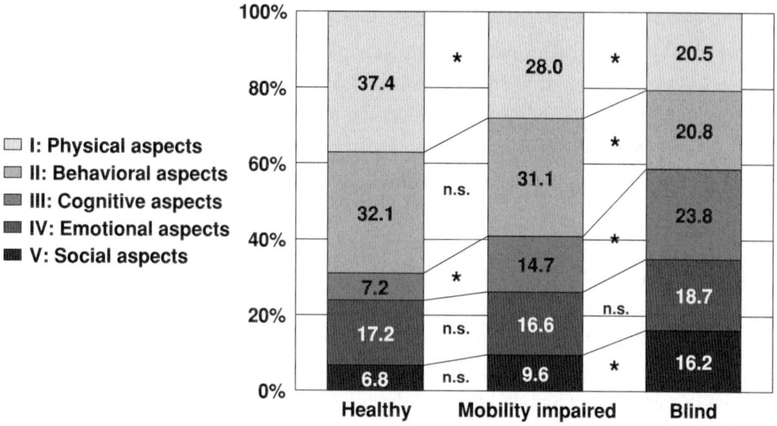

Figure 2. Relative frequencies of meaning of home domains for healthy, mobility impaired, and blind older adults. Note: Evaluation of verbal transcripts and tapes, based on 1,804 statements of N = 126 subjects. Mean number of statements per person amounted to 14.3. Multivariate MANOVA procedure for five domains was conducted to test differences between subgroups (Wilk's lambda = 0.707; F = 4.40 (10, 232); p < 0.05; explained variance: 29.3%). To show differences in detail, univariate simple contrasts were computed for each category between healthy and mobility impaired, as well as between mobility impaired and blind subjects. Reproduced from Oswald 2003, p. 138.*

from competence loss (Oswald, 2003) (Figure 2). The findings demonstrate the benefit of assessing processes of housing-related belonging in great detail to show differences between housing-related identity (e.g. by judging cognitive aspects of meaning as important) and housing-related autonomy (e.g. by judging housing-related behaviour as important) among elders suffering from different types of competence loss.

2.2. *On the Variability of Processes of Housing-Related Agency*

Three processes of housing-related agency are reported. Within the home environment, processes of environmental centralisation are regarded. Second, and in contrast, moving is considered from a motivational perspective with regard to the large scale of environmental agency. Third, facets of establishing p–e fit are introduced.

2.2.1. *Variety of Environmental Centralisation in Relation to Functional Capacities*

Within a sub-sample of healthy and mobility-impaired participants of the "PASA" study, persons were asked to identify their most favourite places at home and to give information on the length of stay as well as to show and report on their posture, line of sight, habits, as well as objects. It was assumed that particularly mobility-impaired older adults demonstrate high levels of environmental centralisation, especially in their most favourite places at home. Examples for those most favourite places and related objects and habits are given in Figure 3.

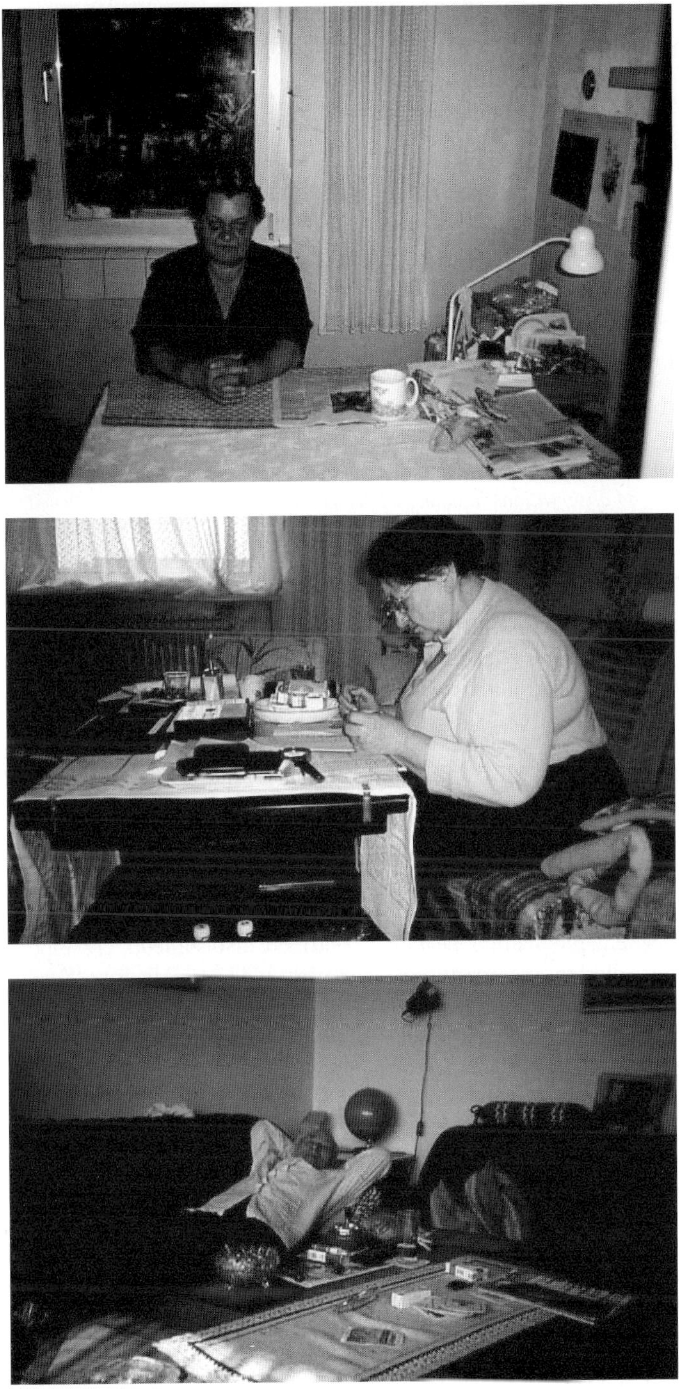

Figure 3. Environmental centralisation at home: some examples.

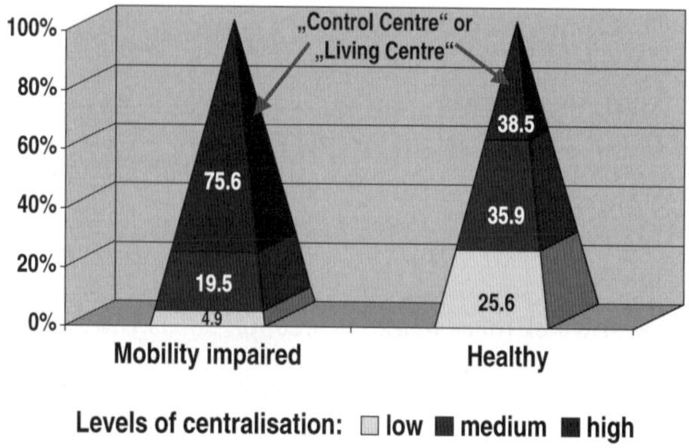

Figure 4. Environmental centralisation at home. Note: High level of centralisation: Single place ("control centre", remain seated); medium level of centralisation: Parts of a room (standing up from seat); low level of centralisation: One room (walking around). Data are based on 84 observations at home, 63–92 years old women and men (Oswald, 1996).

It was found that both mobility-impaired and healthy participants reported tendencies towards environmental centralisation. However, in accordance with our assumptions and former results (Lawton, 1985, 1989), mobility-impaired elders, more often than healthy elders, had high levels of centralisation and created "control centres" at home in terms of spatial extension and behaviour. Findings revealed that they both react to environmental press (docility hypothesis) and actively use environmental richness (proactivity hypothesis) in order to maximize control and autonomy, which seems to be especially effective when confronted with severe competence loss (Figure 4). In addition, qualitative analyses revealed that those places not only serve to enhance control but also reflect the individual biography, and thus contribute to housing-related identity ("living centres", Rubinstein & Parmelee, 1992). Participants mentioned not only essential things (e.g. medication, beverage, food), but also subjectively important objects (e.g. pictures, diaries, memorabilia), memories, plans and feelings for "providing a sense of identity" (Rowles, 1983). In sum, environmental centralisation, as one facet of agency, is instrumental in allowing older adults to maintain autonomy, especially when suffering from mobility impairments, although "living centres" also reflect an aggregation of the dweller's housing-related identity.

2.2.2. Variety of Motivation to Move From Home to Home

Another form of adaptive behaviour is voluntary moving (Oswald & Rowles, in press). The RELOKA study provides evidence on motivations for moving which involved a group of 217 older adults in Germany (60–89 years old) who moved from one home to another within the 3-year period immediately prior to being interviewed (Oswald, Schilling, Wahl, & Gäng, 2002). Using a combined qualitative and quantitative methodology, data on reasons for moving were obtained by assessing responses to open-ended questions supplemented by more in-depth probing of each of the motivating factors identified by the participants. The study differentiated between content (e.g. person, physical environment, social environment) and level of need-related motivations (basic needs, higher-order needs; Carp & Carp, 1984). Basic needs reflect maintenance of personal autonomy with respect to necessary activities of daily living and competencies in everyday life. Higher-order needs reflect more identity-related and development-oriented domains including privacy, comfort, stimulation or favoured personal style and preferences. Evidence emerged showing that participants had multiple reasons for moving, about half of which relate to the satisfaction of basic needs to maintain autonomy and half to higher-order needs. They mentioned, on average, four different reasons for moving. With respect to the content level of motives, physical environment-related motivations were the most prevalent. These included basic housing needs ("I found the apartment was too large to do my daily work") as well as higher-order needs ("We wanted to have a balcony and a view"). In the domain of motives pertaining to the social environment, the differentiation between basic ("My daughter can do the shopping for me now, because she lives just around the corner") and higher-order needs ("I wanted to spend more time with my grandchildren") can also be shown. We conclude that there was rarely one single reason for moving, but rather a set of needs that, in conjunction, lead to relocation. Although the participants in this study varied in health status and basic needs, most reported that higher-order needs were increasingly significant elements in terms of relocation decision making in old age (Oswald et al., 2002). In sum, findings on relocation from home to home in old age show that agency is triggered by basic needs to maintain autonomy (e.g. to reduce physical barriers) as well as by higher-order needs (e.g. to fulfil personal goals), which contribute to identity and well-being in general.

2.2.3. P–E Fit Assessments in Relation to Age and Living in Different Settings

As introduced earlier, establishing p–e fit opens another perspective on housing-related agency for those who are especially at risk in later life, in terms of the congruence level of individual competence or needs and environmental demands or conditions. To address the interaction between housing needs and housing conditions, three housing-related p–e fit indices for basic, higher-order and social aspects of housing were established in the project "Heidelberg 2002" (Oswald et al., 2005). The aim was to describe p–e fit among elders of different ages and in different urban districts. Results revealed differences in the p–e fit indices by district in the domains of higher-order and social housing needs versus conditions. P–e fit was higher in the rich and most scenic neighbourhood, whereas lowest scores were found in the poor and run-down district. Age, however, was important in explaining differences in the domains of basic housing needs versus conditions with highest scores in the older age group in all three districts. Another example of a very detailed p–e fit measure on accessibility at home is the "housing enabler" instrument (Iwarsson & Slaug, 2001), assessed in the European "ENABLE-AGE" study. Aiming at the relationship between environmental press and personal competence, accessibility was characterized as a combination of observed environmental barriers from a total of 188 barriers inside and outside the home with a list of 15 individual functional limitations, resulting in an individual weighted score of housing accessibility in the domains outdoors, entrances, indoors and communication. As will be shown next, p–e fit assessments are not only instrumental to further clarify the variability of processes of agency, but also to explore the relationship of housing-related agency and belonging as well as the processes of p–e exchange in relation to outcomes of housing-related identity and autonomy.

2.3. On the Relationship of Housing-Related Belonging and Agency

To address housing comprehensively with regard to processes of belonging *and* agency, selected findings from the European project "ENABLE-AGE" are presented (Iwarsson et al., 2005). The aim was to explore the relationship between housing-related agency and belonging. The results are based on data from randomly sampled 1,918 very old people 75–89 years old living alone in their private urban homes in Sweden, Germany, the UK, Hungary and Latvia. In a survey study, a wide range of well-proven measurements from various disciplines (e.g. psychology, occupational therapy) was administered within the home of the participants. To address housing-related agency, p–e fit in terms of housing accessibility was assessed (Iwarsson & Slaug, 2001). To address housing-related belonging, a set of quantitative measures were administered, i.e. a questionnaire on usability in the home (Fänge & Iwarsson, 2003), a questionnaire on meaning of home (Oswald, Mollenkopf, & Wahl, 1999), a questionnaire on housing-related control beliefs (Oswald et al., 2003), and a global evaluation of housing satisfaction. Correlative findings show that it is not the number of environmental barriers at home, but accessibility, indicating processes of agency in terms of p–e fit that interplays with different aspects of housing-related belonging. Good accessibility is particularly associated with high scores in perceived usability, high amounts of behavioural aspects of meaning of home (e.g. "being able to change or rearrange things as I please") and low external control beliefs (e.g. "I am not responsible for what happens in my home"). Although there were different levels of accessibility in different European settings, the findings revealed a great amount of comparability of the relationship between aspects of housing-related agency and belonging, simultaneously controlling for basic health and socio-economic status. In sum, the findings reveal a link between housing-related belonging, in terms of usability, behavioural meaning and control beliefs and housing-related agency, in terms of accessibility in very old age, as well as an existing tendency towards structural homogeneity of this relationship in objectively different European sites.

2.4. On the Relationship of Housing-Related Agency, Belonging and a Range of Outcomes

Data from two studies are presented to provide (1) empirical evidence on the interrelations between aspects of housing-related belonging and agency and (2) a set of variables on housing-related autonomy, well-being and housing-related identity. Again, findings from the "ENABLE-AGE" project are instrumental in demonstrating a consistent link between housing-related processes of p–e exchange (agency and belonging) and housing-related autonomy and well-being. To indicate housing-related autonomy, objective and perceived independence in everyday life (ADL) was assessed. To measure cognitive aspects of well-being, life satisfaction and environmental mastery (Ryff, 1989) were evaluated. Measures for emotional aspects of well-being, positive and negative affect (PANAS; Watson, Clark, & Tellegen, 1988) as well as depression (GDS; Yesavage et al., 1983) were assessed. The findings show that both processes of housing-related agency and belonging are related to housing-related autonomy and well-being. Again, it was not the mere number of barriers in the home environment, but housing accessibility that proved important for housing-related autonomy in terms of independence in daily life and well-being. Additionally, behavioural aspects of the meaning of home in particular correlated with autonomy and well-being, indicating housing-related belonging. Those participants with good accessibility (high p–e fit) at home, who perceive their home as useful and valuable for activities (high scores in behavioural meaning and usability), and who think that others or fate are only a little responsible for their housing situation (low external control beliefs), had a better autonomy in daily life (ADL/IADL), a better sense of well-being (environmental mastery) and suffered less from depressive symptoms. Although the level of accessibility, life satisfaction or depression was different in East versus West-European sites included in this study, there was a tendency towards partially comparable patterns of relationships between housing-related processes of p–e exchange and housing-related autonomy and well-being. However, the findings do not address the link between processes of p–e exchange and housing-related identity. Thus, results from the "Heidelberg 2002" study on the relationship between housing-related agency/belonging and housing-related urban identity are finally reported. One aim in this study was to explain urban identity (Urban Identity Scale; Lalli, 1992) in different urban districts with a set of predictors, including aspects of housing-related agency in terms of the mentioned p–e fit indices and aspects of housing-related belonging in terms of place attachment. Results revealed that p–e fit (indicating agency) as well as indoor place attachment (indicating belonging) are especially important in explaining urban identity in different neighbourhoods, independent from the participant's age, gender, finances and housing amenities (Oswald et al., 2005).

3. CONCLUSION

The aim of this chapter is to present findings from a research program on housing in middle and late adulthood driven by the basic assumption that both the processes of housing-related belonging and the processes of housing-related agency contribute to housing-related identity and autonomy and are thus fundamental to ageing in place.

Concerning findings on facets of housing-related belonging, elders differ in their subjective evaluation of home in terms of global ratings of residential satisfaction or place attachment, as well as in detailed meaning of home patterns due to their age, health status or geographic location. As was shown, cognitive and emotional aspects of meaning of home became particularly important when suffering from competence loss. Concerning findings on facets of housing-related agency, processes of environmental centralisation, relocation and establishment of p–e fit reveal variability due to age, health and setting in which people live.

As far as the relationship between housing-related processes of p–e exchange and outcomes of housing-related autonomy and identity is concerned, the findings strengthen the link between belonging and identity, as well as between agency and autonomy. In the ageing process, stability in housing-related belonging, e.g. place attachment scores or meaning of home patterns, contributes most to a continuous housing-related identity, for instance, when facing a severe competence loss or significant amounts of environmental reconstructions (i.e. East versus West German sites after reunification). Regarding housing-related agency, elders have the potential to proactively adapt and change their home environments to enhance accessibility and to maintain housing-related autonomy, either by means of moving from home to home or through environmental centralisation when suffering from diseases. However, it was also shown that both domains are not easy to separate in real life, for instance, when agency-related aspects of meaning of home are mentioned, when older people arrange both essential and non-essential objects within their "living centres" at home, or when elders who move from home to home report motives based on basic needs to maintain autonomy as well as higher-order needs to maintain identity. Comprehensively, results from "ENABLE-AGE" and "Heidelberg 2002" strengthen the link between housing-related agency *and* belonging as well as between housing-related agency and belonging on one hand and housing-related autonomy, identity and well-being on the other. Housing accessibility, indicating agency in terms of p–e fit interplays with different aspects of subjective housing, indicates belonging. Furthermore, processes of housing-related agency *and* belonging were strongly related to *both* housing-related autonomy and well-being at large. Findings on urban identity revealed that housing-related agency, in terms of p–e fit, *and* belonging, in terms of place attachment, are related to urban identity.

Taken together, the findings can be interpreted with regard to a fragmentation of results in environmental gerontology. Home-related individual development in later life may best be understood as a balance between environmental stability and change, with the higher goal of maintaining identity and autonomy. Established patterns of housing-related belonging contribute positively to maintain identity as well as to autonomy. Conversely, processes of housing-related agency in terms of environmental adaptation and proactive change positively contribute to housing-related autonomy, but also contribute to identity (Figure 1). From a broader developmental perspective on the impact of housing on ageing in place, we would argue that "successful" or "healthy" ageing is characterised by *a combination of both processes*, especially in very old age or when suffering from competence loss.

However, this research project emphasised community-dwelling elders, and has so far not been related to institutional settings. Furthermore, housing research in middle and late adulthood needs to strive for a better consolidation of qualitative and quantitative findings, including longitudinal studies, to reflect the full scope of ageing in place reality. Additionally, complex research designs and open-minded practitioners are needed to address simultaneously the functional and the meaningful dimensions of the home to fully understand the concept of housing, especially in old age, and thus to facilitate the necessary adaptations like relocation into purpose-built homes or into special-care units. This approach would lead to new perspectives beyond the classic ways of risk reduction and prevention at home—for example, through the creative development of health-related resources within the field of experiential housing, serving to enhance or to re-establish health outcomes in old age.

AFFILIATION

German Centre for Research on Ageing at the University of Heidelberg

REFERENCES

Altman, I., & Low, S. M. (Eds.). (1992). *Human behavior and environment, vol. 12: Place attachment.* New York: Plenum.

Aragonés, J. I., Francescato, G., & Gärling, T. (2002). *Residential environments. Choice, satisfaction, and behavior.* Westport, CT: Bergin & Gervey.

Baltes, M. M., Maas, I., Wilms, H.-U., & Borchelt, M. (1999). Everyday competence in old and very old age: Theoretical considerations and empirical findings. In P. B. Baltes & K. U. Mayer (Eds.), *The Berlin aging study* (pp. 384–402). Cambridge: Cambridge University Press.

Born, A. (2002). *Regulation persönlicher Identität im Rahmen gesellschaftlicher Transformationsbewältigung* (Regulation of personal identity in the face of societal transformation). Münster: Wasmann.

Bronfenbrenner, U. (1999). Environments in developmental perspective: Theoretical and operational models. In S. L. Friedman & T. D. Wachs (Eds.), *Measuring environment across the life span* (pp. 3–28). Washington, DC: American Psychological Association.

Carp, F. M., & Carp, A. (1984). A complementary/congruence model of well-being or mental health for the community elderly. In I. Altman, M. P. Lawton, & J. F. Wohlwill (Eds.), *Human behavior and environment: Elderly people and the environment* (Vol. 7, pp. 279–336). New York: Plenum.

Fänge, A., & Iwarsson, S. (2003). Accessibility and usability in housing: Construct validity and implications for research and practice. *Disability and Rehabilitation, 25*, 316–325.

Feldman, R. C. (1990). Settlement-identity. Psychological bonds with home places in a mobile society. *Environment and Behavior, 22*(2), 183–229.

Feldman, R. (1996). Constancy and change in attachments to types of settlements. *Environment and Behavior, 28*(4), 419–445.

Galster, G. (1987). Identifying the correlates of dwelling satisfaction. An empirical critique. *Environment and Behavior, 13*, 735–758.

Hidalgo, M. C., & Hernadez, B. (2001). Place attachment: Conceptual and empirical questions. *Journal of Environmental Psychology, 21*, 273–281.

Iwarsson, S., Sixsmith, J., Oswald, F., Wahl, H.-W., Nygren, C., Sixsmith, A., Széman, Z., & Tomsone, S. (2005). The ENABLE-AGE Project: Multi-dimensional methodology for European housing research. In: Vestbro, D. U., Hürol, Y. & Wilkinson, N. (Eds.), *Methodologies in housing research* (pp. 70–90). Gateshead: The Urban International Press.

Iwarsson, S., & Slaug, B. (2001). *Housing enabler. An instrument for assessing and analyzing accessibility problems in housing.* Lund, Sweden: Studentlitteratur.

Kahana, E. (1982). A congruence model of person–environment interaction. In M. P. Lawton, P. G. Windley, & T. O. Byerts (Eds.), *Aging and the environment. Theoretical approaches* (pp. 97–121). New York: Springer.

Lalli, M. (1992). Urban-related identity: Theory, measurement, and empirical findings. *Journal of Environmental Psychology, 12*, 285–303.

Lawton, M. P. (1977). The impact of the environment on aging and behavior. In J. E. Birren & K. W. Schaie (Eds.), *Handbook of the psychology of aging* (pp. 276–301). New York: Van Nostrand Reinhold.

Lawton, M. P. (1982). Competence, environmental press, and the adaptation of older people. In M. P. Lawton, P. G. Windley, & T. O. Byerts (Eds.), *Aging and the environment* (pp. 33–59). New York: Springer.

Lawton, M. P. (1985). Housing and living environments of older people. In R. H. Binstock & E. Shanas (Eds.), *Handbook of aging and the social sciences* (2nd ed., pp. 450–478). New York: Van Nostrand Reinhold.

Lawton, M. P. (1987). Environment and the need satisfaction of the aging. In L. L. Carstensen & B. A. Edelstein (Eds.), *Handbook of clinical gerontology* (pp. 33–40). New York: Pergamon Press.

Lawton, M. P. (1989). Environmental proactivity in older people. In V. L. Bengtson & K. W. Schaie (Eds.), *The course of later life* (pp. 15–23). New York: Springer.

Lawton, M. P. (1998). Environment and aging: Theory revisited. In R. J. Scheidt & P. G. Windley (Eds.), *Environment and aging theory: A focus on housing* (pp. 1–31). Westport, CT: Greenwood Press.

Lawton, M. P., & Nahemow, L. (1973). Ecology and the aging process. In C. Eisdorfer & M. P. Lawton (Eds.), *Psychology of adult development and aging* (pp. 619–674). Washington, DC: American Psychological Association.

Nahemow, L. (2000). The ecological theory of aging: Powel Lawton's legacy. In R. Rubinstein, M. Moss, & M. Kleban (Eds.), *The many faces of aging* (pp. 22–40). New York: Springer.

Neisser, U. (1988). Five kinds of self-knowledge. *Philosophical Psychology, 1*, 35–59.

Oswald, F. (1996). *Hier bin ich zu Hause. Zur Bedeutung des Wohnens: Eine empirische Studie mit gesunden und gehbeeinträchtigten Älteren* (Here I feel at home. On the individual meaning of home: An empirical study with healthy and mobility impaired elders). Regensburg: S. Roderer Verlag.

Oswald, F. (2003). Linking subjective housing needs to objective living conditions among older adults in Germany. In K. W. Schaie, H.-W. Wahl, H. Mollenkopf, & F. Oswald (Eds.), *Aging independently: Living arrangements and mobility* (pp. 130–147). New York: Springer.

Oswald, F., Hieber, A., Wahl, H.-W., & Mollenkopf, H. (2005). Ageing and person–environment fit in different urban neighbourhoods. *European Journal of Ageing, 2*(2), 88–97.

Oswald, F., Mollenkopf, H., & Wahl, H.-W. (1999). *Questionnaire on the meaning of home. Manual.* Unpublished manuscript, German Centre for Research on Ageing.

Oswald, F., & Rowles, G. D. (in press). Beyond the relocation trauma in old age: New trends in today's elders' residential decisions. In H.-W. Wahl, C. Tesch-Römer, & A. Hoff (Eds.), *New dynamics in old age: Environmental and societal perspectives.* Amityville, New York: Baywood Publication.

Oswald, F., Schilling, O., Wahl, H.-W., & Gäng, K. (2002). Trouble in paradise? Reasons to relocate and objective environmental changes among well-off older adults. *Journal of Environmental Psychology, 22*(3), 273–288.

Oswald, F., Schmitt, M., Wahl, H.-W., & Lang, F. (2004). *Contextual and individual predictors of life satisfaction in adulthood and old age.* Poster presented at the poster workshop "Toward integration of contextual resources of development across adulthood and old age" at the XVIIIth Biennial Meeting of the International Society for the Study of Behavioural Development (ISSBD), Ghent, Belgium.

Oswald, F., & Wahl, H.-W. (2001). Housing in old age: Conceptual remarks and empirical data on place attachment. *Bulletin on People–Environment Studies, 19*, 8–12.

Oswald, F., & Wahl, H.-W. (2004). Housing and health in later life. *Reviews of Environmental Health, 19*(3–4), 223–252.

Oswald, F., & Wahl, H.-W. (2005). Dimensions of the meaning of home. In G. D. Rowles & H. Chaudhury (Eds.), *Home and Identity in Late Life: International Perspectives*, (pp. 21–46). New York: Springer.

Oswald, F., Wahl, H.-W., Martin, M., & Mollenkopf, H. (2003). Toward measuring proactivity in person–environment transactions in late adulthood: The housing-related control beliefs questionnaire. *Journal of Housing for the Elderly, 17*(1/2), 135–152.

Oswald, F., Wahl, H.-W., Mollenkopf, H., & Schilling, O. (2003). Housing and life-satisfaction of older adults in two rural regions in Germany. *Research on Aging, 25*(2), 122–143.

Pinquart, M., & Burmedi, D. (2004). Correlates of residential satisfaction in adulthood and old age: A meta-analysis. In H.-W. Wahl, R. Scheidt, & P. G. Windley (Eds.), *Aging in context: Socio-physical environments* (Annual Review of Gerontology and Geriatrics). (pp. 195–222). New York: Springer.

Proshansky, H. M., Fabian, A. K., & Kaminoff, R. (1983). Place-identity. *Journal of Environmental Psychology, 3*, 57–83.

Relph, E. (1976). *Place and placelessness.* London: Pion.

Rowles, G. D. (1983). Geographical dimensions of social support in rural appalachia. In G. D. Rowles & R. J. Ohta (Eds.), *Aging and milieu. Environmental perspectives on growing old* (pp. 111–129). New York: Academic Press.

Rowles, G. D., Oswald, F., & Hunter, E. G. (2004). Interior living environments in old age. In H.-W. Wahl, R. Scheidt, & P. G. Windley (Eds.), *Aging in context: Socio-physical environments* (Annual Review of Gerontology and Geriatrics, 2003) (pp. 167–193). New York: Springer.

Rowles, G. D., & Watkins, J. F. (2003). History, habit, heart and hearth: On making spaces into places. In K. W. Schaie, H.-W. Wahl, H. Mollenkopf, & F. Oswald (Eds.), *Aging independently: Living arrangements and mobility* (pp. 77–96). New York: Springer.

Rubinstein, R. L. (1989). The home environments of older people: A description of the psychological process linking person to place. *Journal of Gerontology, 44*(2), 45–53.

Rubinstein, R. L., & De Medeiros, K. (2004). Ecology and the aging self. In H.-W. Wahl, R. J. Scheidt, & P. G. Windley (Eds.), *Aging in context: Socio-physical environments* (Annual Review of Gerontology and Geriatrics, 2003) (pp. 59–84). New York: Springer.

Rubinstein, R. L., & Parmelee, P. A. (1992). Attachment to place and representation of life course by the elderly. In I. Altman & S. M. Low (Eds.), *Human behavior and environment, vol. 12: Place attachment* (pp. 139–163). New York: Plenum.

Ryff, C. D. (1989). Beyond Ponce de Leon and life satisfaction: New directions in quest of successful ageing. *International Journal of Behavioral Development, 12*(1), 35–55.

Scheidt, R. J., & Windley, P. G. (1985). The ecology of aging. In J. E. Birren & K. W. Schaie (Eds.), *Handbook of the psychology of aging* (pp. 245–258). New York: Van Nostrand.

Sixsmith, J. (1986). The meaning of home: An exploratory study of environmental experience. *Journal of Environmental Psychology, 6*, 281–298.

Sixsmith, A. J., & Sixsmith, J. A. (1991). Transition in home experience in later life. *Journal of Architectural and Planning Research, 8*(3), 181–191.

Stedman, R. S. (2002). Toward a social psychology of place. Predicting behaviour from place-based cognitions, attitude and identity. *Environment and Behavior, 34*(5), 561–581.

Tuan, Y. F. (1980). Rootedness versus sense of place. *Landscape, 24*, 3–7.

Wahl, H.-W. (2001). Environmental influences on aging and behavior. In J. E. Birren & K. W. Schaie (Eds.), *Handbook of the psychology of aging* (5th ed., pp. 215–237). San Diego: Academic Press.

Wahl, H.-W., & Lang, F. R. (2003). Aging in context across the adult life: Integrating physical and social research perspectives. In H.-W. Wahl, R. Scheidt, & P. G. Windley (Eds.), *Aging in context: Socio-physical environments* (Annual Review of Gerontology and Geriatrics, 2003) (pp. 1–35). New York: Springer.

Wahl, H.-W., & Oswald, F. (2004). Wohnen im alter: Bezüge zu autonomie, identität und wohlbefinden (Housing in later life: Relations to autonomy, identity and well-being.). *Public Health Forum, 42*, 11–12.

Wahl, H.-W., & Oswald, F. (in press). Umwelten für ältere Menschen (Environments for older people). In E.-D. Lantermann & V. Linneweber (Eds.), *Enzyklopädie Umweltpsychologie. (Encyclopedia of Environmental Psychology.) Band 2: Spezifische Umwelten und umweltbezogenes Handeln.* Göttingen: Hogrefe.

Wahl, H.-W., Oswald, F., & Zimprich, D. (1999). Everyday competence in visually impaired older adults: A case for person–environment perspectives. *The Gerontologist, 39*(2), 140–149.

Watson, D., Clark, L. A., & Tellegen, A. (1988). Development and validation of brief measures of positive and negative affect: The PANAS scales. *Journal of Personality and Social Psychology, 54*(6), 1063–1070.

Weideman, S., & Anderson, J. R. (1985). A conceptual framework for residential satisfaction. In I. Altman & C. M. Werner (Eds.), *Human behavior and environment, vol. 8: Home environments* (pp. 153–182). New York: Plenum.

Yesavage, J. A., Brink, T. L., Rose, T. L., Lum, O., Huang, V., Adey, M., & Leirer, V. O. (1983). Development and validation of a geriatric depression screening scale: A preliminary report. *Journal of Psychiatric Research, 17*(1), 37–49.

Zingmark, K., Norberg, A., & Sandman, P.-O. (1995). The experience of being at home throughout the life span. Investigation of persons aged from 2 to 102. *International Journal of Aging and Human Development, 41*(1), 47–62.

GRAHAM D. ROWLES

COMMENTARY: A HOUSE IS NOT A HOME: BUT CAN IT BECOME ONE?

1. A HOUSE IS NOT A HOME

Over the past 20 years there has been a proliferation of research on the tantalisingly ambiguous concept of home (Altman & Werner, 1985; Dovey, 2005; Miller, 2001; Rowles & Chaudhury, 2005). Oswald and his colleagues seek to contribute to this literature by making a distinction between two characterisations of home. The first is home *defined objectively in terms of agency*. In essence, the concern here is with the observable functional use of the residential environment as manifest in constructs such as *environmental press/docility*, *environmental richness/proactivity* and *person–environment fit*—"... the full range of objective behaviors". The second is home *defined subjectively in terms of the experience of belonging*. It embraces "... the full range of subjective experiences". Under this rubric, home as belonging is manifest in *residential satisfaction*, *place attachment* and *meaning*. The fundamental separation of the two perspectives stems from a pervasive Janus-like confounding tension in the manner in which we view the phenomenon. What Oswald and his colleagues present as an agency perspective focuses on *looking at* the phenomenon of human habitation of dwellings from a logical empiricist analytical perspective. In contrast, a belonging perspective on home involves an empathic gaze and *phenomenological understanding* of a state of being.

This bifurcation of research on the concept of home is helpful in bringing into sharper focus a tension that has long pervaded work on this topic—an uneasy relationship between objective characterisations of "home" as a dwelling or residential structure and the subjective characterisation of "home" as a state of being at one with one's world. In this brief essay, I take this argument one stage further and use it to reinforce what is obvious to the layman but seems to remain stubbornly ignored by the research community—that a house and a home are entirely different constructs.[1] Indeed, the wisdom of the layman in this regard is clearly encapsulated in the platitude "a house is not a home". The importance of making this critical distinction has been strongly advocated by Amos Rapoport for many years but for some reason his plea has fallen on deaf ears (Rapoport, 1995, 2005). Equating house with home simply reinforces continuing ambiguity in understanding the manner in which individuals identify with their place of residence.

The fuzzy fusion of house and home is reinforced by the real estate industry. Real estate agents are concerned with selling physical structures—apartments or single family dwellings constructed of wood, bricks, mortar and other building materials.

H.-W. Wahl et al. (eds.), The Many Faces of Health, Competence and Well-Being in Old Age, 25–32.

These are physical structures, nothing more. In themselves—they carry no meaning and have no soul. But real estate agents do not advertise houses. Instead, they sell "homes," somewhat disingenuously using a word that evokes a state of being and a host of warm and positive meanings in order to increase the possibility of a sale. Similarly, in American society, the final residence of many frail elders, for many decades was called a nursing *home*. For most residents, such environments were far from being "home". Yet, perhaps as a salve to a societal conscience, the phrase nursing homes was used with the implicit message that it provided the resident with something more than accommodation—that it was a setting that somehow facilitated a sense of being at home. Was this a lexical ploy to absolve society from a sense of guilt at having institutionalised its elders? Only in the past decade has official terminology been changed to the more honest designation—nursing facility, signifying acknowledgement that these structures are not necessarily homes but rather, in and of themselves, merely physical spaces.

At this point, it is important to define both house and home. A house is a physical structure providing shelter and a set of more or less functional spaces to undertake activities of daily living. It is a location from which we customarily venture forth and to which we return, often on a daily basis, as we engage in the cycle of work, rest and play. The layout and design of a residence influences the degree to which it is possible for an individual to undertake these activities within the constraints of his or her level of physical and mental competence. Considered within the framework of ageing/environment theory, certain housing designs are more conducive than others to progressive adjustment to both normative and pathological changes associated with ageing. Environmental gerontologists have identified some distinctive features of such changes. For example, there is a tendency to spend more time in the residence (Baltes, Maas, Wilms, Borchelt, & Little, 1999), an increasingly well documented pattern of environmental centralisation involving the development of "control centres" or "living centres" within the dwelling (Rubinstein & Parmalee, 1992), progressive increase in the significance of the surveillance zone—space within the visual field of the dwelling (Rowles, 1981), and an increased propensity to rearrange furniture to ensure that there are places to hold on to in order to compensate for an increasingly unsteady gait or to remove obstacles to mobility (Pastalan, 1990). In parallel with these insights, there has developed an extensive literature on the design of housing attuned to the changing needs of elders (Frain & Carr, 1996; Golant, 1992; Peace & Holland, 2001; Scheidt & Windley, 1998; Zimmerman, Sloane, & Eckert, 2001). This literature includes work on smart houses (Fisk, 2001; Meyer & Mollenkopf, 2003) and dwellings constructed or adapted according to principles of universal design (Kose, 1998; Story, 1998). The idea is that such behavioural adaptations and environmental design features reduce the possibility or at least delay the need for involuntary relocation and hence facilitate ageing in place (Frank, 2002; Rowles, 1993; Tilson, 1990).

The notion of home is far more emotionally loaded and evocative. I contend that it pertains to an entirely different phenomenon. Home is a sense of being at one with the world that is manifest experientially, as noted by Oswald and his associates, in a sense of belonging. Many commentators and researchers have attempted to identify the elements of belonging that underlie the experience of being at home (Oswald & Wahl, 2005;

Rowles & Chaudhury, 2005; Sixsmith, 1986; Zingmark, Norberg, & Sandman, 1995). Considered in concert, these elements comprise a mélange of experiential dimensions—feelings of familiarity, comfort, security, mastery, ownership and identity—that, together, convey and express a transcendent wholeness and rightness in a person's life. Being "at home" is inherently, and by definition, a positive experiential state. It is a state of being representing what I believe to be a universal human quest.

Most important in the context of this essay, *home is not an inherently place-based concept* but rather a phenomenon that may be manifest in a particular location. Clarifying the fundamental difference between the location-based concept of house and the experience of home is particularly important given the development of recent research suggesting that "home" is not necessarily a positive place: places that are home to some people are places of exclusion to others (Scharf, Phillipson, & Smith, 2005); residences that are the site of abuse or mistreatment are generally not fondly remembered with a sense of belonging but rather as sites of alienation, fear and angst (Chaudhury & Rowles, 2005; Watkins & Hosier, 2005; Weisman, 1994). If we accept that "home" is a universally positive feeling and state of being rather than a location, then, by definition, houses or apartments that foster negative memories of abuse and associations with mistreatment cannot be home, at least inasmuch as they are associated with such emotions and experiences. Complicating this issue, of course, is the more ambiguous situation of a dwelling that is associated with both positive and negative life experiences that on one level is viewed as home and on another may evoke a sense of alienation that is the antithesis of home—homelessness (Watkins & Hosier, 2005).

2. BUT CAN IT BECOME ONE?

Does the conceptual separation of house and home mean that a house cannot become a home? On one level, the answer to this question, of course, is yes, it means precisely that. A dwelling, in and of itself, can never be home. On the other hand, the physical space of a house can nurture or support a sense of home; it can become a symbol of and repository for home and provide cues to sustaining feelings of being "at home". Inasmuch as a resident is able to imbue a house or apartment with positive emotional valence—through the familiarity of a comfortable rhythm and routine of habitual daily use (Rowles, 2000; Seamon, 1980), the attribution of social and personal significance to its spaces (Marcus, 1995, pp. 159–184; Pruchno, Dempsey, Carder, & Koropeckyj-Cox, 1993), the development of emotional identification with its contents (Boschetti, 1995; Paton & Cram, 1992; Whitmore, 2001), and affinity for the history of events that have transpired within its walls (Rowles, 1978; Rowles, Oswald, & Hunter, 2004)—then a house can become the site or locale of home. How does this perspective equate with the experience of belonging as presented by Oswald and his colleagues? Experiencing "satisfaction", developing feelings of "attachment" and finding "meaning" within the walls of a particular structure, reinforced by the presence of artefacts and memorabilia that serve as cues to the evocation of such emotions, transforms a house into the stage upon which a sense of being at home (and belonging) is created. But this sense of "home" is created by the inhabitant not by the dwelling *per se*. Hence, a house that evokes a sense of home and belonging to one person, to a guest or visitor may be meaningless space. To an outsider a house can never be home.

3. SOME IMPLICATIONS: MORE QUESTIONS THAN ANSWERS?

Four fascinating and provocative questions arise from this chapter. First, how do people transform the *space* of a residence into the locus of a sense of *home*? There is a growing literature on the fascinating topic of "home making"—the process through which people move into a residence and over the course of time engage in patterns of habitation that gradually transform that space into a place that evokes a sustaining sense of being at home (Maloney, 1997; Rowles & Watkins, 2003). Studies, to date, suggest that home making involves a repetitive pattern of use of interior space as a rhythm and routine of daily activity is established. This process is complemented by the arrangement of furniture in a manner that maximises a sense of environmental mastery. Gradually, a sense of physical insideness—what Seamon (1980) termed body subject—develops and becomes taken-for-granted as the use of space within the dwelling transitions from the realm of conscious decision-making to implicit and often unconscious routine. The process of habitation and creating a sense of home also involves decorating the space and the selective assembly and display of mementos and artefacts that have meaning to the individual and convey a sense of identity. By surrounding him or herself with such cues, the individual is, usually with intentionality, placed in a setting providing a constant visual bombardment of familiar stimuli that provide a sense of identity through the personal meanings they evoke. We surround ourselves with photographs, books, mementoes and artifacts that convey the essence of how we want to represent and identify ourselves. Over time, our sense of being at home is intensified by the accumulation of an event history of the dwelling as layer upon layer of life experiences accumulate within the space. In sum, we create home. There is a need for much more research to clarify each of these elements of home making. But there are even more challenging questions. How is the process of home making influenced by shared residence with others (a roommate or spouse) who are also trying to create home in the same space? To what extent does the degree to which we own or control the space of the residence influence our ability to create home? Does increasing length of residence result in linear intensification of the sense of being "at home"?

Second, how is the process of creating home affected by relocation? It is important to explore the manner in which elements of being at home are transported, recreated and transformed following relocation in order to identify potential interventions for reducing the stress of both voluntary and involuntary moves. This is particularly important for frail elders with high levels of environmental vulnerability. With each successive move, do people become increasingly adept at the process of transforming the spaces of houses into places that evoke home? There is some evidence that when people relocate there is a tendency to arrange furniture in the same configuration as it was in their previous dwelling (Toyama, 1988). Is this an adaptive strategy harnessed to reduce relocation stress? Are elders who have relocated frequently over their life course at an advantage in comparison with those who have spent the majority of their life in a single dwelling with regard to the ability to create home? In old age does the process of recreating home universally involve the need for adaptation within the framework of moves to more confined spaces with an associated disbandment of the household and divestiture of possessions (Eckerdt, Sergeant, Dingel, & Bowen, 2004; Morris, 1992)?

Third, how does the experience of being at home change with the changing capability of the ageing individual? In what ways does home making and sustaining a sense of home evolve in association with age-related changes in the manner in which the dwelling is inhabited? For example, are there consistent transitions in the experience of home associated with spending more time each day within the dwelling, with processes of environmental centralisation, or as a result of the increasing significance of the surveillance zone?

These questions lead us naturally to the issue of the degree to which there may be developmental trajectories in the experience of home with distinctive manifestations over the life course and especially in old age (Watkins & Hosier, 2005). Is the creation and meaning of home substantively different for an individual as he or she approaches the end of life and frames their experience within an increasing recognition of mortality? To what extent do contemporary theoretical perspectives on the experience of ageing, especially neodisengagement perspectives such as socioemotional selectivity (Carstensen, Isaacowitz, & Charles, 1997), gerotranscendance (Tornstam, 1997) and selection, optimisation and compensation (Baltes, 1997), require us to consider different conceptions of the experience of home and different priorities in the process of home making. Does the meaning and quest for home transform itself and become more intense toward the end of life?

This question leads to the fourth, and perhaps most important question, a question concerned with the existential meaning of home in old age. What is the relationship between being at home and belonging and the antithesis of this experience—being homelessness and alienated? This is far more than merely a question of the manner in which we relate to the dwelling we inhabit. On this level, home is integrally involved with the ongoing quest to make a sense of our lives and to centre ourselves in relation to our place in the universe and a higher spiritual sense of being and identity. As we approach the end of our life the quest for home on this level may become ever more insistent and compelling.

4. CONCLUSION

Oswald and his associates' substantial and provocative contribution not only serves a useful function in helping us distinguish among functional and experiential dimensions of an individual's relationship to his or her residence but also provides an important vehicle for exposing some of the challenges of research in this domain. Their treatise perpetuates a shortcoming of research in this domain by failing to adequately distinguish between house and home—between a location and state of being. By seeking to clarify this distinction, it is my hope that I have been able to reveal the need for an increased emphasis on developing an understanding of how individuals, through the process of their functional and experiential habitation of dwellings are able to create a sense of belonging that translates into the experience of "home" that may be place situated but which is not place dependent. To answer the question posed in the title of this essay, a house, by definition, can never *per se* be a home but it can become the locus of home for an individual inasmuch as it becomes imbued with meaning by that individual and can become a symbol and reflection of a state of being.

AFFILIATION

Graduate Center for Gerontology, University of Kentucky

NOTE

[i] Throughout this commentary I use the terms residence, house and dwelling interchangeably to signify physical structures. The term home will be reserved for the state of being that is the focus of my observations.

REFERENCES

Altman, I., & Werner, C. M. (1985). *Home environments*. New York: Plenum Press.

Baltes, P. B. (1997). On the incomplete architecture of human ontogeny: Selection, optimization and compensation as foundation of developmental theory. *American Psychologist, 52*, 366–380.

Baltes, M. M., Maas, I., Wilms, H. U., Borchelt, M., & Little, T. (1999). Everyday competence in old and very old age: Theoretical considerations and empirical findings. In P. B. Baltes & K. U. Mayer (Eds.). *The Berlin aging study: Aging from 70 to 100*. Cambridge: Cambridge University Press.

Boschetti, M. A. (1995). Attachment to personal possessions: An interpretive study of the older person's experience. *Journal of Interior Design, 21*(1), 1–12.

Carstensen, L. L., Isaacowitz, D. M., & Charles, S. T. (1997). Taking time seriously: A theory of socioemotional selectivity. *The American Psychologist, 54*(3), 165–181.

Chaudhury, H., & Rowles, G. D. (2005). Between the shores of recollection and imagination: Self, aging and home. In G. D. Rowles & H. Chaudhury (Eds.). *Home and identity in late life: International perspectives*. (pp. 3–18). New York: Springer Publishing Company.

Dovey, K. (2005). Home as paradox. In G. D. Rowles & H. Chaudhury (Eds.). *Home and identity in late life: International perspectives* (pp. 361–369). New York: Springer Publishing Company.

Eckerdt, D. J., Sergeant, J. F., Dingel, M., & Bowen, M. E. (2004). Household disbandment in later life. *Journal of Gerontology: Social Sciences, 59B*, S265–S273.

Fisk, M. J. (2001). The implications of smart homes technologies. In Peace, S. M. & Holland, C. (Eds.). *Inclusive housing in an aging society* (pp. 101–124). Bristol, UK: Policy Press.

Frain, J. P., & Carr, P. H. (1996). Is the typical modern house designed for future adaptation for disabled older people? *Age and Ageing, 25*, 398–401.

Frank, J. B. (2002). *The paradox of aging in place in assisted living*. Westport, CT: Bergin & Garvey.

Golant, S. M. (1992). *Housing America's elderly: Many possibilities/few choices*. Newbury Park: Sage Publications.

Kose, S. (1998). From barrier free to universal design: An international perspective. *Assistive Technology, 10*(1), 44–50.

Maloney, M. F. (1997). The meanings of home in the stories of older women. *Western Journal of Nursing Research, 19*(2), 166–176.

Marcus, C. C. (1995). *House as a mirror of self*. Berkeley, CA: Conari Press.

Meyer, S., & Mollenkopf, H. (2003). Home technology, smart homes and the aging user. In K. W. Schaie, H.-W. Wahl, H. Mollenkopf, & F. Oswald (Eds.). *Aging independently: Living arrangements and mobility* (pp. 148–161). New York: Springer Publishing Company.

Miller, D. (Ed.). (2001). *Home possessions: Material culture behind closed doors*. Oxford: Berg.

Morris, B. R. (1992). Reducing inventory: Divestiture of personal possessions. *Journal of Women and Aging, 4*(2), 79–92.

Oswald, F., & Wahl, H.-W. (2005). Dimensions of the meaning of home in later life. In G. D. Rowles & H. Chaudhury (Eds.). *Home and identity in late life: International perspectives* (pp. 21–45). New York: Springer Publishing Company.

Pastalan, L. A. (1990). Designing a humane environment for the frail elderly. In D. Tilson (Ed.). *Aging in place: Supporting the frail elderly in residential environments* (pp. 273–285). Glenview, IL: Scott, Foresman & Company.

Paton, H. C., & Cram, F. (1992). Personal possessions and environmental control: The experiences of elderly women in three residential settings. *Journal of Women and Aging, 4*(2), 61–78.

Peace, S. M., & Holland, C. (2001). *Inclusive housing in an aging society*. Bristol, UK: Policy Press.

Pruchno, R. A., Dempsey, N. P., Carder, P., & Koropeckyj-Cox, T. (1993). Multigenerational households of caregiving families: Negotiating shared space. *Environment and Behavior, 25*(3), 349–366.

Rapoport, A. (1995). A critical look at the concept 'home.' In D. N. Benjamin (Ed.). *The home: Words, meanings and environments* (pp. 25–52). Aldershot, UK: Avebury.

Rapoport, A. (2005). On using 'home' and 'place.' In G. D. Rowles & H. Chaudhury (eds.). *Home and identity in late life: International perspectives* (pp. 343–360). New York: Springer Publishing Company.

Rowles, G. D. (1978). *Prisoners of space? Exploring the geographical experience of older people*. Boulder, CO: Westview Press.

Rowles, G. D. (1981). The surveillance zone as meaningful space for the aged. *The Gerontologist, 21*(3), 304–311.

Rowles, G. D. (1993). Evolving images of place in aging and 'aging in place.' *Generations, 17*(2), 65–70.

Rowles, G. D. (2000). Habituation and being in place. *Occupational Therapy Journal of Research, 20* (Suppl. 1), 52S–67S.

Rowles, G. D., & Chaudhury, H. (Eds.). (2005). *Home and identity in late life: International perspectives*. New York: Springer Publishing Company.

Rowles, G. D., Oswald, F., & Hunter, E. G. (2004). Interior living environments in old age. In H.-W. Wahl, R. J. Scheidt, & P. G. Windley (Eds.). *Aging in context: Sociophysical environments* (Annual Review of Gerontology and Geriatrics, Vol. 23) (pp. 167–194). New York: Springer Publishing Company.

Rowles, G. D., & Watkins, J. F. (2003). History, habit, heart and hearth: On making spaces into places. In K. W. Schaie, H.-W. Wahl, H. Mollenkopf, & F. Oswald (Eds.). *Aging independently: Living arrangements and mobility* (pp. 77–96). New York: Springer Publishing Company.

Rubinstein, R. L., & Parmalee, P. A. (1992). Attachment to place and representation of life course by the elderly. In I. Altman & S. M. Low (Eds.). *Human behavior and environment vol. 12: Place attachment* (pp. 139–163). New York: Plenum Press.

Scharf, T., Phillipson, C., & Smith, A. E. (2005). Ageing in challenging environments: Everyday life in deprived urban communities of England. Paper presented at the 18th International Congress on Gerontology, Rio de Janeiro, Brazil.

Scheidt, R. J., & Windley, P. G. (1998). *Environment and aging theory: A focus on housing*. Westport, CT: Greenwood Press.

Seamon, D. (1980). Body subject, time-space routines, and place ballets. In A. Buttimer & D. Seamon (Eds.). *The human experience of space and place* (pp. 148–165). London: Croom Helm.

Sixsmith, J. A. (1986). The meaning of home: An exploratory study of environmental experience. *Journal of Environmental Psychology, 6*, 281–298.

Story, M. F. (1998). Maximizing usability: The principles of universal design. *Assistive Technology, 10*(1), 4–12.

Tilson, D. (Ed.). (1990). *Aging in place: Supporting the frail elderly in residential environments*. Glenview, IL: Scott, Foresman & Company.

Tornstam, L. (1997). Gerotranscendence: A reformulation of the disengagement theory. *Journal of Aging Studies, 11*(2), 143–154.

Toyama, T. (1988). *Identity and milieu: A study of relocation focusing on reciprocal changes in elderly people and their environment.* Stockholm, Sweden: Department for Building Function Analysis, The Royal Institute of Technology.

Watkins, J. F., & Hosier, A. F. (2005). Conceptualizing home and homelessness: In a NFE course perspective. G. D. Rowles & H. Chaudhury (eds.). *Home and identity in late life: International perspectives* (pp. 197–215). New York: Springer Publishing Company.

Weisman, L. K. (1994). *Discrimination by design: A feminist critique of the man-made environment.* Urbana-Champaign, IL: University of Illinois Press.

Whitmore, H. (2001). Value that marketing cannot manufacture: Cherished possessions as links to identity and wisdom. *Generations, 25*(3), 57–63.

Zimmerman, S., Sloane, P. D., & Eckert, J. K. (2001). *Assisted living: Needs, practices, and policies in residential care for the elderly*. Baltimore: The Johns Hopkins University Press.

Zingmark, K. Norberg, A., & Sandman, P.-O. (1995). The experience of being at home throughout the lifespan: Investigation of persons aged from 2 to 102. *International Journal of Aging and Human Development, 41*(1), 47–62.

HEIDRUN MOLLENKOPF, STEPHAN BAAS, ROMAN KASPAR,
FRANK OSWALD and HANS-WERNER WAHL

OUTDOOR MOBILITY IN LATE LIFE: PERSONS, ENVIRONMENTS AND SOCIETY

This chapter deals with a complex phenomenon: the out-of-home mobility of ageing and aged persons. It is a complex issue because so many different aspects come together in the interaction between persons and their environments. Mobility means the physical ability to move and the realisation of all types of trips and activities outside the home, and it can be motivated by diverse, often inseparably intertwined motives. Trips can be manifested in a goal-directed mode or for its own sake, and they can be performed on foot, by harnessing natural forces or by employing any mechanised or motorised means of transportation. Spatial and traffic conditions as well as the societal conditions for mobility are different. This holds not only for national legislations, traffic policy, level of mechanisation, etc. but also for values, lifestyles or what we call a society's "Zeitgeist". In that sense, mobility is a crucial characteristic of modern societies. And last but not least, all of these conditions are subject to permanent change. Over the course of the 20th century, technological advances—from individual automobiles, public transportation systems and special driving services to trains, ships and airplanes—have made it possible to traverse distances even despite physical or sensory impairments or frailty. As transport technologies improved, the shape of urban and rural settlements has changed as well. The provision of an extended road infrastructure accelerated extensive suburban development and the establishment of industrial and commercial enterprises beyond residential areas. The growing dispersal of travel origins and destinations, in turn, increased the importance of mobility for bridging the widening gap between functional areas. Altogether, these developments led to a continual increase in mobility and travel (World Business Council for Sustainable Development, 2002). Therefore, mobility has become a major condition for ensuring the ability to lead an autonomous life and participate actively in society.

Individual states, resources, and needs change as people age. Ageing is accompanied by an increasing risk of physical disabilities, as well as declining sensory abilities, and hence, restriction of mobility. At the same time, social changes, such as grown children leaving home, retirement and the loss of close confidants, demand a growing measure of mobility if the elderly person is to continue being part of society (Mollenkopf, 1996). Mobility also promotes healthy ageing and delays the onset of frailty (Leventhal, Rabin, Leventhal, & Burns, 2001; Rantanen et al., 2000). Hence, the detailed analysis of outdoor mobility in old age, as well as its potentials and hindrances, is highly relevant for a "good life" (Lawton, 1983) for both today's and tomorrow's ageing population.

H. W. Wahl et al. (eds.), The Many Faces of Health, Competence and Well-Being in Old Age, 33–45.

This complexity of out-of-home mobility explains why we added "persons, environments and society" to our chapter's title. For the same reason, assessing mobility in later life requires interdisciplinary approaches suited to integrating its various micro, meso and macro level facets. As for the micro level of person-related physical, sensory and cognitive competencies and impairments, of individual motivations and behaviour, and of socio-structural aspects like age, gender, education and economic resources, the behavioural and social, as well as medical sciences, are in demand. Sociological theories are also needed concerning the macro level of societal and technological conditions and related developments. Traffic and transport policy and research are just as relevant as urban planning, architecture and vehicle engineering. Further disciplines may be necessary depending on the focus of interest.

The complex context and meaning of outdoor mobility was addressed in several studies at the German Centre for Research on Ageing (DZFA). They focussed on the question of whether older people are able to profit from the wider scope of action provided by modern society, or whether the developments towards a broader range of mobility, resulting also in higher traffic density and increasing distances to be bridged, diminish their abilities to lead their everyday life, keep up social relations and participate in activities outside the home. To answer these questions we first introduce the studies with respect to older adults' possibilities of moving about. Main findings will be presented and discussed from a social science perspective, considering the ecological understanding of person–environment interaction, as well as general societal developments that may impact ageing adults' future options of realising their outdoor-oriented needs.

THE STUDIES ON OUT-OF-HOME MOBILITY

The first data we can use for our research date back to the international project "Keeping the Elderly Mobile—Technology to Meet Their Outdoor Mobility Needs". The objectives of this project were to expand the body of knowledge about the mobility behaviour of elderly people outside the home and about the motives behind that behaviour; to research deeper mobility needs that might exist and the reasons preventing their satisfaction; and to determine which factors complicate the mobility of elderly people or prevent these people from satisfying their desires for mobility (Mollenkopf et al., 2004).

The investigation was conducted in urban regions featuring different settlement and transport infrastructures in Finland (Jyväskylä), eastern and western Germany (Chemnitz and Mannheim) and Italy (Ancona). In each case, middle-sized cities referring to the situation in the respective countries were chosen. In autumn 1995, the first phase of data collection was launched with standardised interviews in the homes of 2,172 older adults and a diary in which the respondents wrote down the circumstances of the trips they realised during three days. The samples were drawn from the population registers of each Municipality Registration Office. The interviewees were selected using stratification by age (55–74 and 75+ years), sex and living area (town centres and intermediate and outskirt parts of the towns). In the second phase, which took place in autumn 1996, the collected data were supplemented by qualitative case studies in order to gather further information about social and technological factors that typically facilitate or frustrate the satisfaction of mobility needs. The comparison between three cities from different parts of Europe made it possible to throw light on the way in which the mobility of elderly people is affected by different infrastructures, the possession of private means of transportation and various cultural traditions.

In 1996, elements of this study were also conducted as part of an investigation in a residential area of Zoetermeer, the Netherlands (Tacken & Caso, 1999). Similarly, an additional study using the same methodological design and instruments as the 1995 study was conducted in two German rural areas in 1999 (Mollenkopf, Oswald, Schilling, & Wahl, 2001; Oswald, Wahl, Mollenkopf, & Schilling, 2003).

In the year 2000 we were able to extend our research both scientifically by including psychological perspectives and geographically by including more countries as well as rural areas. The interdisciplinary project entitled "MOBILATE. Enhancing Outdoor Mobility in Later Life—Personal Coping, Environmental Resources, and Technical Support", funded within the European Commission's 5th Framework Programme, was conducted (in alphabetical order) in Finland, Germany, Hungary, Italy and the Netherlands (Mollenkopf, Marcellini, Ruoppila, Széman, & Tacken, in press).

This project is a European study of how men and women in later adulthood manage their daily commutes and which conditions they feel promote or hinder their ability to get around. An essential focus of research was on how environmental resources impact on the living conditions of older adults in different parts of Europe. Therefore, particular emphasis was placed on the contrast between rural and urban regions. In order to take into consideration the specific national peculiarities, middle-sized cities were chosen in proportion to each country's characteristics. For the same reason, inside rural regions of each country, villages or areas were chosen which can be regarded as characteristic for the respective country. The goal of the research endeavour was to provide a comprehensive and detailed description and explanation of older adults' actual outdoor mobility, to better understand the complex interplay between personal competencies and aspects of the physical and social environments and to identify specific ways to facilitate mobility in later life, paying special consideration to the cultural, geographic and structural differences in the various European regions.

The national samples of men and women in middle and late adulthood (55 years of age or older) were randomly drawn from the respective municipality population registers. The total sample consisted of altogether 3,950 community dwelling elders. They were disproportionately stratified by gender and age (persons aged 55–74 years and 75 years or older, with approximately equal numbers of men and women in each group). Stratification was applied in order to get cell sizes sufficiently large for detailed analyses which would not have been possible with a proportional sampling.

Moreover, in three of the participating countries (eastern and western Germany, Finland and Italy), the study repeated the assessment conducted among the respondents from the urban areas in 1995. Hence, the analysis enabled us to trace the development of ageing individuals, identify changes in the physical and social environment and conduct a comparison of cohorts among the older participants of the study (Mollenkopf et al., 2003; Ruoppila et al., 2003).

The Conceptual MOBILATE Model

In national travel surveys, mobility usually has been defined as locomotion, as a movement in time and space. It is measured in terms of trips or journeys, reported in standardised diary forms. Descriptive information is generally collected and provided on distances, travel modes used, periods of time and the activity pursued at the destination reached (ECMT, 2000; Litman, 2003; Organisation for Economic Co-operation and Development (OECD), 2001). This approach is well suited if one is interested in travel behaviour, travel flow, etc. as it is the case for traffic and transport planning. In modern societies, however, with their high priorities on self-determination, freedom and individuality, out-of-home mobility comprises much more than just the functional means for bridging the distance from a place A to a destination B under certain conditions. The assessment of outdoor mobility of men and women living in modern—or even "post"-modern—societies—should, therefore, include as much as possible these modern aspects of mobility. In the MOBILATE project we used such a holistic concept of mobility.

In general, the MOBILATE model as depicted in Figure 1, proposes that out-of-home mobility is determined by personal (health-related and psychological) and socio-economic factors as well as environmental (structural and regional) conditions and features of the person–environment interaction. Our understanding of out-of-home mobility, going beyond the common notion of trip-making behaviour, simultaneously considers the variety of transport modes used, the diversity of outdoor activities pursued and realised mobility (actual trip-making). In other words, flexibility regarding different

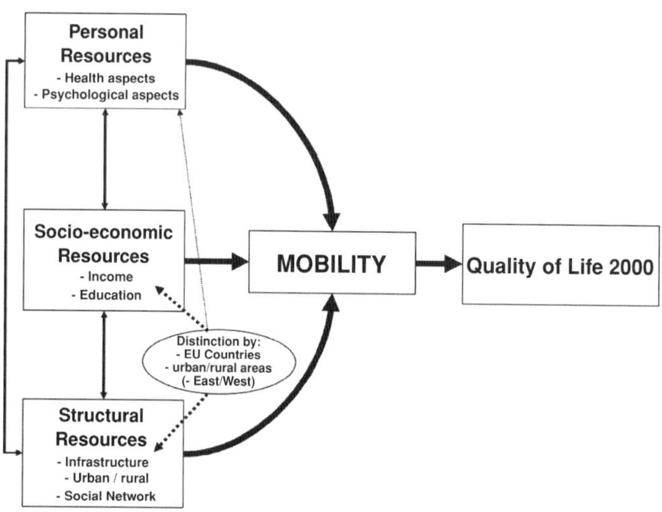

Figure 1. The Underlying Mobility Model.

transport modes and a wide range of leisure time interests as motives for mobility are taken into consideration. "Quality of Life" forms the final outcome within our conceptual model. A high variability of out-of-home mobility is hypothesised to impact individual evaluations of life in general and the experience of positive affect states.

From an environmental gerontology perspective, the key to maintaining outdoor mobility lies within the interaction between each individual and his or her immediate surroundings and significant others. The consideration of living and neighbourhood environments and of social, spatial and technological environments (including transport facilities) is thus crucial for a comprehensive understanding of outdoor mobility. Furthermore, an individual's mobility behaviour can be affected by objective environment-related factors such as failing physical and cognitive abilities and lack of social and financial resources, and by such subjective factors as mental states, attitudes and the assessment of situations and one's own abilities. Standardised questionnaires were used to assess essential features of the community and various kinds of activities and mobility. Demographic and health aspects, social networks and personality measures were assessed as well. If available, internationally acknowledged measures were employed. The concrete travel behaviour or actual mobility was assessed by a mobility diary in which the respondents documented their trips over the course of two days (the days before and after the interview). In the following we will present selected findings that emerged from these projects.

FINDINGS

The significance of mobility in late life can be derived from several indicators. A first one is the high importance older people attribute to moving about outside their homes.

Results (1): The Significance of Out-of-Home Mobility (Case Studies)

When the older adults participating in the case studies were asked what out-of-home mobility means to them, seven main aspects were noted in all cities studied: mobility as a basic emotional experience; mobility as physical movement, as a basic human need; as movement in natural surroundings and observation of nature; as a social need; as an expression of personal autonomy and freedom; as a source of stimulation and diversion; and the possibility to move about as a reflective expression of the life force one still has. "It's everything, it's life!", or "Still being able to take part in social life", were exemplary spontaneous statements (Mollenkopf, Marcellini, Ruoppila, & Tacken, 2004, pp. 126–127). Accordingly, the idea of no longer being able to move about outdoors one day is regarded as terrible. In this respect, "The end. If you can't do anything any more it's like being in prison", "The worst thing that can happen to a person", or "I can't find words for it. It is inhumane" were some characteristic answers.

Results (2) Mobility Patterns of Older Adults (MOBILATE Survey)

Whether elderly men and women are able to satisfy their desires for mobility, how they manage as they go about their daily affairs and how satisfied they are depends

Table 1. Mean number of journeys

	Country											
	Finland		*Germany East*		*Germany West*		*Hungary*		*Italy*		*The Netherlands*	
Variable (M)	*Urban*	*Rural*	*Urban*	*Rural*	*Urban*	*Rural*	*Urban*	*Rural*	*Urban*	*Rural*	*Urban*	*Rural*
Total	1.4	1.2***	0.9	0.9	0.9	1.0	0.9	0.6***	1.2	1.1	0.8	0.5***
No car	1.1	0.9	0.8	0.8	0.7	0.7	0.9	0.6	0.8	0.8	0.7	0.3
Car passenger	1.3	1.1	1.0	0.6	0.8	0.9	0.7	0.6	0.8	0.8	0.7	0.7
Car driver	1.7	1.5	1.0	1.1	1.1	1.2	1.0	0.6	1.5	1.5	0.9	0.6

Note: $^{***}p < 0.001$.

significantly on their state of health, habits and the means of transport available to them. Concerning general patterns of out-of-home mobility among older adults, we found urban–rural differences for all countries under study (Table 1). The share of people who make at least one trip a day is higher among people living in urban areas than among those in the countryside. These differences reach statistical significance for Finland, Hungary, and the Netherlands.

The availability of an automobile clearly influences the mean number of older people's journeys: In almost all regions, the persons who have ready access to a car in their households are generally apt to be more often on the go than those without such a means of transportation. Only in the urban areas of eastern Germany, Hungary and the Netherlands, having a car in one's household did not substantially affect the number of journeys undertaken.

Elderly people whose physical strength and sensory abilities are waning are often in particular need of a car in order to deal with daily demands and to join in social or cultural activities. However, the number of pensioner households that own a car varies greatly according to region, age, gender and size of the household. On average, older persons in Italy most frequently have a car available, followed by the older adults in Finland, Eastern and Western Germany and the Netherlands. A far lower share of the Hungarian elders own a car compared to their western European contemporaries, particularly in the rural areas where access to a car is even lower than in the urban area of this country. In addition to the availability of cars, preconditions for mobility differ with respect to individual health status. When health is impaired, the amount of time spent outdoors during the whole day is clearly lower. People with poor health start later and they go back home earlier (not shown in a table; see Mollenkopf et al., 2004).

Concerning transport modes, walking is on average the most common travel mode of older adults in Europe. Almost half of all trips made by the people who participated in the study were on foot (46%). The car, used as a driver (28.4%) or as a passenger (11.3%), was the second most important mode with altogether 40%; public transport

Table 2. Main transport modes

	Urban areas				Rural areas			
	55–74		75+		55–74		75+	
	Male	*Female*	*Male*	*Female*	*Male*	*Female*	*Male*	*Female*
By foot	37	48	54	62	30	47	46	60
Car	48	28	27	17	51	34	33	26
Public transport	8	15	13	18	5	3	8	4
Bicycle	8	9	6	3	13	16	13	9
Total $N =$	1506	1674	270	471	1494	1363	264	336

Note: Percentages; $N = 7378$ journeys; weighted data; based on diaries.

including all modes (bus, tram, train, taxi or special transport) was used in 8% and the bicycle in 10% of the trips documented in the diaries. Large differences become obvious when one differentiates between urban and rural regions, and socio-structural variables such as age and gender (Table 2).

Driving a car is the main travel mode of younger men (55–74 years) in both urban and rural regions, especially in Italy. The trips of women and of older men are by far more often undertaken by foot or made as car passengers. This is often the case in rural areas, which are characterised by a lack of public transport services. Usually, the availability and accessibility of public transport, as well as the abundance of shops and other facilities, is better in urban than in rural regions. Thus, it is not surprising that in the cities, people travel more by public transport and by foot. Buses and trams (where available) are used mostly by older people, and within each age group, women use this mode more often than men.

The various options for outdoor mobility find expression in the older persons' subjective evaluation of their possibilities to get where they want or need to go. As expected, people are more satisfied in urban areas, and younger persons (55–74 years) are more satisfied than older (75+) persons. In regression analyses, done separately for each region (not shown in a table; see Mollenkopf et al., 2002), we found that biological age is not the critical factor determining the extent of satisfaction with one's mobility options. By contrast, being physically able to move about, being satisfied with the public transport system, and being able to drive a car (and not just to have a car available) were the most important variables in almost all regions studied.

Results (3). The Specific Contribution of Mobility to Older Adults' Satisfaction with Life and Well-being

But now let us see whether our assumption, that in modern society mobility means much more than the practical utility of getting from a place A to a destination B, was right. We had claimed a strong relation between outdoor mobility and modern values such as freedom, self-determination and flexibility. In case this assumption also would hold true for older adults, it should be reflected in a higher subjective quality of life if they were provided with a broad range of transport options and the possibility to pursue a great diversity of outdoor activities in addition to their actual mobility and in addition to basic human conditions such as health and income. As indicator for subjective quality of life, we used a one-item scale assessing satisfaction with life in general (Veenhoven, 1996; Zapf & Habich, 1996) and the positive or negative affect scale (PANAS) (Watson, Clark, & Telegen, 1988) as a measurement of emotional well-being. Regression analyses were carried out separately for each country (for predictor and remarks see Tables 3 and 4).

In view of the findings we have to differentiate our hypothesis: As expected and in accordance with previous studies (for an overview see Diener, Suh, Lucas, & Smith, 1999; Golant, 2004; Veenhoven, 1996), satisfaction with one's health and income was revealed to be the most important predictors of satisfaction with life in general. These aspects contributed substantially to emotional well-being as well, albeit with clearly less impact. As far as the three different components of mobility (options of transport modes, options of outdoor activities and actual mobility) are concerned, they did not contribute substantially to the older persons' satisfaction with life in general. Only in Germany and Italy did a large diversity of activities play a positive role with respect to the cognitive evaluation of life quality. However, subjective mobility related aspects, such as the importance of being out (in three out of the five participating countries) and satisfaction with the possibilities to pursue leisure time activities (in all regions studied), were significant predictors of satisfaction with life, thus supporting our notion of a more comprehensive understanding of mobility.

The impact of the mobility indicators increases when considering the emotional aspects of quality of life. A great diversity of outdoor activity options, in particular, contributes significantly to positive affect, even more so than satisfaction with health and income. Actual mobility in terms of trips made plays a positive role in the German and Hungarian regions, and a broad range of transport options is an important additional predictor of well-being in Finland. As is the case in regard to general life satisfaction, outdoor orientation and satisfaction with leisure activities explain emotional well-being as well, each in at least three of the countries.

Altogether the findings confirm that actual mobility, measured in terms of trips made, does not play a decisive role in explaining older adults' quality of life. Against our assumption, the impact of a broad range of transport modes used is limited as well. However, performing a great diversity of outdoor activity options and/or the satisfaction with one's opportunities to be active contribute substantially to both satisfaction with life in general and positive affect. Hence, subjectively important activities are obviously the prime motive of outdoor mobility, whereas the trips made and the transport modes used seem to be the functional means to achieve these goals. The strong impact of being able to pursue activities for satisfaction with life and emotional well-being supports the hypothesis that in modern society older adults' quality of life is largely affected by these mobility aspects, featuring values such as self-determination, flexibility and the freedom to get where and to do what one wants to do.

Table 3. Predictors of satisfaction with life

	Standard β-weights				
	Finland	*The Netherlands*	*Germany*	*Hungary*	*Italy*
Region (1 = urban; 2 = rural)					0.12**
East/West (1 = east; 2 = west)					
Age			0.05*		
Gender (1 = male; 2 = female)	0.11***				
Diversity of network				0.15***	0.09*
Satisfaction with health*	0.20***	0.34***	0.23***	0.29***	0.29***
Satisfaction with income*	0.48***	0.20***	0.34***	0.28***	0.30***
Satisfaction with leisure activities*	0.21***	0.21***	0.23	0.15***	0.22***
Wish for more outdoor activities (0 = no; 1 = yes)					
Importance of being out†		0.15***	0.10***	0.09*	0.02
Options of transport modes‡					
Options of outdoor activities¶			0.09***		0.11*
Actual mobility§					
N	584	571	1476	548	599
Model r^2	0.4755	0.3815	0.4790	0.3218	0.3573

Note: MOBILATE survey 2000; MOBILATE diary 2000.
* $p < 0.01$.
** $p < 0.01$.
*** $p < 0.001$.
*Self-evaluation rating on an 11-point rating scale, higher scores indicating higher satisfaction.
†Self-evaluation rating on an 11-point rating scale, higher scores indicating higher importance.
‡Sumscore ranging from 0 (no transport mode used, respondent is immobile) to 13 (all transport modes are used).
¶Standardised sumscore ranging from 0 (no outdoor activity purposed) to 1 (all asked outdoor activities pursued).
§Mean number of trips per person and day.

Table 4. Predictors of subjective well-being (positive affect)

	Standard β-weights				
	Finland	*The Netherlands*	*Germany*	*Hungary*	*Italy*
Region (1 = urban; 2 = rural)			−0.23***	0.12**	
East/West (1 = east; 2 = west)					
Age	−0.30***		−0.09***		−.23***
Gender (1 = male; 2 = female)		0.10**		0.08*	
Diversity of network			0.15***	0.13**	
Satisfaction with health*	0.13**		0.11***	0.13**	0.11**
Satisfaction with income*		0.09*			
Satisfaction with leisure activities*	0.09*	0.09*		0.17***	0.28***
Wish for more outdoor activities (0 = no; 1 = yes)					0.09*
Importance of being out†	0.09*		0.09***	0.18***	
Options of transport modes‡	0.13**				
Options of outdoor activities¶	0.19***	0.19**	0.32***	0.18***	0.19***
Actual mobility§			0.13***	0.12**	
N	565	535	1438	491	597
Model r^2	0.4101	0.1569	0.3817	0.3077	0.4184

Note: MOBILATE survey 2000; MOBILATE diary 2000.
*$p < 0.01$.
**$p < 0.01$.
***$p < 0.001$.
*Self-evaluation rating on an 11-point rating scale, higher scores indicating higher satisfaction.
†Self-evaluation rating on an 11-point rating scale, higher scores indicating higher importance.
‡Sumscore ranging from 0 (no transport mode used, respondent is immobile) to 13 (all transport modes are used).
¶Standardised sumscore ranging from 0 (no outdoor activity purposed) to 1 (all asked outdoor activities pursued).
§Mean number of trips per person and day.

CONCLUSIONS AND OUTLOOK

With today's increasing functional and spatial separation of the occupational and private spheres of life, and of commercial, residential and leisure domains, mobility has become an ever more important aspect of ensuring the ability to lead one's everyday life, keep up social relations and take part in every kind of activity outside one's own four walls. Mobility and the use of the transport system, whether by foot or with private or public means of transportation, in order to get where one wants to go are therefore major prerequisites for maintaining quality of life. Due to the increasing risk of a decline of physical and sensory competences in old age, the growing population of older people will find it difficult to maintain the requisite levels of mobility and, by this, social well-being. Such difficulties are exacerbated by unfavourable environmental and technological conditions. But our first and perhaps most important finding is: The decline of outdoor mobility in old age, well-known from many other studies, is not an entirely voluntary retreat from the world.

In view of these findings, the question arises on what consequences the increasing number of older car owners will exert on the possibilities and preferences of aging adults to be on the go. In Europe, elderly people—at least currently—are far less "automobile" than in the USA (Rosenbloom, 2000). This will change, however, in the coming years when the generation of people for whom driving a car has become a matter of course reach retirement age. The greater availability of private cars may expand the elderly persons' scope of movement and action. At the same time, individual advantages may be accompanied by societal disadvantages, as the use of motorised means of transportation is a major cause of environmental degradation, of increasing noise and air pollution. The growing volume and density of traffic that results also increases the potential hazards of older adults' travel. Traffic congestion, particularly in urban centres, has reached the extent that may unsettle elderly people and keep them from venturing out. Moreover, as a person ages, the risk of his or her having an accident grows in relation to driving performance (and hence in relation to the exposure to danger). Walking or biking are not good alternatives either: Elderly people are very vulnerable as unprotected road users (Schlag, 2003).

At the same time, the mobility needs of older adults will be supported further by technological advances at various levels. Easier access to expeditious and convenient modes of transportation will enable almost unlimited mobility and change our very definition of what is "near" or "far". These examples clearly illustrate both the new freedom and flexibility of travelling and the dangers of isolation in a modern hermitage due to the new reliance upon technology. It is an open question whether the formidable technical possibilities will lead older adults to stay at home more or to get out and about more—both of which are possible.

Hence, two parallel, but opposing tendencies can be observed: On the one hand, opportunities—especially technologically supported options—for being on the go in old age increase substantially. On the other hand, the inter-related trends of urban decentralisation, decreasing public transport services, dispersal of travel origins and destinations and increasing automobile use mutually reinforce each other. As a result, elderly people who do not have the alternative of using a personal automobile or ICT applications may come to suffer structural discrimination if important elements of the infrastructure, basic services and recreation facilities continue to depend on personal transportation and remain concentrated either in city centres or in remote areas. This is particularly salient for elderly people whose life space gradually but steadily contracts because of changes in their physical and sensory abilities. As our findings show, being able to continue leading independent lives, maintain social contact and take advantage of recreational activities are great needs in old age (see also Schaie, 2003).

Ensuring older persons more opportunities for participation in their social, built-up and natural environments despite the physical handicaps, possible financial constraints and social, technological and spatial barriers that exist in their world, would thus greatly contribute to their quality of life and well-being. Therefore, the question of whether and how external conditions and demands of the environment can be harmonised with individual needs and resources will be a societal and political topic in the years to come.

AFFILIATION

The German Centre for Research on Ageing at the University of Heidelberg

REFERENCES

Diener, E., Suh, E. M., Lucas, R. E., & Smith, H. L. (1999). Subjective well-being: Three decades of progress. *Psychological Bulletin, 125*, 276–302.

European Conference of Ministers of Transport (ECMT). (2000). Transport and aging of the population. Report of the 112th round table on transport economics, held in Paris on 19th–20th November 1998. Paris Cedex, France: OECD Publications.

Golant, S. M. (2004). The urban–rural distinction in gerontology: An update of research. In H.-W. Wahl, R. J. Scheidt, & P. G. Windley (Eds.), *Aging in context: Socio-physical environments* (Annual Review of Gerontology and Geriatrics, 2003) (pp. 280–312). New York: Springer Publishing.

Lawton, M. P. (1983). Environment and other determinants of well-being in older people. *The Gerontologist, 23*(4), 349–357.

Leventhal, H., Rabin, C., Leventhal, E. A., & Burns, E. (2001). Health risk behaviours and aging. In J. E. Birren & K. W. Schaie (Eds.), *Handbook of the psychology of aging* (pp. 186–214). New York: Academic Press.

Litman, T. (2003). Measuring transportation: Traffic, mobility and accessibility. *The ITE Journal, 73*(10), 28–32.

Mollenkopf, H. (1996). Social integration of elderly people in industrialised societies: An introduction. In Mollenkopf, H. (Ed.), *Elderly people in industrialised societies* (pp. 13–22). Berlin: Edition sigma.

Mollenkopf, H., Marcellini, F., Ruoppila, I., Baas, S., Ciarrocchi, S., Hirsiaho, N., et al. (2003). The MOBILATE follow-up study 1995–2000. Enhancing outdoor mobility in later life: Personal coping, environmental resources, and technical support. (DZFA Research Report No. 14). Heidelberg: German Centre for Research on Ageing (DZFA).

Mollenkopf, H., Marcellini, F., Ruoppila, I., Széman, Z., & Tacken, M. (Eds.) (in press). *Enhancing mobility in later life—Personal coping, environmental resources, and technical support.* The out-of-home mobility of older adults in urban and rural regions of five European countries. Amsterdam: IOS Press.

Mollenkopf, H., Marcellini, F., Ruoppila, I., Széman, Z., Tacken, M., Kaspar, R., et al. (2002). The role of driving in maintaining mobility in later life: A European view. *Gerontechnology, 1*(4), 231–250.

Mollenkopf, H., Marcellini, F., Ruoppila, I., Széman, Z., Tacken, M., & Wahl, H.-W. (2004). Social and behavioural science perspectives on out-of-home mobility in later life: Findings from the European project MOBILATE. *European Journal of Ageing, 1,* 45–53 (DOI: 10.1007/s10433-004-0004-3).

Mollenkopf, H., Marcellini, F., Ruoppila, I., & Tacken, M. (Eds.) (2004). *Ageing and outdoor mobility: A European study.* Amsterdam: IOS Press.

Mollenkopf, H., Oswald, F., Schilling, O., & Wahl, H.-W. (2001). Aspekte der außerhäuslichen Mobilität älterer Menschen in der Stadt und auf dem Land: Objektive Bedingungen und subjektive Bewertung. *Sozialer Fortschritt,* 50(9–10), 214–220.

Organisation for Economic Co-operation and Development (OECD). (1985). *Traffic safety of elderly road users.* Paris: Road Transport Research (OECD).

Oswald, F., Wahl, H.-W., Mollenkopf, H., & Schilling, O. (2003). Housing and life satisfaction of older adults in two rural regions in Germany. *Research on Aging, 25*(2), 122–143.

Rantanen, T., Harris, T., Leveille, S. G., Visser, M., Foley, D., Masaki, K., et al. (2000). Muscle strength and body mass index as long-term predictors of mortality in initially healthy men. *Journal of Gerontology: Medical Sciences, 55 A,* M168–M173.

Rosenbloom, S. (2000). Report by the chairperson (United States). In European Conference of Ministers of Transport (ECMT) (Ed.), *Transport and aging of the population* (Report of the 112th round table on transport economics) (pp. 7–42). Paris Cedex, France: OECD Publications.

Ruoppila, I., Marcellini, F., Mollenkopf, H., Hirsiaho, N., Baas, S., Principi, A., et al. (2003). The MOBILATE cohort study 1995–2000: Enhancing outdoor mobility in later life. The differences between persons aged 55–59 years and 75–79 years in 1995 and 2000 (DZFA Research Report No. 17). Heidelberg: German Centre for Research on Ageing (DZFA).

Schaie, K. W. (2003). Mobility for what? In K. W. Schaie, H.-W. Wahl, H. Mollenkopf, & F. Oswald (Eds.), *Aging independently. Living arrangements and mobility* (pp. 18–27). New York: Springer Publishing.

Schlag, B. (2003). Safety and accidents among older drivers: The German perspective. In K. W. Schaie, H.-W. Wahl, H. Mollenkopf, & F. Oswald (Eds.), *Aging independently: Living arrangements and mobility* (pp. 205–219). New York: Springer Publishing.

Tacken, M., & Caso, O. (1999). Elderly and outdoor mobility in a Dutch new town: Zoetermeer-Meerzicht. In Tacken, M., Marcellini, F., Mollenkopf, H., & Ruoppila, I. (Eds.), *Keeping the Elderly Mobile. Outdoor Mobility of the Elderly: Problems and Solutions* (pp. 75–86). Delft: Delft University Press.

Veenhoven, R. (1996). Developments in satisfaction-research. *Social Indicators Research, 37,* 1–46.

Watson, D., Clark, L. A., & Telegen, A. (1988). Development and validation of brief measures of positive and negative affect: The PANAS scales. *Journal of Personality and Social Psychology, 6,* 1063–1070.

World Business Council for Sustainable Development (WBCSD). (2002). *Mobility 2001—World mobility at the end of the twentieth century and its sustainability.* Available from www.wbcsdmobility.org.

Zapf, W., & Habich, R. (Eds.). (1996). *Wohlfahrtsentwicklung im vereinten Deutschland* (Welfare development in Germany after unification). Berlin: Edition sigma.

JON E. BURKHARDT

COMMENTARY: MOBILITY—A KEY TO UNDERSTANDING AND IMPROVING TRANSPORTATION SERVICES FOR SENIORS AND OTHERS

Dr. Mollenkopf and her associates have made a vital contribution to our understanding of the often used but seldom well-defined concept of mobility (Mollenkopf, Baas, Kaspar, & Wahl, 2004). Like the proverbial blindfolded scientists investigating an elephant, most previous researchers have tended to focus on small pieces of a much larger whole; Dr. Mollenkopf's team of authors offers a broader and more integrated perspective.

Many authors have noted trends in many countries regarding spatial dispersion of homes and economic activities, leading to a corresponding dispersion of travel origins and destinations (Burchell et al., 1998). A substantial contribution of the research of Mollenkopf and her associates is the recognition that not responding the growing disparities between individuals who can readily access transportation services and those persons who cannot is indeed a societal form of *structural discrimination*. In order to ensure that seniors and others have full access to the goods and services of modern societies, it is vital to pay much more attention to the issue of mobility than it has received to date.

Using nearly a decade of research, beginning in 1994 with sponsorship of the Social Science Research Centre Berlin and continuing in 2000 with the MOBILITATE project sponsored by the European Commission, Mollenkopf and associates asked older adults residing in the cities studied what mobility meant to them. The results identified seven main aspects of mobility:

- Physical movement [a basic human need],
- A basic emotional experience,
- Movement in natural surroundings and observation of nature,
- A social need,
- An expression of personal autonomy and freedom,
- A source of stimulation and diversion,
- A reflective expression of one's personal life force.

These findings correlate nicely with Metz's seminal article that discusses the need for an operational definition of mobility (Metz, 2000). In that article, Metz argues for the following "qualitative elements of mobility":

- travel to achieve access to desired people and places;

H.-W. Wahl et al. (eds.), The Many Faces of Health, Competence and Well-Being in Old Age, 47–52.

- psychological benefits of movement—getting "out and about";
- exercise benefits;
- involvement in the local [wider] community;
- potential travel—knowing that a trip could be made even if it is not.

Metz notes that the last four items are "destination-independent" benefits, which is to say that they are benefits that can be considered to be "incidental" to the purpose of accessing specific destinations and persons. Metz's psychological, exercise and social benefits form close parallels to those found by Mollenkopf, and knowing that a trip could be made even if it is not is arguably a good expression of personal autonomy and freedom. Metz also quotes Bly who noted that "the extent to which physical travel satisfies some inherent social need, and provides amenity value separate from the activity at the destination, has not yet been adequately measured" (Bly et al., 1995).

The measurement process undertaken by Mollenkopf and associates should create significant improvements in our understanding of what mobility means for seniors. Mobility problems of seniors in the United States may be even more common than in Europe due to the overwhelming reliance in the States on automobiles as the primary (and often, sole) means of transportation, even for seniors. In 1997, Straight showed that the median number of trips by drivers in the United States who are 75 years of age or older is three times that of nondrivers 75 years of age or older and that half of these nondrivers take two or fewer trips per week (Straight, 1997). In 2004, Bailey found that 21% of Americans 65 and older do not drive (Bailey, 2004), and that more than 50% of nondrivers 65 and older (3.6 million Americans) stay home on any given day because they lack transportation options. They make fewer trips to doctors, shops and restaurants and to family or social activities. According to Bailey, seniors tend to make good use of public transportation services where they are available, but 34% of Americans (many of whom live in suburban and rural areas) report that they have no public transportation services available to them in their community (Burkhardt, McGavock, Nelson, & Mitchell, 2002; Pucher and Renne, 2003). Added to this concern is the fact that 3.5 million Americans *never leave their home*; 1.9 million of these are persons with disabilities (US DOT, 2003).

An extremely useful avenue for future research would appear to be measuring the detailed impacts of a loss of mobility. Mollenkopf and associates touch on this issue, but its full explication is likely to require a serious longitudinal study involving detailed travel diaries over a number of years. Their reports of the dramatic expression of personal desires to remain mobile are mirrored by other results in the United States (Burkhardt, Berger, Creedon, & McGavock 1998; Stutts, 1996). Comments regarding stopping driving reported by seniors in the United States have included (Burkhardt et al., 1998):

> "The end of the world, I would think so."
>
> "I would crawl right into myself."
>
> "I would be unhappy, very unhappy. I think most people would.... [If I had to stop driving] I'd get out and walk if I could walk."

> "That would be a pretty hard pill to swallow."
>
> "Well, it would be bad, make it bad. I go... [lots of places now]. But if I couldn't drive, I'd have to pester someone or starve, one or the other."
>
> "I think that would be the end of my independence. Because if I'm feeling low in spirits, I get in the little red thing [my car] and go over to the shopping centre and they know me.... Things like that perk me up again. Psychologically, it's a very important thing."

These comments suggest an important distinction in perspectives in Europe and the United States: Mollenkopf and associates report that "the idea of being no longer able to move about outdoors one day is regarded is terrible" and that "walking is clearly the most common mode of travel of older adults in Europe". Mollenkopf's interviewees seemed to be able to identify mobility in terms of "getting around", while mobility in the United States too often means driving. Mollenkopf's subjects reported driving for 28.4% of their trips and riding in a car as a passenger for 11.3% of their trips; in the United States, comparable figures for seniors are driving for more than 45% of their trips and riding in a car as a passenger for 43% of their trips.

A detailed catalogue of the consequences of low mobility or of losing the mobility that one once had, still needs to be created. In a majority of cases, mobility—whether measured in quantitative or qualitative terms—declines (Burkhardt, 1999). Fewer trips will be taken, shorter distances will be travelled, fewer or no trips will be taken under certain conditions, and the older person will be more often travelling according to the schedules and convenience of others instead of their own desires. Some of the consequences of mobility losses could be expected to include

- a loss of independence and greater dependence on others;
- personal identity issues; a decline in self-esteem;
- decreases in life satisfaction;
- an increase in social isolation;
- depression and reduced physical and emotional health;
- extra efforts and costs for families and communities.

It must be noted that it requires a great deal of planning for an older person to get to and from a destination without personally driving. This was shown in focus groups with elders 70 years and older (Burkhardt et al., 1998), including some of who had reduced or ceased driving. Mobility changes that were mentioned with some frequency by seniors who were reducing their driving including having to plan your life around other people's schedules and the reduction or total loss of recreational activities, such as going out to eat, movies, and socialisation, especially at night. Still, very few individuals will make no trips at all, and most persons will find a way to make "necessary" trips, even if at higher monetary and psychological trip costs.

After driving, the most common transportation mode is riding in a car as a passenger. Asking for and accepting rides from family and friends is difficult for an older person, particularly a person raised in the tradition of independence and self-sufficiency. As one older woman stated: "You really get humble, you hate to ask". Seniors who do not drive are hesitant to ask for additional rides because they are often unable to reciprocate by providing a ride or other services. Some seniors are able to meet their basic transportation needs of grocery shopping, medical appointments and other basic errands reasonably well after stopping driving if they possess specific resources or had made certain accommodations.

The concept that "life depends on driving" is less prevalent when other travel options are available; many European cities are superior to their U.S. counterparts in the variety of travel options that they offer. Persons who have access to a well-developed public transportation system and can live in close proximity to the kinds of shopping and recreational opportunities that appeal to seniors feel that a car was not a necessity to live an active life. They can control their own mobility choices and make reasoned choices about driving or not driving.

Certainly in the United States, the older person who reduces or ceases driving bears the brunt of the mobility changes that occur, in terms of monetary, social, psychological and emotional costs (Burkhardt, 1999). When it is not possible to maintain previous connections established by our elderly citizens, society suffers from the lack of access to the expertise of these older adults, as well as from the loss of their productivity as workers and volunteers. Thus, there are many reasons to take steps to reduce the potential mobility losses associated with the reduction or cessation of driving.

The subjects studied by Mollenkopf and associates reported little correlation between mobility and life satisfaction: "... three different components of mobility ... did not contribute substantially to the older person's satisfaction with life in general". To be sure, the finding that satisfaction with one's income and health has a large influence on overall life satisfaction measures is not at all surprising. But Mollenkopf's finding of little correlation should by no means be taken as "proof" of the unimportance of mobility: one suspects that further research involving quantitative measures of *mobility losses* could actually show important correlations with life satisfaction. For example, Marottoli's work (Marottoli, de Leon, Williams, Berkmall, & Tinetti, 1995) demonstrates a relatively strong correlation between loss of mobility and depression. Considering Marottoli's and Mollenkopf's works at the same time, it seems that further research should perhaps focus more on mobility losses rather than upon measures of mobility. This might be a crucial avenue for further research.

What can we conclude about mobility? What could we call its significant impacts on individual lives? Among the many potential impacts on seniors and others, mobility

- provides access to economic opportunities and needed goods and services;
- provides freedom and independence; reduces the need to depend on (inconvenience) others;
- offers comfort in dependability: the knowledge that rides are there when needed;
- generates social interaction, personal stimulation and emotional satisfaction; reduces isolation and loneliness;
- saves money;
- avoids unnecessary institutionalisation.

Mobility is clearly multidimensional, as noted by Mollenkopf's seven main aspects of mobility—as a basic emotional experience, as physical movement, as a basic human need, as movement in natural surroundings and observation of nature, as a social need, as an expression of personal autonomy and freedom, as a source of stimulation and diversion and as a reflective expression of one's personal life force. Mollenkopf's seven aspects are more personal and emotional than those described in other research, which has focused more on mobility's economic impacts, thus significantly expanding previous conceptions of mobility. Combining the knowledge of all these sources will considerably enhance our ability to understand and measure mobility for citizens of many countries.

Our ability to open up the benefits of modern societies to all citizens who have difficulties access transportation services—seniors, persons with disabilities, persons with low incomes, youth and others—requires an emphasis on firm understandings of mobility. We need to concentrate on the needs of seniors and others with special transportation needs by examining their mobility options, measuring the outcomes of service programs and providing transportation plans for regional and local governments. Investments in mobility make good economic sense, provide needed access, provide wide personal and community benefits and help address the forthcoming challenges of societies that are rapidly aging.

For too long, we've taken the "if we build it, they will come" approach to all modes of transportation. While that may work for as much as 90% of persons who might use any transportation mode, the 10% who are left out become severely disadvantaged by their inability to access all the components of modern society. Concepts of universal design need to become an automatic component of all our transportation modes. The level of access offered to transportation services for persons with special needs, including the elderly, the disabled and the working poor—collectively referred to as "the transportation disadvantaged"—should be seen as a measure of a society's true commitment to raising the living standards of all of its citizens. We need to ensure that transportation is a facilitator, not a barrier, to the independence that people want and need, because it is more cost effective for any society to have mobile citizens, with (nearly) everyone in charge of their own lives. The paper by Mollenkopf and associates contributes significantly to our ability to bring the issue of mobility for seniors and others to the forefront of attention in society.

AFFILIATION

WESTAT, Rockville, MD, USA

REFERENCES

Bailey, L. (2004) *Stranded without options*. Surface Transportation Policy Project, Washington, DC.

Bly, P. H., Hunt, P. B., Maycock, G., Mitchell, C. G. B., Porter, J., & Allsop, A. (1995). *Future scenarios for inland surface transport* (TRL Report 130). Transport Research Laboratory, Crowthorne.

Bureau of Transportation Statistics. (2003). *Transportation difficulties keep over a half million disabled at home*. Washington, DC: U.S. Department of Transportation.

Burchell, R. W., Shad, N. A., Listokin, D., Phillips, H., Downs, A., Seskin, S., Davis, J. S., Moore, T., Helton, D., & Gall, M. (1998). *The costs of sprawl—revisited, TCRP Report 39*. Transit Cooperative Research Program. Washington, DC: Transportation Research Board, The National Academies (contains a large list of references).

Burkhardt, J. (1999). Mobility changes: their nature, effects, and meaning for elders who reduce or cease driving. In *Accessible transportation and mobility 1999. Transportation Research Record 1671*. Washington, DC: Transportation Research Board.

Burkhardt, J. E., Berger, A. M., Creedon, M. A., & McGavock, A. T. (1998). *Mobility and independence: Changes and challenges for older drivers*. Prepared by Ecosometrics, Incorporated for the US Department of Health and Human Services and the National Highway Traffic Safety Administration.

Burkhardt, J., McGavock, A. T., Nelson, C. A., & Mitchell, C. G. B. (2002). *Improving public transit options for older persons: TCRP Report 82*. Transit Cooperative Research Program. Washington, DC: Transportation Research Board, The National Academies.

Marottoli, R. A., de Leon, C. M., Williams, C. W., Berkmall, L. F., & Tinetti, M. E. (1995). Consequences of driving cessation among elderly individuals. *Journal of the American Geriatrics Society, 43*, SA6.

Metz, D. H. (2000). Mobility of older people and their quality of life. *Transport Policy, 7*, 149–152.

Mollenkopf, H., Baas, S., Kaspar, R., & Wahl, H.-W. (2004). *Outdoor mobility in later life: Persons, environments and society*. Presented to the Conference on The Many Faces of Health, Competence and Well-being in Old Age, Heidelberg, Germany.

Pucher, J. & Renne, J.L. (2003). Socioeconomics of urban travel: evidence from the 2001 NHTS. *Transportation Quarterly, 57*, 3.

Straight, A. (1997). *Community transportation survey*. Washington, DC: American Association of Retired Persons.

Stutts, J. (1996). *Older driver functional disabilities and road safety*. Paper presented at the Expert Panel Conference on Safety and Mobility Issues of Older Driver, Leesburg, VA.

HANS-WERNER WAHL,[1] VERA HEYL,[1] STEFANIE BECKER,[2]
OLIVER SCHILLING[1] and HEIDRUN MOLLENKOPF[1]

AGE-RELATED LOSS IN VISION: A CASE TO LEARN ABOUT AGEING IN CONTEXT

1. TOWARDS A CONTEXTUAL UNDERSTANDING OF AGE-RELATED VISION LOSS: A GENERAL FRAMEWORK

The term context, as used in the ageing literature, has many facets (see Dannefer, 1992; Wahl & Lang, 2004). When we use this term in relation to age-related vision loss, we predominantly refer to the following aspects. First, vision loss does not operate in a vacuum but must always be seen in the whole concert of resources available to the ageing individual. Second, vision loss is a prototypical case of a resource loss with direct consequences in terms of person–environment transactions. Third, vision loss deserves attention in regard to the specific lifespan context in which it is appearing.

Figure 1 depicts the conceptual framework used to address these different contextual aspects in a simultaneous manner.

To begin, we feel that the understanding of age-related vision loss can profit from a dialectic between the experience of vision loss as a major development-constraining condition and the assumed capacity for proactivity (Lawton, 1989). Developmental constraints can be identified on the level of core person characteristics, for instance, by putting pressure on the preservation of the self in both positive behavioural and emotional outcomes. Furthermore, developmental constraints also come with increased vulnerability for the visually impaired individual with respect to the sociophysical and physical-spatial environments. The concept of proactivity emphasises that dealing with vision loss both as an internal and as an external resource adjustment is an active process, which can best be understood by merging general adaptational models of development with ecology models explicitly pointing to the role of person–environment relations in ageing (Wahl & Weisman, 2003). For example, a general adaptational model such as the Heckhausen and Schulz (1995) Life-span Theory of Control argues that maintaining primary control, that is, investing time and effort in the attainment of major life goals, is particularly at risk as people age. The case may be even stronger in the situation of severe vision loss, in which the primary control motivation is in special need of being backed by active compensation such as accepting that certain goals in life are no longer attainable. Hence, proactivity assumes that ageing individuals faced with vision loss are not "pawns" of their loss experience; instead, they actively strive to use remaining resources on the inter- and extrapersonal level to counteract the developmental threat as much as possible. Proactivity is also in operation when it comes to the regulation of the person–environment system (Lawton, 1989, 1999). For example, in

H.-W. Wahl et al. (eds.), The Many Faces of Health, Competence and Well-Being in Old Age, 53–64.

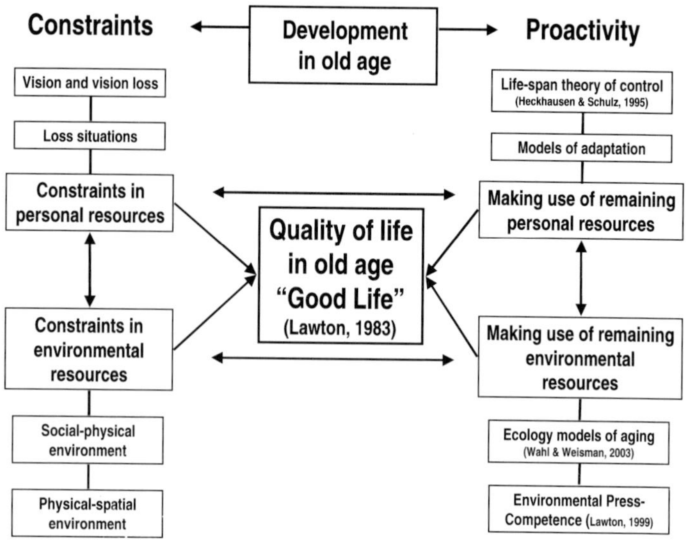

Figure 1. Conceptual framework of age-related vision loss.

the event of vision loss, narrowing down one's out-of-home action range to a rather limited area around one's home echoes proactivity in terms of reducing one's sociospatial life space, and simultaneously enhancing one's sense of control within this downsized "world". This also means that proactivity frequently comes with a Janus face, offering at the same time gain and loss to the ageing individual (see also Baltes, 1987).

The given interplay between experiencing vision loss as a major developmentally constraining condition and counteracting this experience in terms of proactivity may lead to dramatic interindividual differences in what remains possible in terms of the "good life" (Lawton, 1983), seen as the ultimate global outcome in our conceptual framework. We prefer the term "good life" in contrast to other terms, such as "successful" ageing, because the connotation of "success" seems problematic when referring to major loss situations such as severe vision impairment. Also, Lawton's (1983) term has been explicitly defined as the result of person–environment transactions, including the physical-spatial environment, which fits well with our contextual understanding of vision loss.

Finally, an important assumption is that our theoretical framework is not restricted to severe loss of vision and can, at least in principle, also be generalised to address normal age-related vision loss in a contextual perspective. One question arising from such a view is how normal vision change is related to change in cognition, activity and well-being and whether a robust pattern of such relations exists, for example, across samples from different countries. However, we also assume that such a potentially robust developmental pattern will become more dependent on additional intra- and extrapersonal resources, when very severe vision impairment occurs. That is, normal age-related vision loss does not dramatically alter person–environment relations and thus depends only marginally on the specific characteristics of a given "environmental press" (Lawton, 1999; Lawton & Nahemow, 1973). In the case of severe vision loss, the "good life" is strongly related to existing or threatened person–environment fit or else misfit between personal functioning and environmental challenges, and thus substantially adds to the explanation of variations in "good life" outcome variables, such as basic and instrumental activities in daily living (ADL-IADL) and the exertion of leisure activities (Lawton, 1983; Lawton & Nahemow, 1973).

2. METHOD

Due to the fact that this work aims to synthesise major aspects of a whole research program that addressed the psychosocial role of age-related vision loss, we will provide here only a brief description of the methods used in this research (see original papers cited below for more details). We regard a mix of cross-sectional and prospective studies as most promising in order to address major implications of our theoretical framework. For instance, learning about the behavioural, social and emotional consequences as well as about robust relations with other mediating or outcome variables can be successfully achieved by relying on cross-sectional work. Addressing the causal role of adaptational dynamics, in terms of proactivity, of course presumes longitudinal data.

We rely on rather small samples of visually severely impaired elders (in the range below 100 participants) allowing for high data density. Also, in order to address the question of what is specific for the experience of vision loss in terms of behavioural and emotional outcomes, we included unimpaired elders and elders suffering from other types of chronic conditions such as severe mobility loss. We used rather large samples up to more than 1,000 participants, when exploring links between normal age-related vision change and variables such as cognition and out-of-home activities. All of these data stem from community-residing older adults roughly between the age of 55 and below 100 years; the assessment of vision function is always based on an objective screening of visual acuity and not only on subjective vision data. In addition, controlled intervention research based on pre- and postintervention control group designs has also begun to take place more recently.

In accordance with what frequently has been done in the general literature in the field, we have included in our research a scope of eye diseases and focused on their functional–psychosocial consequences (e.g. Wahl, Schilling, Oswald, & Heyl, 1999). We have also addressed the special case of age-related macular degeneration (AMD), which is the most frequent cause of vision loss in later life (e.g. Wahl, Becker, Burmedi & Schilling, 2004).

3. RESULTS

Results are presented in three sections. First, we address severe vision loss and add empirical substance to major elements of our theoretical framework. Because severe vision loss was the major focus of our work so far, reported findings will mainly deal with this aspect. Second, we proceed to normal age-related vision loss and address the question of how this relates, in combination with other resources, to the "good life" in behavioural and emotional terms. Third, we briefly touch upon on data of two pilot evaluation studies aimed to translate our findings into psychosocial intervention.

3.1. Severe Age-Related Vision Loss in Context: A Selection of Findings

With respect to the development-constraining character of the experience of severe vision loss, our findings replicate and extend what already has been reported in earlier studies, that is, how the experience of vision loss is a major developmental threat to the individual affected by this stress experience and also its impact on personal resources (Wahl et al., 1999). In accordance with many other studies (e.g. Horowitz, 1994; see Burmedi, Becker, Heyl, Wahl, & Himmelsbach, 2002a,b for a general review), we found that the impact of severe vision loss on the activities of daily living is quite dramatic, as compared to unimpaired elders, specifically in the case of ADL-IADL. Impact is even more pronounced in the situation of blindness as compared to severe visual impairment.

Also important is that we have controlled in these analyses for confounders such as age, sex, household situation, education and self-reported health in these data. As can also be seen, implications of severe vision loss on the "good life" are less dramatic when it comes to well-being, particularly when compared to the well-being consequences of another major chronic condition, that is, mobility impairment. However, the impact of severe vision loss, specifically blindness, on day-to-day functioning has been found to be stronger than the experience of mobility impairment.

Long-term consequences of the experience of vision loss were observed up to 7 years in our studies (Heyl & Wahl, 2001a,b). As we have found, behavioural and, still more pronounced, emotional consequences tend to increase over time and thus remain a development challenge for those affected across long-term intervals. Major factors explaining interindividual differences in outcomes over time are comorbidity and the speed of progression of the vision loss.

Adaptational dynamics at the psychological level also play a major role and seem to operate in a causal manner when it comes to the explanation of differential outcomes, reflecting in a sense processes of what has been coined proactivity in our conceptual framework. In a recent study with AMD patients observed over a 1-year interval, we have addressed this by making use of the Life-span Theory of Control suggested by Heckhausen and Schulz (1995). As was found, selective primary control was quite important for outcomes such as ADL, IADL and positive and negative emotions (see Figure 2). As can be seen in Figure 2, those high in selective primary control were higher in ADL, IADL, positive emotions and, at least tentatively, lower in negative emotions, keeping their higher level across the 1-year observation period, which contrasts with those low in this control modality (see also Wahl et al., 2004). These relationships were not affected by the progression of visual impairment over time.

According to our conceptual framework, additional contextual perspectives on age-related vision loss demand the explicit consideration of person–environment dynamics and the accompanying developmental constraints. With respect to the living environment, a detailed assessment of the physical home environment was done by use of a

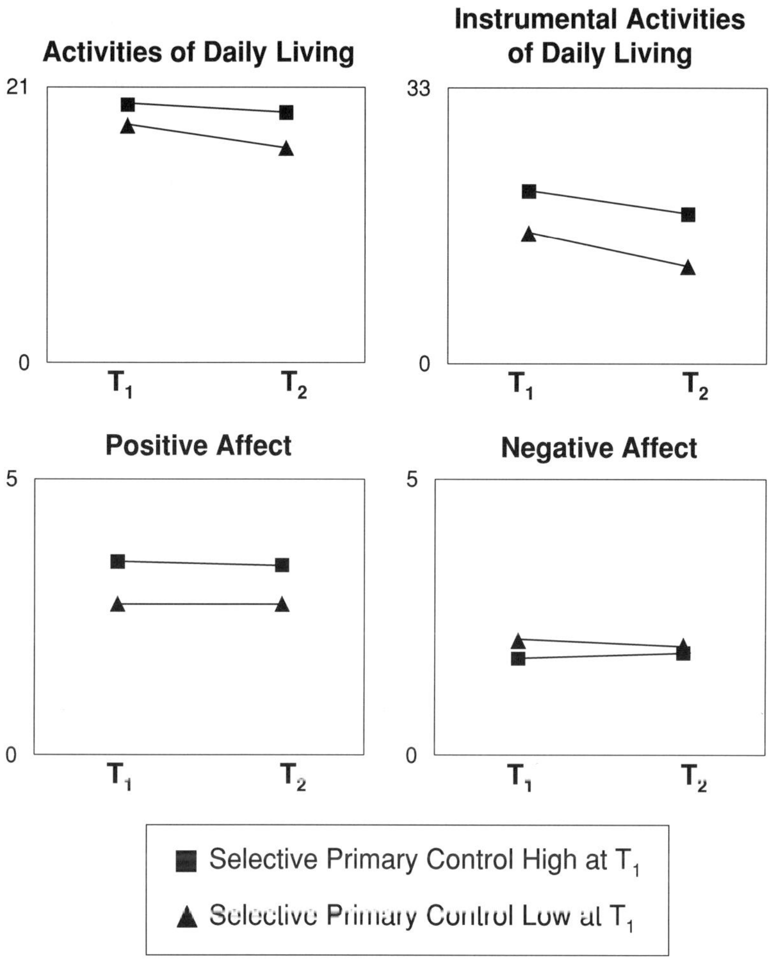

Figure 2. Role of selective primary control for major outcomes in visually impaired elders. Note: N = 71, participants 60 years and older and suffering from age-related macular degeneration. T1–T2: 1-year observation interval.

standardised and reliable walk-through procedure (Wahl, Oswald, & Zimprich, 1999). Next, different degrees of vision loss (blindness, severe visual impairment, no vision impairment) were correlated with different person–environment fit situations that were then linked to self-reported performance in everyday competence. It was found that the existence of a person–physical environment misfit situation and lowered everyday competence (specifically IADL exerted in the home environment) were substantially associated in case of both blindness and severe vision loss, whereas this was not true regarding the unimpaired group. This supports the well-known but empirically underanalysed docility hypothesis with which Lawton (e.g. Lawton & Nahemow, 1973) has assumed that loss in basic functioning, such as vision impairment, is linked to increased vulnerability for "environmental press". In contrast, unimpaired elders were not much affected by such "environmental press" in their home environments.

However, environmental press seems not only to be passively tolerated in a reactive manner, but there is reason to assume the existence of person–environmental proactivity on this level as well. A fine-tuned analysis of compensation efforts based on the coding of verbal reports in relation to the conductance of day-to-day activities revealed a full range of person- and environment-related strategies aimed to reduce person–environment fit gaps (Wahl, Oswald, & Zimprich, 1999). For example, we have observed pronounced adjustment of one's behaviour in terms of using other senses ("latent skills", in general terms) or simplifying the conductance of normal household-related activities, which in turn supports the assumption of proactivity. It seems that such compensation within the home environment also comes with what Lawton (1985) has coined "density of control" or the creation of "control centres". By this means a significantly reduced action potential in conjunction with a range of compensations adds to the "good life" by maintaining relatively high control in a reduced world, which is a strategy we have labelled as "winning by losing" in the case of visually impaired elders. This may also echo the Janus-faced character of proactivity in the situation of severe vision loss, as stated earlier, as part of the expectation driven by our theoretical framework.

3.1.1. Conclusion I

Seen from a lifespan development point of view, as suggested in our theoretical framework, severe vision loss operates as a major developmental constraining condition and threatens behavioural, social and emotional adaptation and thus the "good life" in old age (Lawton, 1983). Also, reduced everyday competence and well-being in visually impaired elders come in conjunction with an increased vulnerability to "environmental press" (Lawton & Nahemow, 1973). However, this remains a one-sided picture of the "real" dynamics, as long as ageing individuals' proactivity on both the personal and the person–environmental level is not taken into consideration. One pathway to demonstrate this fundamental human tendency is the Life-span Theory of Control suggested by Heckhausen and Schulz (1995). This approach is specifically promising because vision loss can be seen not only as a loss of environmental control (Wahl et al., 2004), but control dynamics also lie at the heart of the regulation of person–physical environment relations (see findings best interpreted as tendencies towards "density of control" or creating "control centers"; Lawton, 1985). Nevertheless, an important task of future research is to also test the potential of alternative adaptational models such as Brandtstädter and Renner's (1990) distinction between assimilation and accommodation in order to better understand the experience and outcome of severe vision loss (Boerner, 2004).

3.2. Normal Vision Loss in Context: A Selection of Findings

Additional contextual understanding of age-related vision loss emerges when we turn to the situation of normal vision loss. Although the vision loss itself is important, it

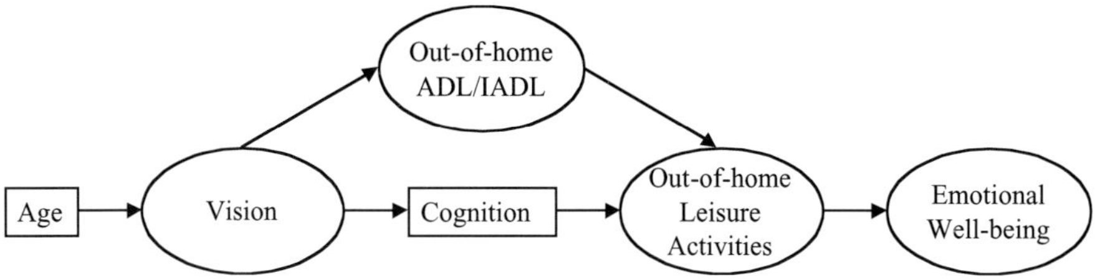

Figure 3. A robust model of age, visual, cognition, out-of-home activities and well-being. Note: Cognition is based on the digit symbol test.

must be seen within the context of other resources in order to achieve a more realistic picture of the ongoing dynamics in terms of person and environment-related resources and their impact on the "good life". In line with work emerging from the Berlin Aging Study (BASE; Marsike, Klumb, & Baltes, 1997), we analysed the role of vision on out-of-home activities on the basic level (ADL-IADL out of the home) as well as on a more expanded level (leisure out-of-home). We have selected out-of-home activities because the challenge to counteract uncontrollable environmental press is higher outside of the "safe" home environment and thus the role of functional losses such as vision impairment should become particularly crucial (see also Wahl, Heyl, & Schilling, 2002). Additionally, we considered cognitive performance as a major driver of such relations. With these variables considered in simultaneous manner, we were able to identify a rather robust pattern of interrelations across different countries (Figure 3). The data set of the study "Enhancing Outdoor Mobility in Later Life: Personal Coping, Environmental Resources, and Technical Support" (MOBILATE), which also involved a vision screening, was used for this purpose (Mollenkopf, Baas, Kaspar, Oswald, & Wahl, in press).

A path model with vision mediating the role of calendar age on out-of-home ADL-IADL as well as on cognition was identified. However, no direct "influence" of vision on outcomes, such as expanded out-of-home leisure activities and well-being, was needed in order to achieve a good model fit in a cross-country perspective that included samples from Finland, East and West Germany, as well as Italy. In fact, the standardised path coefficients are surprisingly similar across the samples from those regions and countries (see Table 1).

3.2.1. Conclusion II

Our findings support, in combination with other work (e.g. Lang, Rieckmann, & Baltes, 2002; Marsike et al., 1997), the notion that not only severe vision loss but also "normal" vision loss plays a substantial role for maintaining the "good life" in old age. Caution is of course in place when it comes to causal explanations of the observed relations and satisfactory model fit results. Given that our data so far are cross-sectional, and taking into consideration the general state of discussion in this field of inquiry (specifically in regard to the link between vision and cognition; see Wahl & Heyl, 2003, for review),

Table 1. Testing the basic vision model with respect to its robustness across sociocultural contexts: results of structural equation modelling

	Standardised path coefficients			
	Finland (n = 610)	*East Germany (n = 768)*	*West Germany (n = 751)*	*Italy (n = 600)*
Age → Vision	−0.72	−0.72	−0.72	−0.72
Vision → ADL/IADL	0.73	0.73	0.73	0.73
Cognition → Leisure	0.71	0.59	0.60	0.73
Vision → ADL/IADL	0.52	0.51	0.51	0.52
Cognition → Leisure	0.31	0.36	0.35	0.30
Leisure → Well-being	0.66	0.66	0.66	0.65

Note: $\chi^2 = 697.20$, df $= 157$, $p < 0.05$, root mean squared error of approximation = 0.036, Tucker–Lewis index) = 0.989, comparative fit index = 0.993; all participants aged 55 years and older.

we interpret these dynamics in terms of a mixed causal model. On the one hand, the similar decline trajectory of vision and cognition likely reflects a "common cause" (see also Lindenberger & Baltes, 1994), that is, an age-related alteration of the neural architecture at large; on the other hand, we expect, informed by the literature on *severe* vision loss addressed in the foregoing section, that the relation of vision and cognition to out-of-home activities can be interpreted in a causal manner and that this is also likely with respect to their role in relation to well-being.

In sum, *objective* vision alterations are part of the "normal ageing" process exerting its role "early" in the causal pathways. Seen against our theoretical framework, the development-constraining role of normal vision loss operates more in the background of the "normal" ageing process. This must be qualified further based on findings supporting the view that *subjective* evaluations of vision can directly impact on well-being as was found in the BASE (Smith, Fleeson, Geiselmann, Settersten, & Kunzmann, 1999). When objective vision loss becomes quite severe as in the occurrence and progression of AMD, it likely takes over as a direct cause of loss in behavioural and emotional outcomes, making its developmental-constraining role most obvious in day-to-day life.

3.3. Using Findings for Psychosocial Intervention with Visually Impaired Older Adults

Parallel to our more basic research, we have recently begun to use our findings in order to plan intervention and to serve the mostly unmet psychosocial needs of many visually impaired older adults. In terms of our conceptual framework, many older adults are left alone with the developmental constraints caused by their vision loss and the challenge to strengthen their proactivity as much as possible frequently does not take place.

To be sure, we are not the first to address this need in an empirically controlled manner (see, for example, Brody et al., 2002). However, we believe that we are able to offer quite a direct link between basic findings and application and add by this means to an evidence-based approach in the intervention field. First, we have developed a respective psychosocial group intervention program tailored to five sessions distributed across 5 weeks and provided a first successful pilot evaluation of the program (see Birk et al., 2004, for the details). We also tested for a minimal intervention tailored to only three group sessions distributed across 3 weeks. In addition, we tested in this study for differential effects of an emotion-focused versus problem-focused group intervention approach (Wahl, Holz, Kämmerer, & Becker, 2004). We found that adaptation to vision loss increased only in the problem-focused intervention group, while depression decreased only in the emotion-focused group. Although these findings are promising and speak to the usefulness of psychosocial intervention, two major limitations also deserve mentioning. First, we found that dropout persons were significantly worse off than the participants both in emotional and behavioural measures. Hence, a major challenge to intervention research, as well as clinical psychosocial practice, is to reach those who are likely to possess the strongest demand in terms of emotional and behavioural burden due to their vision loss. Second, a follow-up study conducted 3 months after baseline revealed that training gains completely disappeared once again, which supports the view that psychosocial intervention must cover quite a substantial period and intensity to show sustainable effects in the longer run.

3.3.1. Conclusion III

It is an important and necessary step to make better use of existing research findings on age-related vision loss in creating psychosocial intervention programs while evaluating the potential of these programs in a rigorous empirical manner. A major driving force to do so is that psychosocial needs of visually impaired elders are hardly met in the day-to-day clinical practice of medical eye treatments. In sum, data coming from the scarce intervention research in the field (e.g. Brody et al., 2002; Dahlin-Ivanoff, 2000) as well as our own findings generated so far (Birk et al., 2004; Wahl, Holz, et al., 2004) support the view that a group intervention setting is a promising tool in this regard, but long-term outcomes of such intervention deserve stronger attention in this area of inquiry.

4. FROM VISION IN CONTEXT TO AGEING IN CONTEXT

Vision loss provides a promising research paradigm to underline the notion that good ageing deserves the engagement of a variety of adaptational processes drawing upon both intra- and extrapersonal resources in response to developmental challenges (Featherman, Smith, & Peterson, 1990). The occurrence of severe and progressive vision loss, as in the case of AMD, may even be seen as a simulation of accelerated ageing, in which intrapersonal and environmental resources have to be reorganised in quite a short time. We also followed this kind of thinking in our recent application of the Life-span Theory of Control Approach (Heckhausen & Schulz, 1995; Wrosch, Schulz, & Heckhausen, 2004) to AMD, in which we have also shown that compensatory control efforts increase over a 1-year time interval (Wahl, 2004).

In addition, we believe that addressing the development-constraining condition of vision can highlight the demand to use and apply the term context in ageing research to the social and physical-spatial environment. While the social surrounding has traditionally found much attention in the ageing literature, this is less true regarding the physical-spatial context. Going further, research on vision loss may also add to the need to no longer let the "social relations" field (e.g. Antonucci, 2001) and "ecology" field (e.g. Wahl, 2001) stand side by side; instead, both of these major environmental spheres demand strong integrative perspectives as people age (Wahl and Lang, 2004). Take for example the shrinkage in action range due to age-related loss in vision as has also been found in our research (not addressed in detail in this chapter; Wahl, 1998). On the one hand, such reduction of life space is adaptive and enhances the feeling of being in control in downsized settings. On the other hand, "adaptation" of this kind at the physical-spatial level frequently comes with major loss experiences in the social domain and sometimes with the feeling of no longer being part of day-to-day community life or even an active or "valuable" citizen. Research on vision loss can thus deepen the more general understanding of proactivity in ageing. In particular, it seems to lie at the heart of human development in later life that proactivity comes with a Janus face, that is, gains and losses tend to operate increasingly hand in hand while people age (Baltes, 1987).

AFFILIATIONS

[1]*The German Centre for Research on Ageing, University of Heidelberg*

[2]*Institute of Gerontology, University of Heidelberg*

REFERENCES

Antonucci, T. C. (2001). Social relations. An examination of social networks, social support, and sense of control. In J. E. Birren & K. W. Schaie (Eds.), *Handbook of the psychology of aging* (5th ed., pp. 427–453). San Diego: Academic Press.

Baltes, P. B. (1987). Theoretical propositions of life-span developmental psychology: On the dynamics between growth and decline. *Developmental Psychology, 23*, 611–626.

Birk, T., Hickl, S., Wahl, H.-W., Miller, D., Kämmerer, A., Holz, F., et al. (2004). Development and pilot evaluation of a psychosocial intervention program for patients with age-related macular degeneration. *Gerontologist, 44*, 836–843.

Boerner, K. (2004). Adaptation to disability among middle-aged and older adults: The role of assimilative and accommodative coping. *Journal of Gerontology: Psychological Sciences, 59*, P35–P42.

Brandtstädter, J., & Renner, G. (1990). Tenacious goal pursuit and flexible goal adjustment: Explication and age-related analysis of assimilative and accommodative strategies of coping. *Psychology and Aging, 5*, 58–67.

Brody, B. L., Roch-Levecq, A.-C., Gamst, A. C., Maclean, K., Kaplan, R. M., & Brown, S. I. (2002). Self-management of age-related macular degeneration and quality of life: A randomized controlled trial. *Archives of Ophthalmology, 120*, 1477–1483.

Burmedi, D., Becker, S., Heyl, V., Wahl, H.-W., & Himmelsbach, I. (2002a). Behavioral consequences of age-related low vision: A narrative review. *Visual Impairment Research, 4*, 15–45.

Burmedi, D., Becker, S., Heyl, V., Wahl, H.-W. & Himmelsbach, I. (2002b). Emotional and social consequences of age-related low vision: A narrative review. *Visual Impairment Research, 4*, 47–71.

Dahlin-Ivanoff, S. (2000). *Development and evaluation of a health education programme for elderly persons with age-related macular degeneration*. Gothenburg, Sweden: Göteborg University.

Dannefer, D. (1992). On the conceptualization of context in developmental discourse: Four meanings of context and their implications. In D. L. Featherman, R. M. Lerner, & M. Perlmutter (Eds.), *Life-span development and behavior* (Vol. 11, pp. 83–110). Hillsdale: Erlbaum.

Featherman, D. L., Smith, J., & Peterson, J. G. (1990). Successful aging in a "post-retired" society. In P. B. Baltes & M. M. Baltes (Eds.), *Successful aging: Perspectives from the behavioral sciences* (pp. 50–93). New York: Cambridge University Press.

Heckhausen, J., & Schulz, R. (1995). A life-span theory of control. *Psychological Review, 102*, 284–304.

Heyl, V., & Wahl, H.-W. (2001a). On the long-term psychosocial adaptation to vision loss in the later years. In H.-W. Wahl & H.-E. Schulze (Eds.), *On the special needs of blind and low vision seniors: Research and practice concepts* (pp. 77–83). Amsterdam: IOS Press.

Heyl, V., & Wahl, H.-W. (2001b). Psychosocial adaptation to age-related vision loss: A six-year perspective. *Journal of Visual Impairment and Blindness, 95*, 739–748.

Horowitz, A. (1994). Vision impairment and functional disability among nursing home residents. *The Gerontologist, 34*, 316–323.

Lang, F. R., Rieckmann, N., & Baltes, M. M. (2002). Adapting to aging losses: Do resources facilitate strategies of selection, compensation, and optimization in everyday functioning? *Journal of Gerontology: Psychological Sciences, 57B*, P501–P509.

Lawton, M. P. (1983). Environment and other determinants of well-being in older people. *The Gerontologist, 23*, 349–357.

Lawton, M. P. (1985). Activities and leisure. In C. Eisdorfer, M. P. Lawton, & G. L. Maddox (Eds.), *Annual review of gerontology and geriatrics* (pp. 127–165). New York: Springer.

Lawton, M. P. (1989). Environmental proactivity and affect in older people. In S. Spacapan & S. Oskamp (Eds.), *The social psychology of aging* (pp. 155–164). Newbury Park: Sage.

Lawton, M. P. (1999). Environmental taxonomy: Generalizations from research with older adults. In S. L. Friedman & T. D. Wachs (Eds.), *Measuring environment across the life span* (pp. 91–124). Washington, DC: American Psychological Association.

Lawton, M. P., & Nahemow, L. (1973). Ecology and the aging process. In C. Eisdorfer & M. P. Lawton (Eds.), *The psychology of adult development and aging* (pp. 619–674). Washington, DC: American Psychological Association.

Lindenberger, U., & Baltes, P. B. (1994). Sensory functioning and intelligence in old age: A strong connection. *Psychology and Aging, 9*(3), 339–355.

Marsike, M., Klumb, P., & Baltes, M. M. (1997). Everyday activity patterns and sensory functioning in old age. *Psychology and Aging, 12*, 444–457.

Smith, J., Fleeson, W., Geiselmann, B., Settersten, R. A., & Kunzmann, U. (1999). Sources of well-being in very old age. In P. B. Baltes & K. U. Mayer (Eds.), *The Berlin aging study. Aging from 70 to 100* (pp. 450–471). Cambridge: Cambridge University Press.

Wahl, H.-W. (1998). "Der Raum ist eingefallen"—Alterskorrelierte Sehbeeinträchtigung als Lebenskrise und Herausforderung an Bewältigungsressourcen [Age-related vision impairment as life crisis and coping challenge]. *Zeitschrift für Klinische Psychologie, 27*, 111–117.

Wahl, H.-W. (2001). Environmental influences on aging and behavior. In J. E. Birren & K. W. Schaie (Eds.), *Handbook of the psychology of aging* (5th ed., pp. 215–237). San Diego: Academic Press.

Wahl, H.-W. (2004). Sehverlust im höheren Lebensalter aus Person-Umwelt-Perspektive: Befunde und Anwendungsimplikationen [Vision loss in old age from a person-environment persepctive: Findings and implications for application]. In Verband der Blinden- und Sehbehindertenpädagogen und -pädagoginnen (VBS) (Ed.), *"Qualitäten". Rehabilitation und Pädagogik bei Blindheit und Sehbehinderung. Kongressbericht* (pp. 88–121). Würzburg: Edition Bentheim.

Wahl, H.-W., & Heyl, V. (2003). Connection between vision, hearing, and cognitive function in old age. *Generations, 27*, 39–45.

Wahl, H.-W., & Lang, F. R. (2004). Aging in context across the adult life: Integrating physical and social research perspectives. In H.-W. Wahl, R. Scheidt, & P. G. Windley (Eds.), *Aging in context: Socio-physical environments (Annual Review of Gerontology and Geriatrics, 2003)* (pp. 1–35). New York: Springer.

Wahl, H.-W., & Weisman, G. D. (2003). Environmental gerontology at the beginning of the new millennium: Reflections on its historical, empirical, and theoretical development. *The Gerontologist, 43*, 616–627.

Wahl, H.-W., Becker, S., Burmedi, D., & Schilling, O. (2004). The role of primary and secondary control in adaptation to age-related vision loss: A study with macular degeneration. *Psychology and Aging, 19*, 235–239.

Wahl, H.-W., Heyl, V., & Schilling, O. (2002). The role of vision impairment for the outdoor activity and life satisfaction of older adults: A multi-faceted view. *Visual Impairment Research, 4*, 143–160.

Wahl, H.-W., Holz, F., Kämmerer, A., & Becker, S. (2004). Psychosoziale Beratung und Versorgung von älteren Menschen mit altersabhängiger Makuladegeneration. Entwicklung, Durchführung und Evaluation einer modellhaften Intervention [Psychosocial counseling and support for older persons with macular degeneration]. Heidelberg: Deutsches Zentrum für Alternsforschung.

Wahl, H.-W., Oswald, F., & Zimprich, D. (1999). Everyday competence in visually impaired older adults: A case for person-environment perspectives. *The Gerontologist, 39*, 140–149.

Wahl, H.-W., Schilling, O., Oswald, F., & Heyl, V. (1999). Psychosocial consequences of age-related visual impairment: Comparison with mobility-impaired older adults and long-term outcome. *Journal of Gerontology: Psychological Sciences, 54B*, P304–P316.

Wrosch, C., Schulz, R., & Heckhausen, J. (2004). Health stress and depressive symptomatology in the elderly: A control-process approach. *Current Directions in Psychological Science, 13*, 17.

AMY HOROWITZ

COMMENTARY: AGE-RELATED LOSS IN VISION: A CASE TO LEARN ABOUT AGING IN CONTEXT

In the preceding chapter, Dr. Wahl and colleagues have provided an overview of a multifaceted research programme on age-related vision loss conducted at the German Centre for Research on Ageing at the University of Heidelberg. The scope of this research programme is extremely impressive, not only for its specific contributions to the study of vision loss in later life, but also for informing the more general phenomenon of ageing in context. As such, this commentary begins with a brief discussion of the major contributions of this research programme to understanding psychosocial adaptation to age-related vision loss, and then addresses some specific issues raised in the chapter.

One of the most basic, but critical, contributions of this research is that it drew attention to a long ignored area of study. At a time when gerontologists were overlooking, the implications of sensory impairments for life quality, and those studying adjustment to vision impairment were ignoring the elderly, Wahl and colleagues highlighted the importance of studying vision impairment as a prototypical disability of later life; that is, vision impairment as an age-related developmental challenge which propels the older adult to activate his/her internal and external resources to maintain well-being. The message that was clearly conveyed was that the study of age-related vision loss would have important implications for the general study of late-life disability as well.

Second, and of paramount significance, has been his contribution in bringing a theoretical perspective into what had been a largely atheoretica field. In particular, Dr. Wahl was the first to identify the Life Span Theory of Control (Heckhausen & Schulz, 1995) as a theoretical framework with crucial relevance for understanding how visually impaired older adults address daily challenges and strive to balance and rebalance control in their everyday lives. Because the experience of vision loss in later life tends to constitute a major threat to one's sense of competence and control, as well as being typically characterised by gradual onset and progressive deterioration, it is an age-related loss that poses increasing and continuously changing adaptational challenges requiring a process-oriented approach represented by the Life Span Theory of Control. Based on this framework, research teams at both the German Centre for Research on Aging at the University of Heidelberg and the Arlene R. Gordon Research Institute of Lighthouse International (http://www.lighthouse.org) were able to collaborate and develop similar study designs, eventually providing an unparalleled opportunity to not only contribute to the theoretical understanding of adaptational processes in later life, but to explore cross-national comparisons as well.

H.-W. Wahl et al. (eds.), The Many Faces of Health, Competence and Well-Being in Old Age, 65–70.

Dr. Wahl's third major contribution is that he has brought the unique, and critical, perspective of an environmental gerontologist to broaden the scope of research in the field to include questions related to person–environment transactions and person–environment fit. His substantive findings pointing to the greater salience of person–physical environment misfit for everyday competence of visually impaired older adults, as compared to the unimpaired elderly, has been one of the few empirical tests of Lawton's theory of environment press.

There were several criteria issues raised in the Wahl et al. paper, with space allowing for discussion of only the few which are highlighted in the sections below.

1. VISION IMPAIRMENT AS A PROTOTYPICAL VERSUS AN EXTRAORDINARY EVENT

The research programmes in both Heidelberg and New York have approached vision impairment in later life as a prototypical age-related disability because of its especially robust relationships with both physical functioning and psychological well-being (Burmedi, et al., 2002a,b; Horowitz, 2003; Horowitz & Reinhardt, 2000). Not only does vision impairment consistently emerge as a risk factor for disability in the research literature (Burmedi et al., 2002a), but also it has been identified as one of the "big three" conditions, along with stroke and arthritis, having the most pervasive implications for everyday functioning (Ford et al., 1988; Verbrugge & Patrick, 1995). Given the well-documented relationship between disability and depression in later life (Bruce, 2001), it is thus not surprising that vision impairment is also a very strong risk factor for poorer psychological well-being, and especially for significant depressive symptomatology.

The effect on functional competence, however, is not the only pathway by which vision impairment affects the "good life". It can be proposed that it is also important to look at the characteristics of vision impairment in later life that uniquely influence the elder's *subjective* experience of this impairment.

One of the most distinctive characteristics of a vision loss is the intense fear it evokes. Loss of vision is seen as an extraordinary traumatic event that threatens the very identity of the individual. Why would this be the case, more so than for other disabilities? Simply, there are pervasive social attitudes, myths and stereotypes that surround "blindness" in Western culture that are not necessarily attached to other disabilities—age-related or otherwise. In mythology, religious and popular literature, loss of vision has been historically associated with punishment for sin, with the abject beggar and with the loss of autonomy. One only needs to mention Oedipus Rex to conjure up images of blindness as retribution. Children are introduced to these stereotypes early in life through the many fairy tale characters that inevitably lose and then regain their sight to reach a "happy ever after" ending (Horowitz, 2004). These stereotypes define current attitudes of the general public. For example, in the United States, public opinion polls have found that other physical disabilities, such as mobility limitations and hearing impairment, are more tolerable than "blindness", (The Lighthouse Inc., 1995), and that blindness ranked fourth, following only AIDS, cancer and Alzheimer's disease, as the illness most feared by

Americans of all ages, primarily because of its association with complete helplessness and dependency (National Society to Prevent Blindness, 1984). Fears about the loss of autonomy, and the move from independence to dependence, then, become central to understanding individual reactions and meanings ascribed to a vision problem. That is, the older adult whose mobility is limited by a vision loss may have a totally different subjective experience than an older adult with the same objective functional limitation, but as a result of arthritis. Thus, the concept of "illness representations" reflecting the subjective meanings individual attach to their specific health conditions, is an important one to incorporate in research focussing on adaptational processes of older adults facing a variety of health-related developmental challenges.

2. NORMAL VISION CHANGES VERSUS AGE-RELATED VISION IMPAIRMENT

The goal of integrating research addressing normal vision changes with that focussing on the functional and psychosocial implications of age-related vision impairment in later life is one of the central themes of the Wahl et al. paper. However, I would suggest that this may not only be a goal difficult to attain, but one that may not be necessarily desirable. Rather, there is a pressing need to clearly distinguish the implications of normal age-related changes in vision from the experience of vision impairment caused by age-related eye disorders, in both our research designs and presentation of findings.

Age-related vision changes involving major visual functions, such as acuity, contrast and adaptation to dark, typically begin in midlife, progress gradually allowing for gradual accommodation, and, most importantly, can be functionally corrected by regular prescription lenses. A person experiencing these normal age-related changes would be very unlikely to characterise their vision change as a challenge to either their functional or emotional well-being (even if, for some, it may symbolise the onset on the aging process). The study of these normal vision changes, and their relationship with other neurological functions such as cognition, can tell us much about what Rowe has called "usual" aging (Rowe & Kahn, 1987). However, because these normal changes do not result in significant functional limitations, they are not consistent with the conceptual underpinnings of adaptational research that is concerned with how people interpret and address constraints that can have potentially significant implications for well-being.

In contrast, vision impairments are the result of disease processes and are not correctable by glasses or medical/surgical interventions. Furthermore, even in the case of age-related eye diseases, there is likely a threshold of impairment that must be crossed before adaptational processes are fully engaged. These visual impairments typically, over time, have functional consequences for everyday living, and, as discussed earlier, also have a strong subjective component that interacts to influence psychological well-being. While there are important overlapping and complimentary interests in these two areas of study, it is critical that each carefully distinguish whether they are addressing normal vs. disease processes. The question of whether they can be fully integrated within a common conceptual framework remains to be answered.

3. THE IMPORTANCE OF EXAMINING AGING IN CONTEXT

The work of Wahl and his colleagues is distinguished by the emphasis on a contextual view of vision and vision loss. As was stressed in the preceding chapter, we cannot treat vision loss as operating in a vacuum. Rather the experience of this developmental constraint must be examined within a context of comorbidity, remaining resources and proactivity in their use, and how they interact to influence the "good life" in old age. Our research findings from a Lighthouse International study of depression among 584 visually impaired older adults strongly support this contextual perspective (Horowitz, Reinhardt, Brennan, & Raykov, 2003). Findings indicate that objective clinical indicators of vision impairment do not have a direct effect on functional disability, but only an indirect one through subjective evaluations of vision loss severity. This suggests that the extent to which clinical impairments result in functional disability depends, in part at least, on the way the impairment is perceived. Similarly, clinical vision impairment had no direct relationship with depression, which supports the growing body of research indicating that objective measures of disease severity are only weakly, if at all, related to mental health outcomes (Horowitz & Reinhardt, 2000). Rather, the link between physical impairment and mental health outcomes is primarily through the extent of disability that the impairment causes. What we found to be most interesting is that functional disability did *not* have a significant *direct* effect on depression, as would be expected, but an indirect one that was fully mediated by personal and social resources. Thus, high functional disability does not always lead to high depression, in that high levels of personal and social resources are protective and can combat the negative effects of disability. These findings clearly support the need to account for the context—personal, social and environmental—in which older adults confront development constraints as they age in order to understand the pathways to the "good life".

4. THE APPLICABILITY OF THE LIFE SPAN THEORY OF CONTROL TO THE STUDY OF AGE-RELATED VISION IMPAIRMENT

Lastly, the applicability of the Life Span Theory of Control to the study of adaptation to age-related vision impairment deserves further examination, both in terms of how the theory frames the empirical work and how the empirical work may further contribute to theory development.

The Life Span Theory of Control has been applied to examine the maintenance of one's sense of competence in the face of the losses and challenges that typically occur in later life through the use of both primary and secondary control strategies. Whereas primary control is aimed at changing the external environment by active action, secondary control is more concerned with adaptation of the self. Further, the dimensions of selection and compensation are considered as core processes of adaptation so that both primary and secondary control modes can involve selective as well as compensatory strategies (Heckhausen & Schulz, 1995).

The findings presented in the Wahl et al. paper highlight the importance of primary control strategies, with those high on selective primary control having better functional status, as well as higher positive affect, both at baseline and the one year follow-up.

These findings support the theory's propositions regarding the importance of primary control for goal achievement. It is also interesting to note from these data that the use of primary control strategies by *both* those initially high and low in their use at baseline, decreased substantially over time when examined in the context of activities of daily living (ADL) and instrumental ADL (IADL) functioning. This, in turn, highlights the developmental aspect of the life span control theory, reflecting ongoing adaptational transactions in response to changing circumstances. That is, over time, when personal losses exceed both available internal and external resources for goal attainment, primary and selective secondary control strategies may become less successful and the shift to self-protective compensatory secondary strategies becomes more adaptive.

The challenge of reading for an older person with macular degeneration, using comments from participants in the Lighthouse study of control strategies and mental health, is presented to illustrate this process over time. First, the person may keep trying to read as before, by taking more time and trying to concentrate harder, representing a *selective primary control strategy* of focussing internal resources through, for example, time and effort (*"I'm just pressing my whole strength and will power into reading").* This person may support his or her efforts by thinking how important and enjoyable it is to read, representing *a selective secondary control strategy* to strengthen internal motivation ("*My head tells me read, read, its good for you, you'll love it*").

If vision loss progresses and reading becomes impossible, the person may decide to use optical devices, representing a *compensatory primary control strategy* which involves the use of external resources to make up for limitations in a person's physical or mental capabilities. (*"I hadn't been able to read the newspaper until I got the machine (Closed Circuit TV) and then last week we set it up and I read the whole paper and I was thrilled*"). However, if the visual disability further progresses and the devices do not help with reading anymore, the person may now devalue the goal of reading and turn to other things he or she can do, representing a *compensatory secondary strategy* where the person disengages from the original goal and re-evaluates his or her priorities. (*"there's nothing I can do about that (not reading). So I try to just not dwell on that. I listen to the radio. I go and watch the TV; get on the phone and talk to a friend, things like that*").

While both research programmes have put a strong emphasis on understanding the dynamic nature of the adaptational process over time, Lighthouse research has taken a somewhat different approach in examining ADL–IADL functioning in the context of these adaptational processes. Whereas the programme at the German Centre on Ageing has primarily examined functional ability as an outcome, we primarily conceptualise it as a predictor which drives the use of different control strategies. These two approaches, however, are not necessarily mutually exclusive as there are inevitable reciprocal effects over time. However, given the view that well-being is primarily a subjective rather than objective phenomenon with subjective assessments of life conditions mediating the effects of the objective situation on indicators of well-being, we hypothesize that control strategies will have a stronger influence on the individual's *satisfaction* with how they are functioning, as outcome, than on their objective functional status.

To conclude this commentary, I would like to strongly concur with Wahl et al. in the call for carefully controlled intervention studies that test evidence-based approaches designed to maximise both physical and psychosocial functioning of older persons confronting an age-related vision loss. The pilot work described in Wahl et al. is breaking new ground in empirically linking different focussed interventions to their logical outcomes; that is problem-focussed group interventions influencing more vision-specific outcome measures, while emotion focussed approaches having their effect on more global measures of affective status. Yet, as has been acknowledged, there is a long road ahead, especially since treatment effects were not maintained over time. Further, one cannot overstate the importance of targeting interventions to individuals who, in fact, evidence distress in the adaptational process. There is great variability in both adaptational processes and their outcomes among older adults who confront developmental losses. Many older adults are amazingly resilient, maximising available internal and external resources to establish a successful person–environment fit in the broadest sense. Others are not so successful. Our challenge as applied researchers is to identify the adaptational strategies implemented by older adults, and better understand why some elders are better able to implement these strategies than others—and ultimately to target, adapt and evaluate interventions to meet the specific needs of the individual.

AFFILIATION

Arlene R. Gordon Research Institute, Lighthouse International

REFERENCES

Bruce, M. L. (2001). Depression and disability in late life: Directions for future research. *American Journal of Geriatric Psychiatry, 9,* 102–112.

Burmedi, D., Becker, S., Heyl, V., Wahl, H., & Himmelsbach, I. (2002). Emotional and social consequences of age-related low vision. *Visual Impairment Research, 4 (1)*, 47–71.

Burmedi, D., Becker, S., Heyl, V., Wahl, H. W., & Himmelsbach, I. (2002). Behavioral consequences of age-related low vision. A narrative review. *Vision Impairment Research, 4 (1)*, 15–45.

Ford, A. B., Folmar, S. J., Salmon, R. B., Medalie, J. H., Roy, A. W., & Galazka, S. S. (1988). Health and function in the old and very old. *Journal of the American Geriatrics Society, 36 (3)*, 187–197.

Heckhausen, J., & Schulz, R. (1995). A life-span theory of control. *Psychol. Rev., 102 (2)*, 284–304.

Horowitz, A. (2003). Depression and vision and hearing impairments in later life. *Generations, 27,* 32–38.

Horowitz, A. (2004). The prevalence and consequences of vision impairment in later life. *Topics in Geriatric Rehabilitation, 20 (3)*, 185–195.

Horowitz, A., & Reinhardt, J. P. (2000). Mental health issues in visual impairment: Research in depression, disability, and rehabilitation. In B. M. Silverstone, M. Lang, R. Rosenthal, & E. Faye (Eds.), *The Lighthouse handbook on vision impairment and vision rehabilitation: Vol. II. Vision rehabilitation* (pp. 1089–1109). New York: Oxford University Press.

Horowitz, A., Reinhardt, J.P., Brennan, M., & Raykov, T (2003, November). *Mediating the disability-depression link: The role of personal and social resources.* Paper presented at the Annual Scientific Meeting of the Gerontological Society of America, San Diego, California.

Lighthouse Inc. (1995). The Lighthouse National Survey on Vision Loss: The experiences, attitudes and knowledge of middle-aged and older Americans New York: The Lighthouse Inc.

National Society for the Prevention of Blindness (1984). Survey '84: Attitudes towards blindness prevention. *Sight-Saving, 53,* 14–17.

Rowe, J. W., & Kahn, R.L. (1987). Human aging: Usual and successful. *Science, 237,* 143–149.

Verbrugge, L. M., & Patrick, D. L. (1995). Seven chronic conditions: Their impact on US adults' activity levels and use of medical services. *American Journal of Public Health, 85,* 173–182.

PART II

FOCUSING ON PSYCHOLOGICAL RESEARCH—CONTRIBUTIONS TO HEALTH, COMPETENCE, AND WELL-BEING IN OLD AGE

ANDREAS KRUSE

INTRODUCTION: DEVELOPMENTAL PERSPECTIVES IN THE SECOND HALF OF LIFE

By way of introduction to the subject area of "adult development", I would like to refer to the following three papers. In my view, each of these contributions touches on a specific aspect of development. I shall discuss each aspect respectively with recourse to a central theory of developmental psychology; thereafter, I shall classify each respective contribution according to the appropriate theory. Three central theoretical positions will be addressed here since I consider them to be fundamental to developmental psychology, but also particularly central to the understanding of the three papers that follow. The initial theoretical position to be discussed is one which considers development in the context of life structures and subjectively meaningful relationships in the world of the individual. Further, a theoretical position will be stated which connects the aleatory of development with the continuity of development. Finally, a theoretical position will be outlined which views the ability of an individual to attain transcendency, understood in the sense of achieving change of perspective, as a significant basis for development.

1. DEVELOPMENT IN THE CONTEXT OF LIFE STRUCTURES AND SUBJECTIVE MEANINGFUL RELATIONSHIPS

In one of Daniel Levinson's formulations of adult development, presented in 1986, the concept of life structure is introduced, through which he describes the underlying pattern or design of a person's life at a given time. Levinson clarifies the meaning of this concept by contrasting it with the concept of personality structure: Theories of the latter are described as ways of conceptualising answers to the question "What kind of person am I?" whereas theories of the former are described as conceptualising answers to another concrete question, i.e. the question "What is my life like now?". Constituting a "mediating zone between personality structure and social structure", the concept of life structure takes both a developmental and a socialisation perspective on human development: "Because the life structure is not solely a property of the individual, its evolution cannot be understood from an intraorganismic, developmental perspective. Because the life structure is not simply a matter of externally imposed events and roles, its evolution cannot be understood simply from a socialisation perspective. It is necessary, instead, to create a new perspective that combines development and socialisation and that draws equally on biology, psychology and social sciences, as well as on the humanities" (Levinson, 1986, p. 13). The central components of the life structure make up the subjectively meaningful relationships of the individual to "various others" in the

H.-W. Wahl et al. (eds.), The Many Faces of Health, Competence and Well-Being in Old Age, 73–79.

external world. The "various others" can take the form of people, a group, an institution, a culture, a particular place. According to Levinson, significant relationships require the following condition as a starting point: there is a high level of investment of the self in the relationship, and furthermore, the self experiences enrichment in the relationship, for example, encouragement and stimulation, and the self can adjust itself further from the effect of this enrichment. Consequently, the following central conclusion can be drawn—I quote: "The central components are those that have the greatest significance for the self and the evolving life course".

Schmitt and Kliegel's paper on the topic: "The influence of marital support on marital satisfaction: Are there age age and gender differences?" includes empirical findings of which the relevance to developmental psychology can, in my view, be effectively highlighted by Levinson's concept of development. Schmitt and Kliegel show that, above all, the quality of marital support is significant to marital satisfaction. In so doing, their chosen operationalisation of the characteristic "quality of marital support"—in the sense of shared activity in the marriage as well as reciprocity of commitment—demonstrates similarity to the concept of "significant relationships with various others". Like Levinson, the authors favour a perspective on relationships that combines the developmental and the socialisation perspective. When they investigate antecedents or predictors of characteristic marital relationships they take into account properties of the person as well as aspects of the sociocultural world. A further result of this study indicates that there are no recognisable differences in middle and late adulthood with regard to the influence of quality of marital support on marital satisfaction. It can also be interpreted from this result that marital relationships display in principle a significant component of life structure—which, in the case of positive quality (and this refers specifically to the case of experienced reciprocity), exerts a positive influence on self-realisation and, with that, on further self-adjustment. However, in the case of negative quality (and this refers specifically to the case of an experienced lack of reciprocity), it exerts a negative influence on the self. I believe that Marina Schmitt's study contains a remarkable additional potential for further research in developmental psychology, by integrating it within Levinson's theoretical formulation, and then, in further longitudinal analyses, posing the question: to what extent marital relationships have an effect on the further development of the self. Since Marina Schmitt's empirical analysis itself comes from a longitudinal study, this approach gives rise to interesting perspectives.

2. THE CONNECTION OF THE ALEATORY OF DEVELOPMENT WITH THE CONTINUITY OF DEVELOPMENT

The thesis introducing the factor of chance or the aleatory of development originates from Kenneth Gergen. This author contrasts the "aleatory change template" with two other major theoretical forms within the developmental domain, i.e. the "stability template" and the "template of ordered change". Gergen argues that the stability template—with the Freudian theory of character formation as a classical example—is challenged by numerous empirical studies suggesting that "whatever habits are acquired during development they do not generally seem to persist across diverse circumstances" (Gergen, 1977, p. 143). Referring to the template of ordered change—with Piagetian theory as a classical example—he states that "in the case of both cognitive and moral development, ample evidence for 'regression' or reversal in sequence has been discovered, and such evidence raises serious questions concerning the predictive capability of the basic theoretical structures" (Gergen, 1977, p. 146). In contrast, the aleatory change template is characterised by the assumption "that there is little about human development that is 'preprogrammed'; that is we enter the world with a biological system that establishes the limits or range of our activities but not the precise character of the activities themselves" (Gergen, 1977, p. 148). Which happy and unhappy events we experience, which people we meet, which ideas we become acquainted with: all this involves an element of chance. Kenneth Gergen emphasises that in the theoretical reconstruction of courses of development we often look for causal and meaningful connections and in so doing overlook factors of chance. Any relationship between two variables might be moderated by a complex (sometimes even unique) interplay of additional variables that vary with sociohistorical circumstances: "In the broadest sense it may be said that the determining confluence is subject to chance, and thus aleatory in nature" (Gergen, 1977, p. 149). However, it would be wrong to view development as the result of chance events alone. It is necessary to consider the way in which people subjectively interpret events and how they attempt to come to terms with them. The factor of continuity is found in the way events are interpreted and overcome (Kruse & Schmitt, 2004; Thomae, 1996).

In their paper on the topic "Stressful life events, protective factors, and depressive disorders in middle adulthood", Voss, Stegmann and Schröder raise the question to what extent burdensome life events at an early age cause increased vulnerability in a person, which can contribute to an increased risk of depressive illness with the occurrence of further burdensome events in the present. This problem can also be considered within the context of the aleatory and continuity of development: which developmental conditions prevail in childhood and youth, which life events occur in childhood and youth: to a large extent this is beyond the influence of the child or young person ("aleatory"). And yet, these developmental conditions and life events exert great influence on the individual's personality and give his or her experience and behaviour a particular direction ("continuity"). Typus melancholicus, as defined by the Heidelberg psychiatrist Tellenbach (1961), can be interpreted as the outcome of developmental conditions and experiences, which were not only restrictive but experienced as burdensome by the individual. More common than the predominance of a depressive disorder throughout the biography of the individual is, however, an increased vulnerability which only leads to a depressive disorder when burdensome life events occur. Obviously, the occurence of burdensome life events is beyond the control potential of the individual. Consequently, coping successfully with critical life events, developmental tasks and challenges has been conceptualised as reflecting person-environment-constellations instead of coping strategies, availability of resources or personality (Staudinger, Marsiske, & Baltes, 1995). This perspective, already proposed by Rutter in the context of his concept of vulnerability and resilience (Kruse & Schmitt, 2004; Rutter, 1990), is confirmed in Voss, Stegmann and Schröder's paper. They classify current burdensome life events as a trigger function for the occurrence of depressive disorders in those people who have already been confronted with burdensome events in childhood and youth.

Our own research on reminiscence of traumatic experiences in former Jewish emigrants and extermination camp survivors (Kruse & Schmitt, 1999, 2000) indicates that stressful memories in Holocaust survivors often can neither be predicted from specific characteristics of the sociohistorical context nor from individual coping patterns. Instead, spontaneously and unexpectedly occurring memories were reported in 143 of the 248 interviews. Despite considerable effort, the majority of people were unable to separate swastikas, stars of David, SS symbols or xenophobic slogans as the "scrawling of some reprobates and scatterbrains" from the public opinion prevailing in the country concerned. Even if these people in general were convinced that they were not exposed to any "real threat", the sight of signs, emblems or slogans awoke stressful memories which inevitably resulted in anxiety states despite all the efforts made in the concrete situation "to follow one's own senses". Spontaneous memories also occurred frequently in situations in which the subjects themselves could not find any cause for the intruding memories. These situations in particular were frequently felt to be particularly stressful because of the impression of having no control over one's own feelings and hence of being exposed helplessly to the situation. Proceeding from the aleatory change template it seems appropriate to conclude that occurrence of stressful memories depends on a magnitude of biographical and context-specific factors and as such might be characterised as aleatory in nature.

In the research of Voss, Stegmann and Schröder, long-term pathogenic effects of critical life experiences are less frequent than expected. They explain barely 10% of variance in psychic and psychosomatic disorders, which has already been clearly demonstrated in the contributions published in Fisher and Reason's (1988) "Handbook of life stress, cognition and health". This shows that the majority of people come to terms with, or master, problems and losses caused by critical life events on their own or with social support. This also clearly indicates that the subjective evaluation of losses, problems and gains, rather than the actual events themselves and their objective consequences, prove central to their effect (see also Kruse, 2005). This evaluation is affected by the extent to which the individual is convinced he or she can responsibly organise his or her own life situation even under burdensome conditions; such a conviction provides a protective effect, as Voss, Stegmann and Schröder demonstrate.

In our own investigations of psychosomatic illness and into coping with illness in old and very old age, we were able to show clearly the protective influence of a sense of coherence (Schneider, Driesch, Kruse, Wachter, & Heuft, 2003; Schneider et al., 2004; Schneider, Kruse, Nehen, Senf, & Heuft, 2000). The outcome established in our longitudinal studies, coming to terms with severe chronic illness, is decisively influenced by a sense of coherence—broadly speaking according to Antonovsky (1979)—demonstrates similarities to Voss, Stegmann and Schröder's reported findings, where, above all, the feeling of self-efficacy provides a protective function in coping with current psychic demands.

At this point, the aleatoric factor comes into play: our own investigations demonstrated that not only the burdensome events experienced in childhood and youth but also the support experienced from significant others exert a great influence on the extent of success in coping with burdensome events in old and very old age. Even in this case, there is a remarkable similarity to the results of Voss, Stegmann and Schröder.

3. THE ABILITY OF ATTAINING TRANSCENDENCY—IN THE SENSE OF CHANGE OF PERSPECTIVE—AS A BASIS FOR DEVELOPMENT

In the 1930s, the philosopher John Dewey attempted to understand what artists experience when they pose a challenge to themselves. A photograph of Matisse, found in his collection, shows Matisse viewing one of his early masterpieces with a look of aversion. Matisse appeared to fear getting stuck in mere repetition. Dewey took up the theme of self-criticism in his book "Art as Experience" (Dewey, 1934/1967). In this book, he put forward the theory that willingness to "let go"—in his terminology, critical revision of "tacit" knowledge and, if necessary, its purpose—forms a significant prerequisite for individual development. In it, a specific attitude towards the self comes to the fore which emphasises that a significant potential for development is to be found in crises, whereby crises in this context are interpreted as calling into question existing knowledge.

A similar statement, and one central to the understanding of development, is to be found in David Hume's "A Treatise of Human Nature". Here, this crisis is outlined as follows: "For my part, when I enter most intimately into what I call myself, I always stumble on some particular perception or other, of heat or cold, light or shade, love or hatred, pain or pleasure" (Hume, 1978, p. 252). In this case, David Hume's concept of stumbling is used as a description of calling into question knowledge taken for granted.

Here I see philosophical precursors of an understanding of development upon which the works of the psychologist Robert Peck are based. The contribution of Robert C. Peck to the understanding of psychological development in the second half of life proceeds from the impression that Erikson's eighth crisis, i.e. ego integrity vs. despair, refers to a major issue of life after 30 (Peck, 1955). Specifically, Peck proposed to divide this crisis into several stages that represent "quite different kinds of psychological learning at different stages in the latter half of life". Concerning old age, Peck distinguishes between three stages or issues, which may occur in different sequences. The first issue "ego-differentiation vs. work-role preoccupation" refers to the impact of vocational retirement, usually in the sixties. With the second issue, "body transcendence vs. body preoccupation" it is recognised that even if physical decline can be observed in most cases mental and social powers may actually increase in old age. The third issue "ego-transcendence vs. ego-preoccupation" refers to the "appearance of the certain prospect of personal death" (Peck, 1955, p. 48) as "one of the new and crucial facts of old age". Peck used the concept of transcendency to clarify that people have to achieve a change of perspective when dominant values and goals no longer agree with currently existing biological, psychological and social developmental demands.

In the paper authored by Rott, Jopp, d'Heureuse and Becker, entitled "Predictors of well-being in very old age", the concept of the evaluation of life, as developed by Lawton (Lawton, et al., 1999; Lawton, et al., 2001), comes to the fore. The authors investigate possible changes in evaluation of life in very old people in the final years or months before death and raise the question, whether a significant reduction in positive evaluation of life—this also includes the expression of the will to live in this evaluation—can be recognised in the run-up to death. They report an outcome in their study which, in my view, is fundamental to the understanding of development—here in the sense of change of perspective: in the run-up to death, no clear deterioration of evaluation of life and no reduction of will to live has been discerned. The authors explain this finding in the following way: if the frame of reference for evaluation of life can be changed successfully—particularly with regard to positively evaluated biographical events coming to the fore and negatively evaluated events being put to the back of the conscious mind—it is then more likely that even in the run-up to death, people will achieve a fundamentally positive evaluation of their life. Let it also be emphasised that we attained similar findings and observations in our own investigations into the experience of finality amongst tumour patients in the end stage of their illness. Rott, Jopp, d'Heureuse and Becker's paper demonstrates very clearly a change of perspective—also with regard to the critical calling into question of "knowledge taken for granted" and, if necessary, its revision. This change of perspective forms a basis for the further development of people—even at the end of life.

Let it be pointed out here that the Heidelberg philosopher, Gadamer (2003), in his last lecture before his death—which addressed the nature of pain—clearly emphasised that the experience of pain can very likely stimulate a change of perspective: according to Gadamer (2003) it can encourage people to become much more conscious of the abilities, interests and events which for each individual summon up happiness, meaning and mental health. Before the occurrence of a borderline situation, these positive aspects of our life are perhaps not really consciously acknowledged; now—with the occurrence of a borderline situation—becoming aware of these positive aspects is essential for the preservation of the will to live.

AFFILIATION

Institute of Gerontology, University of Heidelberg

REFERENCES

Antonovsky, A. (1979). *Health, stress, and coping.* San Francisco: Josse-Bass.

Dewey, J. (1934/1967). Art as experience. In J. A. Boydston (Ed.), *John Dewey—The collected works.* Carbondale: Southern Illinois University Press.

Fisher, S., & Reason, J. (Ed.) (1988). *Handbook of life stress, cognition and health.* Chichester: Wiley.

Gadamer, H. G. (2003). *Der Schmerz.* Heidelberg: Universitätsverlag Winter.

Gergen, K. (1977). Stability, change, and chance in understanding human development. In H. Reese (Ed.), *Life-span developmental psychology* (pp. 136–158). New York: Academic Press.

Hume, D. (1978). *A treatise of human nature.* (Edited by L. A. Selby-Bigge). Oxford: Clarendon Press.

Kruse, A. (2005). Biografische Aspekte des Alter(n)s: Lebensgeschichte und Diachronizität. In U. Staudinger & S. -H. Filipp (Eds.), *Enzyklopädie der Psychologie* (pp. 1–38). Göttingen: Hogrefe.

Kruse, A., & Schmitt, E. (1999). Reminiscence of traumatic experiences in (former) Jewish emigrants and extermination camp survivors. In A. Maercker, M. Schützwohl, & Z. Solomon (Eds.), *Post-traumatic stress disorder. A lifespan developmental perspective* (pp. 155–176). Seattle: Hogrefe & Huber.

Kruse, A., & Schmitt, E. (2000). *Wir haben uns als Deutsche gefühlt.* Darmstadt: Steinkopff.

Kruse, A., & Schmitt, E. (2004). Differentielle Psychologie des Alterns. In K. Pawlik (Ed.), Enyzklopädie der Psychologie—Differentielle Psychologie und Persönlichkeitsforschung: Theorien und Anwendungsfelder der Differentiellen Psychologie (pp. 533–570). Göttingen: Hogrefe.

Lawton, M., Hoffman, C., Kleban, M., Ruckdeschel, K., Winter, L., & Moss, M. (2001). Valuation of life: A concept and a scale. *Journal of Aging and Health, 13,* 3–31.

Lawton, M., Moss, M., Hoffman, C., Grant, R., Ten Have, T., & Kleban, M. (1999). Health, valuation of life, and the wish to live. *Gerontologist, 39,* 406–416.

Levinson, D. J. (1986). A conception of adult development. *American Psychologist, 41,* 3–13.

Peck, R. C. (1955). Psychological developments in the second half of life. In J. E. Anderson (Ed.), *Psychological aspects of ageing. Proceedings of a conference on planning research* (pp. 44–49). Washington, DC: American Psychological Association.

Rutter, M. (1990). Psychosocial resilience and protective mechanisms. In J. Rolf, A. S. Masten, D. Cicchetti, K. H. Nuechterlein, & S. Weintraub (Eds.), *Risk and protective factors in the development of psychopathology* (pp. 181–214). Cambridge: Cambridge University Press.

Schneider, G., Driesch, H., Kruse, A., Wachter, M., & H[illegible], G. ([illegible]). [illegible]tive body complaints as an indicator of somatization in elderly patients. *Psychosomatics, 44,* 91–99.

Schneider, G., Kruse, A., Driesch, G., Wachter, M., Nehen, H. G., & Heuft, G. (2004). What influences self-perception of health in the elderly? The role of objective health condition, subjective well-being and sense of coherence. *Archives of Gerontology and Geriatrics, 39,* 227–237.

Schneider, G., Kruse, A., Nehen, H. G., Senf, W., & Heuft, G. (2000). The Prevalence and Diagnostics of Subclinical Depressive Syndromes in Inpatients 60 Years and Older. *Psychotherapy & Psychosomatics, 69,* 251–260.

Staudinger, U. M., Marsiske, M., & Baltes, P. B. (1995). Resilience and reserve capacity in later adulthood: Potentials and limits of development across the life span. In D. Cicchetti, & D. J. Cohen (Eds.), *Developmental psychopathology, Vol. II: Risk, disorder and adaptation* (pp. 801–847). New York: Wiley.

Tellenbach, H. (1961). *Melancholie.* Berlin: Springer-Verlag.

Thomae, H. (1996). *Das Individuum und seine Welt.* 3. Auflage. Göttingen: Hogrefe.

MARINA SCHMITT[1] and MATTHIAS KLIEGEL[2]

THE INFLUENCE OF MARITAL SUPPORT ON MARITAL SATISFACTION: ARE THERE AGE AND GENDER DIFFERENCES?

Social support—as a substantial resource for any individual—is a central construct in psychology. Accordingly, there is an abundant supply of literature concerning its definition, its psychological and structural aspects, its effects on different dependent variables (e.g. self-efficacy, physical and mental health, subjective well-being), and its role as a buffer between stressful life-events and psychological disorders (Antonucci, 2001). Although social support is of great importance for close relationships, Julien and Markman (1991) pointed out that "researchers have virtually ignored the role of the support that spouses get from each other in determining marital outcomes" (p. 549). Previous studies addressing predictors of marital satisfaction have mainly focused on the influence of socio-economic factors and personality traits on marital satisfaction. While socio-economic factors seem to play a minor role in determining marital satisfaction (Feeney, Noller, & Ward, 1997), personality traits have been shown to be the most prominent stable dispositional factors influencing marital satisfaction in younger couples (Bouchard, Lusier, & Sabourin, 1999; Russell & Wells, 1994).

Concerning the effects of marital support, Cutrona (1996) differentiated four ways in which support from the spouse maintains and increases marital satisfaction. First, marital support helps the individual to avoid emotional retreat, isolation and depression in stressful phases. Second, marital support prevents the escalation of conflicts and the turn to destructive behaviour in the case of marital conflicts. Third, supportive communication strengthens the emotional bonds between both spouses, and fourth, leads to a positive experience in the marital relationship. Based on empirical analyses, Pasch and Bradbury (1998) pointed out that asking for support and granting support depends on marital satisfaction, and has a predictive effect on the development of marital satisfaction.

Besides general effects of marital support on marital satisfaction, existing research indicates gender-specific relations. Many studies have shown that women's perception of marital support is more strongly related to marital satisfaction and subjective well-being than that of men (Acitelli & Antonucci, 1994 or for an overview Gagnon, Hersen, Kabacoff, & van Hasselt, 1999). As Barbee et al. (1993) pointed out, women evaluate supportive behaviour as more satisfying than men do. Additionally, women regard social and interpersonal competencies of their husbands to be of great importance to marital satisfaction because they might feel released from the burden to assume responsibility for marital changes and conflicts. Thus, it seems reasonable to expect a stronger predictive power of supportive behaviour for marital satisfaction among women compared

H.-W. Wahl et al. (eds.), The Many Faces of Health, Competence and Well-Being in Old Age, 81–92.

to men. Concerning reciprocity, Sprecher (1992) and Goodman (1999) point out that women suffer much more from an unbalanced exchange of support than men do.

Surprisingly, previous studies focusing on the role marital support plays in marital satisfaction neglected long-term marriages in middle and old adulthood (Gagnon et al., 1999), which have to face several distinct developmental challenges (Hayslip & Panek, 2002). In midlife (defined as the period in life between 40 and 60 years of age), the couple is often confronted with the empty nest situation and has to cope with the changing physical and sexual abilities and attractiveness, and therefore has to develop an adjusted couple identity as well as new interaction patterns (Gagnon et al., 1999). Additionally, a mutual re-definition of the social relationships with their own parents, adult children, friends and acquaintances takes place in middle adulthood (Demick, 2002). But in old age (defined as the period in life above age 60), too, couples have to face several changes: after retirement, husbands are expected to spend more time on domestic chores (Dorfman, 1992; Lee & Shehan, 1989; Ward, 1993) and therefore couples have to re-develop old and/or find new activities to share (Feeney et al., 1997). Older couples have to meet different challenges such as mastering role changes after retirement, coping with declining health, mental or physical illness of either spouse, need for care, or illness or death of friends (Askham, 1994). We thus assume that marital support may help the individual to cope with these changes and challenges, thereby increasing marital satisfaction.

So far, existing research has not explicitly examined age effects on marital support. Thus, no clear predictions concerning age-related patterns can be derived and our study is mostly exploratory at this point. Reviewing the reported developmental tasks, however, one can assume that long-term relationships in both age groups have to rely on marital support to master these challenges. On the other hand, following socio-emotional selectivity theory (Carstensen, 1992), a narrowing of social networks combined with increasing emphasis placed on significant relationships across the adult life span presumably promotes greater emotional intimacy within the marital dyad in later years and might lead to more supportive behaviour in older couples. As Cobb (1976) pointed out, especially in long-term marriages, marital support may indicate how much an individual is loved, appreciated and cared for by the spouse. Moreover, since health- and retirement-related problems, as well as defining new daily activities, are some of the central issues for older couples, sufficient socio-economic resources in old age might support the couples' adaptation to these challenges.

The objective of the present study is to integrate and extend these findings on the influence marital support has on marital satisfaction into middle and old age. Our main hypothesis was that marital support would be the strongest predictor of marital satisfaction in long-term relationships. This stands in contrast to findings from short-term relationships which point out the role of socio-economic status and stable personality traits as predictors of marital satisfaction. We assume that, since long-term married couples have to deal with different changes and challenges, marital support would be helpful and would lead to higher marital satisfaction. In terms of gender differences, our hypothesis is in line with the existing studies pointing to a stronger relation between marital support and marital satisfaction in women as compared to men. Concerning differences between middle-aged and older adults, our study is more explorative because no clear predictions concerning age-related patterns of marital support can be derived from the literature. Therefore, after controlling for socio-economic variables and stable dispositional personality traits, we investigate the age- and gender-related effects of marital support indicators in predicting marital satisfaction in persons living in long-term marriages in middle and old adulthood.

1. METHOD

1.1. Participants

The participants in this study are a sub-sample of the Interdisciplinary Longitudinal Study of Adult Development (ILSE). The sample was stratified by age and gender. Addresses of 4,800 participants were obtained from the respective local registries. On the basis of this listing, addresses were randomly drawn from this pool and the persons were contacted. This procedure was followed until samples of 500 participants from East and West Germany of each age group were obtained. Half of the data from each age group were collected in the former East Germany (Leipzig), and half in West Germany (Heidelberg, Mannheim, Ludwigshafen). In both age groups, 52% were men. Because of the longitudinal design of the study, men were purposely oversampled. With the reliance on a random drawing from central registries addresses, and based on comparisons with the family status, income, and housing status of the same age groups of the overall population in Germany, our sample is largely representative of the German-speaking population of Germany and comparable with other samples used in longitudinal studies (Martin, Grünendahl & Martin, 2001).

The sub sample used in this analysis consists of those ILSE participants who lived in long-term marriages (i.e. they were married at least six years). Data from $N = 330$ middle-aged adults ($n = 176$ men and $n = 154$ women, born 1950–1952, mean age: 44.2 years) were compared to $N = 258$ older persons ($n = 159$ men and $n = 99$ women, born 1930–1932, mean age: 63.0 years). As in other representative samples including older participants, more men compared to women of the same age range lived in long-term marital relationships. This may be due to the fact that the likelihood of being widowed at this stage of life is higher for women compared to men (Carr, 2004). No couples were included in the sample. Table 1 presents an overview of the sample characteristics.

As to the German population, the sample shows significant differences in educational and financial resources. About 67% of the older participants have received only ≤9 years of education, as have 32% of the middle-aged participants. Twice as many older adults report low monthly incomes as compared to middle-aged participants. In both age groups, 85% are in their first marriage, and about 13% in their second. Only 2% are married for the third or fourth time. Middle-aged adults married significantly earlier in their life than older adults did. As could be expected, the duration of current marriage was significantly longer in older compared to middle-aged adults. While middle-aged adults are married for about 19 years, older adults are married for

Table 1. Sample characteristics

	Middle-aged adults		*Older adults*		
	Men (n = 176)	*Women (n = 154)*	*Men (n = 159)*	*Women (n = 99)*	*Differences*
Monthly income (%)					
<1025 €	2.3	2.4	7.0	3.1	Age: $\chi^2(2) = 64.6^{***}$;
1026–2050 €	30.9	41.0	63.1	71.1	Gender: $\chi^2(2) = 3.1$
>2050 €	66.9	56.6	29.9	25.8	
Education (%)					
≤9 Years	29.7	33.8	66.0	67.7	Age: $\chi^2(2) = 70.3^{***}$
>9 Years	70.3	66.2	34.0	32.3	Gender: $\chi^2(2) = 0.03$
Age at current marriage					
M	26.4	24.4	28.2	26.3	Age: $F = 23.7^{***}$
SD	5.6	6.3	8.3	8.5	Gender: $F = 10.9^{***}$
Number of marriages					
M	1.2	1.2	1.2	1.1	Age: $F = 0.6$
SD	0.5	0.4	0.4	0.4	Gender: $F = 0.9$
Duration of current marriage					
M	18.5	20.9	35.4	36.2	Age: $F = 882.6^{**}$
SD	5.0	4.6	7.5	8.7	Gender: $F = 8.8^{**}$
Number of children					
M	1.8	1.5	2.1	2.0	Age: $F = 16.3^{***}$
SD	1.0	0.8	1.4	1.3	Gender: $F = 3.8$
Age of children					
M	16.0	18.4	34.5	36.1	Age: $F = 1128.6^{***}$
SD	5.3	4.4	8.3	5.0	Gender: $F = 14.0^{***}$

$^{*}p < 0.05$.
$^{**}p < 0.01$.
$^{***}p < 0.001$.

about 35 years. Additionally, older adults have significantly more and older children than middle-aged adults. Even though men and women are within the same age range, women were younger when they married, their marriages last longer and their children are older. No gender differences concerning the existence of children occurred (93% of the men and 90% of the women have at least one child).

1.2. Instruments

The main data collection tool was an extensive semi-structured interview developed to assess the participants' subjective life situation in different domains (Lehr & Thomae, 1987). To assess the quality of the interview-ratings, selected parts of the interviews were compared with a standard rating. All interviewers reached a minimum of 80% agreement with the standard rating. The average agreement with the standard rating was 88.4%, and the average inter-rater correlation was $r = 0.95$ (Martin et al., 2001).

1.2.1. Marital Satisfaction

Concerning marital satisfaction, the participants were first asked how satisfied they were with the *joint activities* and with *intimacy/sexuality* in their marriage. Their answers were scored by the interviewers on a 5-point rating scale ranging from "completely unsatisfied" (1) to "completely satisfied" (5). Additionally, they were asked about the amount of stress they feel in their marriage. *Perceived marital stress* was assessed by the interviewers on a 5-point rating scale ranging from "no perceived stress" (1) to "high perceived stress" (5). In a next step, a factor-analysis including the participants' satisfaction with marital activity, satisfaction with intimacy/sexuality and perceived marital stress was conducted. This factor analysis revealed one factor with an eigenvalue above one and an explained variance of 69%.

1.2.2. Marital Support

Concerning marital support, the interview covered people's activities in their role as spouse, the amount of given and received support, as well as an assessment of the perceived reciprocity using information on instrumental, emotional and informational support. Concerning *marital activity*, the participants were asked about joint activities with their partner in everyday life, similarities they share with their partner and the amount of exchange and communication about their experiences and feelings. Marital activity was rated on a 5-point rating scale ranging from "no contact" (1) to "deep feeling of belonging together, unity, almost all activities are planned together and carried out" (5). The amount of mutual marital support was measured by asking the participants about the areas in which they give or receive support or help. Then they were asked about the amount of given and received support. *Given support* was rated on a 5-point rating scale ranging from "almost no given support for the spouse, neither instrumental, emotional, nor informational" (1) to "regularly given support in three areas of social support or strong support in at least two areas" (5). The ratings of *perceived support* were scored accordingly. *Perceived reciprocity* rating was based on information concerning the give-and-take relation in the marital relationship ranging from "very strong differences between give and take, very unbalanced relationship" (1) to "very strong balance between give and take" (5).

1.2.3. Socio-Economic Status Variables

As socio-economic status variables, net income per household, education and the number of children measured in a socio-economic questionnaire were included in the analysis. The participants categorized their net income per household on a 3-point rating scale with low income (<1025 €), medium income (1026–2050 €) and higher income (>2050 €).

1.2.4. Stable, Dispositional Personality Traits

The German version of Costa and McCrae's (1992) NEO-Five-Factor Inventory (NEO-FFI; Borkenau & Ostendorf, 1993) was used to measure neuroticism, extraversion, openness, agreeableness and conscientiousness.

2. RESULTS

In the first part of this section, age and gender differences concerning marital satisfaction and marital support are described. In a next step, results of stepwise regression analyses to examine the role of marital support in predicting marital satisfaction after controlling for socio-economic status and personality are presented.

2.1. Age and Gender Differences in Marital Support and Marital Satisfaction

With respect to marital satisfaction, a 2 × 2 (age group × gender) analysis of variance (ANOVA) revealed no age and gender differences in satisfaction with marital role and with intimacy. Slight but nevertheless significant age and gender differences occurred concerning perceived stress in marriage: Women reported more stress in their marital relationship than men, and middle-aged persons reported more marital stress than older persons (see Table 2). In the overall factor score on marital satisfaction, no age and gender differences have been obtained.

Concerning marital support, the ANOVAs confirm the necessity to conduct an age- and gender-specific examination. As summarized in Table 2, there are considerable gender effects in given support, received support and perceived reciprocity. In fact, women report giving more and receiving less marital support than men. Accordingly, they perceive reciprocity in their marital relation as less balanced than men do. Results also show main age differences in given and received support as well as reciprocity, indicating lower perceived reciprocity and less given and received support in older adults. Concerning marital activity, we found an age × gender interaction that reveals significantly less marital activity in men only among the older adults.

2.2. Relational Differences in the Prediction of Marital Satisfaction

To examine the role of marital support in predicting marital satisfaction after controlling for SES and personality, we conducted stepwise regression analyses. The factor score of marital satisfaction was included as the dependent variable. In the first step, the SES variables (i.e. net income per household, educational attainment and number of children) were included. In the second step, the "big five" stable dispositional personality traits were taken into account. In the third step, marital support variables (i.e. marital activity, given and received support and reciprocity) were included. In order to investigate age and gender effects, four separate stepwise regression analyses have been conducted.

Results of the stepwise regression analyses (see Table 3) show that socio-economic variables did not play a role in predicting marital satisfaction. Stable, dispositional personality traits contributed slightly but significantly to predicting marital satisfaction, particularly in middle-aged individuals. Most importantly, in all four age and gender groups support-specific variables explained the greatest part of variance in marital satisfaction.

Table 2. *Descriptive statistics and analyses of variance for marital satisfaction and marital support variables*

	Middle-aged adults		*Older adults*		*Differences*		
	Men ($n = 176$) *M (SD)*	*Women* ($n = 154$) *M (SD)*	*Men* ($n = 159$) *M (SD)*	*Women* ($n = 99$) *M (SD)*	$F_{(gender)}$	$F_{(age)}$	$F_{(gender \times age)}$
Marital satisfaction							
Satisfaction with marital activity	4.1 (0.9)	3.9 (1.1)	4.1 (0.8)	4.0 (0.9)	0.0	3.0	0.9
Satisfaction with intimacy	3.5 (1.0)	3.5 (1.1)	3.3 (1.1)	3.5 (1.1)	1.2	1.7	2.0
Perceived stress	2.2 (0.9)	2.3 (1.1)	2.0 (0.9)	2.2 (1.1)	4.8*	5.6*	0.1
Marital satisfaction (Factor score)	0.02 (1.0)	−0.2 (1.1)	−0.0 (0.9)	−0.1 (1.1)	1.5	0.1	0.6
Marital support							
Marital activity	4.1 (0.8)	4.0 (0.8)	3.8 (0.8)	4.1 (0.8)	1.8	2.8	7.8**
Given support	4.1 (0.8)	4.4 (0.7)	3.9 (0.8)	4.2 (0.7)	20.5***	9.4**	0.2
Received support	4.2 (0.9)	3.8 (1.0)	4.0 (0.8)	3.7 (1.0)	4.5***	4.2*	0.2
Reciprocity	4.4 (0.8)	4.2 (1.0)	4.3 (0.8)	4.0 (1.2)	8.1**	4.9*	0.1

* $p < 0.05$.
** $p < 0.01$.
*** $p < 0.001$.

Table 3. *Summary of stepwise regression analyses for variables predicting marital satisfaction*

	Middle-aged adults				*Older adults*			
	Men (n = 176)		*Women (n = 154)*		*Men (n = 159)*		*Women (n = 99)*	
	β	ΔR^2	β	ΔR^2	β	ΔR^2	β	ΔR^2
Step 1: Socio-economics								
Income	0.06	0.03	0.04	0.01	−0.07	0.01	−0.11	0.06
Education	−0.10		−0.03		−0.01		0.05	
Number of children	0.08		0.09		0.05		0.08	
Step 2: Personality								
Neuroticism	−0.03	0.10**	−0.13*	0.17***	−0.12	0.03	−0.15	0.11
Extraversion	0.01		0.01		−0.06		−0.10	
Openness	−0.03		−0.03		−0.08		0.02	
Agreeableness	0.07		−0.03		−0.12		−0.05	
Conscientiousness	0.13		0.11		0.05		0.08	
Step 3: Marital support								
Marital activity	0.38***	0.32***	0.36***	0.44***	0.26**	0.32*	0.22*	0.47***
Given support	−0.06		0.20**		−0.08		−0.12	
Received support	0.18*		−0.10		0.33***		0.28*	
Reciprocity	0.27***		0.50***		0.22**		0.41***	
Total R^2		0.45*		0.62***		0.36*		0.64*

Note: β are taken from a model that includes all 12 variables.
$^{*}p < 0.05$.
$^{**}p < 0.01$.
$^{***}p < 0.001$.

However, there were gender differences concerning the amount of explained variance. In both age groups, the amount of explained variance was higher in the female than in the male group: For men in midlife, including marital support variables in the analysis led to an increase in explained variance of 32% up to 45% overall explained variance. For men in old age, results show an increase in explained variance of 32% up to 36%. For middle-aged and older women the increase in explained variance as well as the total amount of explained variance is much higher (middle-aged women: increase in explained variance of 44% to 62%; older women: increase in explained variance of 47% to 64%).

When looking at the single indicators of marital interaction, perceived reciprocity played the most important role in predicting marital satisfaction for women of both age groups ($\beta = 0.41$ for older women and $\beta = 0.50$ for middle-aged women). For older men, the amount of received support was one of the most important indicators, while for middle-aged men marital activity played the major role. While given support contributed significantly to the prediction of marital satisfaction in middle-aged women and received support did not, the reverse is true for middle-aged men. Concerning age differences in single indicators, marital activity seemed to be more important for middle-aged than for older adults.

3. DISCUSSION

The aim of our study was to describe the relations between marital support and marital satisfaction and to investigate possible age and gender differences in these relations. In contrary to existing research which points to a decline in marital satisfaction in old age (Lee & Shehan, 1989), our results show moderate to high levels of marital satisfaction in long-term marriages. One reason might be that couples living in long-term relationships have developed certain behaviours to prevent negative developments or the escalation of conflicts. Another reason might be that due to selection effects the marriages of persons with lower marital quality ended in divorce or separation. As to age and gender differences in marital support, results show less marital support in women and older adults and underline the necessity of an age and gender specific examination.

Data lead us to make three major conclusions: First, the socio-economic status seems to play no role at all in the mechanisms that underlie marital satisfaction in middle-aged and old adults living in long-term marriages. This is in contrast to previous findings analysing younger adults living in short-term marriages as well as in contrast to the idea that, since health- and retirement-related problems are some of the central issues for older adults in general, sufficient socio-economic resources in old age might support older adults' and therefore also older couples' adaptation to these challenges. In our study, however, socio-economic variables show restricted variance because >90% of the participants reported medium or high levels of income. Thus, one can assume that, among those with low income, many children and low education, socio-economic resources might play a more crucial role as a potential stressor.

Goodman, C. C. (1999). Reciprocity of social support in long-term marriage. *Journal of Mental Health and Aging, 5*, 341–357.

Hayslip, B., Jr., & Panek, P. E. (2002). *Adult development and aging* (3rd ed.). Malabar, FL, US: Krieger Publishing Company.

Julien, D. & Markman, H. J. (1991). Social support and social networks as determinants of individual and marital outcomes. *Journal of Social and Personal Relationships, 8*, 549–568.

Lee, G., & Shehan, C. L. (1989). Retirement and marital satisfaction. *Journal of Gerontology, 44B*, 226–230.

Lehr, U., & Thomae, H. (1987). *Formen seelischen Alterns: Ergebnisse der Bonner Gerontologischen Längsschnittstudie (BOLSA)* [Patterns of Aging: Results of the Bonn Gerontological Longitudinal Study (BOLSA)]. Stuttgart, Germany: Enke Verlag.

Martin, M., Grünendahl, M., & Martin, P. (2001). Age differences in stress, social resources, and well-being in middle and older age. *Journal of Gerontology, 56B*, 214–222.

Pasch, L. A., & Bradbury, T. N. (1998). Social support, conflict, and the development of marital dysfunction. *Journal of Consulting and Clinical Psychology, 2*, 219–230.

Russell, R. J. H. & Wells, P. A. (1994). Personality and quality of marriage. *British Journal of Psychology, 85*, 161–168.

Sprecher, S. (1992). How men and women expect to feel and behave in response to inequity in close relationships. *Social Psychology Quarterly, 55*, 57–69.

Ward, R. A. (1993). Marital happiness and household equity in later life. *Journal of Marriage and the Family, 55*, 427–438.

PASQUALINA PERRIG-CHIELLO

COMMENTARY: CHANGED GENDER ROLES AND THEIR IMPACT ON MARITAL SUPPORT AND SATISFACTION

Long-term marriage is a rather new phenomenon in our society. If only a few decades ago "golden weddings" (50 years of marriage) were rare happenings, this is not the case any longer. Due to longer life expectancy, today's elderly couples have the perspective of a partnership, which may span five to six decades. These cohorts married at a relatively young age (compared to today's young persons) and were raised according to a rather strong value system in which divorce or separation were very seldomly used as a means of solving marital problems. Objective divorce barriers (e.g. financial dependency for women) as well as subjective ones (strong family values, religious convictions) are possible main reasons, which is why the large majority of today's elderly couples are still together and are now facing this totally new and challenging experience—the experience of long-term marriage (Fooken, 2002).

The challenge of a long-term intimate relationship points to the fact that this long period needs a continuous redefinition of the relationship's function and meaning. This redefinition process is not a specificity of old age; it becomes crucial and necessary for even the majority of middle-aged individuals. In fact, middle-aged persons have to cope with a variety of personal and familial transitions, most of which are associated with substantial role changes (such as departure of children, beginning health problems, dismissals, anticipation of retirement). It is a period beyond child rearing, a period of balancing, and of new orientation, which can be associated with considerable spousal stress. However, in contrast to older cohorts, middle-aged persons seem to have an increasingly lower threshold for divorce in response to marital problems and stress (Perrig-Chiello & Perren, 2005).

There is also increasing empirical evidence that for all age groups, and especially in old age, mutual social and emotional support between loving partners is a crucial variable in adapting to these specific developmental tasks and problems and in explaining marital satisfaction (Goodman, 1999). With advancing age, the definition of a new intimacy and interdependence becomes crucial, as it is during a time when physical and social resources steadily begin to decrease while losses increase.

Positive effects of mutual social and emotional support have even been shown in the case of difficult contextual conditions such as caregiving. Perceived marital functioning and relationship quality in the past can indeed have a moderating effect on the actual inequity of the caregiving setting in a partnership. Caregivers who were in a close relationship with the care recipient before the onset of the illness report feeling less burdened and depressed than those who were not (Williamson & Shafer,

H.-W. Wahl et al. (eds.), The Many Faces of Health, Competence and Well-Being in Old Age, 93–98.

1998). In the same vein, results from a study by Wright & Aquilino (1998) revealed that past and actual reciprocity of emotional support between 110 caregiving wives (mean age 69.98 years) and husbands who received care was linked to lower levels of caregiving burden and higher levels of marital happiness for wives. Among the 100 non-caregivers of the same age, exchange of emotional support with their husbands was also related to higher marital satisfaction, but the effects were smaller than in the caregiving group.

In addition, the particular importance of marital support in the second half of life is mirrored by the far-reaching negative effects in those cases where mutual support is lacking, e.g. in the case of marital separation, divorce or widowhood. The results of the Swedish Twin Study of Ageing showed impressively that bereaved twins experienced significantly more depressive symptoms, more feelings of loneliness and less life satisfaction than their married co-twins. For the long-term widowed, loneliness continued to be a real problem and was associated with lower life satisfaction, particularly for women. The negative effects were stronger in young-old than in old-old persons (Liechtenstein, Gatz, Pedersen, Berg & McClearn, 1996). There is also empirical evidence that positive retrospective reports of marital support and marital satisfaction can buffer the impact of widowhood. In a study by Howard (2000), the retrospective reports of marital satisfaction and support of 65 recently widowed women, aged 60–80 years, were significantly correlated with their levels of grief.

This short review shows that since Julien & Markman's 1991 statement, after which "researchers have virtually ignored the role of support that spouses get from each other in determining marital outcomes" (p. 549), things have changed impressively. In the last few years this research gap has increasingly been studied, especially in the middle-aged, but also in older couples (Fooken, 2002; Rogers & Amato, 2000).

The research presented in this volume by Drs Schmitt and Kliegel—which I was invited to comment here—is a good example. As the authors state, during the second half of life, the role of partner has to be redefined in a substantial way due to the very different developmental tasks associated with aging. In their contribution they aim to describe the relation between spousal social support and marital satisfaction, as well as at examining age and gender differences, in the influence of social support on marital satisfaction. Their main hypothesis is that marital support may help to cope with the different challenges of old age and might increase marital satisfaction. Cross-sectional interview data of two age-cohorts, persons in middle age (mean age 44.2 years) and old age (mean age 63.0 years), are reported. It is expected that marital support would be the strongest predictor of marital satisfaction; furthermore, age and gender differences are predicted.

Summing up, the results presented by Schmitt and Kliegel show indeed several age and gender differences: Women reported more marital stress than men and middle-aged persons more marital stress than older persons. Furthermore, main effects of gender were found for given and received support as well as for perceived reciprocity. With respect to marital support, women report giving more and receiving less than men. Accordingly, they perceive the reciprocity in the marital relation as less balanced than men do. The main effect of age suggests lower perceived reciprocity and less given and received support in older adults. Concerning the predictors of marital satisfaction by social support, no age differences resulted. However, a gender-specific effect was found, indicating that women's marital satisfaction was more reliant upon spousal support than men's.

First, let's discuss the *age effects*: At first glance it might be astonishing that older adults report lower reciprocity and less given and received support than middle-aged persons. Based on a socio-cultural and socio-historical context, one would expect just the contrary: In the oldest cohort mutual support and solidarity should be stronger than in middle-aged persons. One reason for this assumption is a difference in life experiences in the two cohorts. The older cohort experienced the second world war with the associated necessity to rely on one another, whereas the middle-aged persons, the baby-boomers, experienced the 60s, with their loosening of strong values and role expectations on the one hand, and an increase in individualism on the other hand. A second argument for the expected higher reciprocity in the elderly is the assumption that the increased vulnerability (due to increasing health problems) would enhance the necessity of mutual support in the older cohort. How do we explain this apparently discrepant result? Should we rather expect just the opposite, in the sense, that the younger generation was more socialized toward a model of companionship and reciprocal help in a partnership?

Results from a Swiss study comparing young, middle-aged and old couples confirmed the findings in the ILSE-Study presented by Schmitt and Kliegel, which suggest that this latter hypothesis might be the correct one. In the Swiss study the amount of the reported emotional and instrumental support by the partner, as well as the perceived efficacy of the support, was highest in the young (younger than 30 years) and lowest in the old group (50–80 years) (Bodenmann & Widmer, 2000).

Considering the fact that the results of this study, as well as of the study of Schmitt and Kliegel, derive from cross-sectional data, we suggest speaking of cohort-effects rather than of age-effects. Recent decades have indeed brought fundamental changes in the understanding of gender-roles and marital relationships. Since the 1960s/1970s, both women and men have become less traditional in the understanding of these roles (more equity in the division of household labour, more egalitarian power relations, etc.).

This has been illustrated very well in a study by Rogers and Amato (2000) who interviewed two cohorts of long-term married couples. The first marriage cohort consisted of individuals who had gotten married between 1964 and 1980 ($N = 1,119$) and were interviewed in 1980, whereas the second marriage cohort consisted of individuals married between 1981 and 1997 ($N = 312$) and interviewed in 1997. Compared with the earlier cohort, the more recent cohort reported less traditional gender-role attitudes and a greater share of housework on the part of husbands, as well as a more egalitarian share of influence in marriage. However, the higher level of mutual support in the younger cohort was not associated with higher marital satisfaction; just the opposite was the case. Members of the younger cohort reported significantly more marital discord than members of the older one. These results suggest that marital satisfaction is not directly linked to the amount of mutual support, but could rather be an outcome of a more complex interaction (e.g. with gender-roles).

In the case of the ILSE-study, the results presented by Schmitt and Kliegel showed main effects for *age and gender* concerning perceived marital stress: Middle-aged persons report more marital stress than older persons, and women more than men. The reported results also reveal main effects for gender in given and received support and perceived reciprocity. With respect to marital support, women report giving more and receiving less from their partners, and women perceive the reciprocity in the marital relation as less balanced than men.

The very same results also were found in the Swiss study mentioned above (Bodenmann & Widmer, 2000): Here in all age groups women—from very young to old—were less satisfied with the support from their partners and perceived a larger imbalance between given and received support.

In a study of our own with a representative Swiss sample of middle-aged persons (Perrig-Chiello & Sturzenegger, 2001), we found the same results: Men were significantly more satisfied with their partnership than women and they reported receiving more support from their partners. Considering the familial and extra-familial social network, men in our study were more partner-centred, whereas women had more extensive and intensive social contacts (with their children, parents, friends).

There is a further remarkable gender difference concerning the perceived quality of relationships: Whereas the quality of relationships with their children and partners ranks highest in men, in women the two first ranks are assigned to their children and their best friend (Perrig-Chiello & Sturzenegger, 2001). Additional empirical evidence comes from a study by Pearson (2000) where it was shown that marital satisfaction increases in men the longer they are married, while decreasing in women.

These consistent results show that men and women seem to have different perceptions of marriage or relationships. How can this difference be explained? Findings from qualitative studies suggest that this gender difference might reflect the willingness of husbands to idealize the situation and to deny existing tensions, as well as the wives' greater willingness to recognize problems and press for changes (Huyck, 1999). Another qualitative study, the Midwest "Parkville" Study by Huyck and Gutmann (1992), focused on the reasons why in long-term marriages women are more disappointed by their relationship than men. The main factors that contributed to their disappointment were centred on a sense that the husband was perceived as too "dependent" and needing care, rather than the strong protector idealized at the beginning of the relationship. Furthermore, the passivity and disinterest of men in exploring the wider world and finally their unwillingness to explore the possibilities of change in the relationship were mentioned.

Different research results indicate that, even though men are more partner-centred than women, satisfying relationships in general and a close intimate partnerships in particular, are apparently of crucial importance to women, much more so than for men (Moen, 2001). Men—especially in older age—seem to have a more functional approach to relationships (e.g. the need to have somebody who cares) and are more confident and less worried than women concerning their partnership. A possible reason for this could be that the experience of divorce and remarriage or new partnership varies by gender. Men tend to marry and remarry much easier than women in the second half of life.

As a matter of fact, in the last decades an increasing number of divorces in long-term partnerships were observed in western countries. This means that an increasing number of divorces occur in middle age, and that consequently women of this age group are more likely to be alone (Cain, 1988; Perrig-Chiello, 2004). All these findings might explain on the one hand the fact that the middle-aged group in the ILSE-Study reported significantly more marital stress than the older age group, and on the other hand, that women are more concerned about their partnership (and report less marital satisfaction) than men.

Finally, a last comment: The results from regression analyses presented by Schmitt and Kliegel suggest that women's marital satisfaction is more reliant upon marital support than it is for men. Is it possible that reciprocity and support are not so predictive for marital satisfaction in men, because of their gender-specific (may be also cohort-specific) role-expectations? As it was stated above, since men of these cohorts have a more functional approach to partnership, support and care from their wives could be an expected "normality" for them.

To sum up, Schmitt and Kliegel's presentation showed that—even though substantial advances have been made in the research on social support and marital satisfaction in long-term partnerships—further research is needed to understand this phenomenon and to disentangle age, cohort and gender differences. Longitudinal and intervention studies as well as qualitative approaches could shed light on the dynamics of this fascinating new phenomenon of long-term marital relationships.

AFFILIATION

University of Berne, Institute of Psychology

REFERENCES

Bodenmann, G., & Widmer, K. (2000). Stressbewältigung im Alter: ein Vergleich von Paaren jüngeren, mittleren und höheren Alters (Coping in elderly couples: A comparison with young and middle-aged couples). *Zeitschrift für Gerontologie und Geriatrie, 33,* 217–228.

Cain, B. S. (1988). Divorce among elderly women: a growing social phenomenon. *Social Casework, 69*(9), 563–568.

Fooken, I. (2002). Wege in die "Lieblosigkeit"—Lebensverlaufsmuster und seelische Gesundheit bei Männern und Frauen im Kontext von Scheidungen und Trennungen nach langjährigen Ehen. In M. Peters & J. Kipp (Eds.), *Zwischen Abschied und Neubeginn. Entwicklungskrisen im Alter* (pp. 157–172). Giessen: Psychosozial Verlag.

Goodman, C. C. (1999). Reciprocity of social support in long-term marriage. *Journal of Mental Health and Aging, 5*(4), 341–357.

Howard, S. P. (2000). Spousal bereavement in older women: The impact of self-esteem and retrospective reports of marital satisfaction and marital support on adjustment. *Dissertation Abstracts, International Section, 60* (8B), 4226.

Huyck, M. E. (1999). Gender roles and gender identity in midlife. In S. L. Willis & J. D. Reid (Eds). *Life in the middle. Psychological and social development in middle age* (pp. 209–234). San Diego: Academic Press.

Huyck, M. H., & Gutmann, D. L. (1992). Thirtysomething years of marriage. Understanding experiences of women and men in enduring family relationships. *Family Perspectives, 26,* 249–265.

Julien, D., & Markman, H. J. (1991). Social support and social networks as determinats of individual and marital outcomes. *Journal of Social and Personal Relationships, 8,* 549–568.

Liechtenstein, P., Gatz, M., Pedersen, N. L., Berg, S., & McClearn, G. E. (1996). A co-twin-control study of response to widowhood. *Journal of Gerontology: Psychological Sciences, 51B*(5), 279–289.

Moen, P. (2001). *The gendered life course.* In R. H. Binstock (Ed.), *Handbook of Aging and the Social Sciences* (pp. 179–196). San Diego: Academic Press.

Pearson, V. (2000). The experience of distress. *Hong-Kong Journal of Psychiatry, 10*(2), 11–15.

Perrig-Chiello, P. (2004). Soziale Integration im Spiegelbild lebenszyklischer Uebergänge. In Ch. Suter (Hrsg.). *Sozialbericht 2004 Schweiz* (pp. 129–154). Zürich: Seismo.

Perrig-Chiello, P., & Perren, S. (2005). Biographical transitions from a midlife perspective. *Journal of Adult Development*, 12, 3, 163–181.

Perrig-Chiello, P., & Sturzenegger, M. (2001). Social relations and filial maturity in middle-aged adults: contextual conditions and psychological determinants. *Zeitschrift für Gerontologie und Geriatrie, Special Issue "Ageing in Europe", 34,* 21–27.

Rogers, S. J., & Amato, P. R. (2000). Have changes in gender relations affected marital quality? *Social Forces, 79*(2), 731–753.

Williamson. G. M., & Shafer, D. R. (1998). Implications of communal relationships theory for understanding loss among family caregivers. In J. H. Harvey (Ed.), *Perspectives of loss: a sourcebook* (pp. 173–187). Philadelphia: Taylor & Francis.

Wright, D. L., & Aquilino, W. S. (1998). Influence of emotional support exchange in marriage on caregiving wives' burden an marital satisfaction. *Family Relations. Interdisciplinary Journal of Applied Family Studies, 47* (2), 195–204.

ELKE VOSS[1], ANNE-KATRIN STEGMANN[1] and JOHANNES SCHRÖDER[2]

STRESSFUL LIFE EVENTS, PROTECTIVE FACTORS AND DEPRESSIVE DISORDERS IN MIDDLE ADULTHOOD

Depression is projected to become the leading cause of disability and the second leading contributor to the global burden of disease by the year 2020 (Murray & Lopez, 1996; WHO, 2002). According to prevalence rates of the most recent epidemiological surveys, nearly one in five persons will develop a depressive disorder once in her lifetime (Wittchen, Müller, Schmidtkunz, Winter, & Pfister, 2000). Depression comprises a major public health problem that causes severe distress and dysfunction, and that also constitutes both social and economic burdens for families, communities and society (Klerman & Weisman, 1992; Lepine, Gastpar, Mendlewicz, & Tylee, 1997).

In the meantime, considerable research has established a significant association between depressive disorders and stressful life events (SLEs) (e.g. Brown & Harris, 1978, 1989), which generally holds true for both clinical and community samples and for persons of all ages and groups (Brilman & Ormel, 2001; Farmer & McGuffin, 2003; Kessing, Agerbo, & Mortensen, 2003). The research findings support the idea that biological as well as psychosocial factors are causally related to depression (e.g. Paykel, 2003).

Following the vulnerability model of Brown and Harris (1978, 1989), the role adverse childhood events play in the development of a depressive disorder can be seen in the creation of enduring intrapsychic vulnerabilities (such as disturbed or insecure attachment styles, helplessness and low self-esteem) that lead to heightened emotional reactivity to adult stress (Harris, Brown, & Bifulco, 1990; Rutter, 1989). Some childhood adversities are associated with an increased risk of early onset depression and prior depression is associated with a high recurrence risk (Angst, 1988). These results imply that the relationship between childhood adversities and adult depression may also be due to the mediating influence of earlier depression (Rutter, 1989). But what is omitted in the vast majority of earlier studies is a separation of the impact of childhood adversities on current depression into (a) effects on first onset and (b) illness course in individuals with a lifetime history of depression (Kessler, 2000).

Furthermore, up to now there has been no definite agreement in research findings about the time interval of the depressogenic effect. Kessler and Magee (1993) found that the adverse effects of some distal events (early parental death, absence of a close

H.-W. Wahl et al. (eds.), The Many Faces of Health, Competence and Well-Being in Old Age, 99–113.

relationship, family mental illness and family violence) showed differential decreases over time. These decreases could be interpreted as evidence that young people who are able to pass through their teenage years without becoming depressed are either free of the depressogenic effects of some early experiences for the rest of their lives (in case of early parental death and absence of a close relationship) or their risk of a subsequent onset is greatly diminished (in case of family mental illness and violence). Because of the limitations of their study, Kessler and Magee (1993) stated a need to replicate such patterns.

In his review on resilience research, Blum (2002) summarised specific personal characteristics as well as characteristics in the family and the extended environment, which could act as counterbalancing forces to stressful events. Especially high self-efficacy, and internalised locus of control were found to be the key protective factors in resilient young people. Further sources of resilience were an external facilitative environment, having a sense of value or positive self-esteem, as well as feeling connected to others.

The role of more recent SLEs is seen in provoking or triggering the onset of a depressive episode in vulnerable individuals. The specific nature of such provoking agents was seen in that they largely involved experiences of loss involving humiliation, entrapment or death (Brilman & Ormel, 2001; Harris, 1996). Specific events or highly related clusters of events have been shown to be more important in relation to depression than a sum of SLEs (Brown & Harris, 1989). However, whether SLEs are strictly precipitating factors or may also be a consequence of the disease is less clear.

With recurrent episodes, the role of adverse recent events might diminish. This is hypothesised to result from a sensitisation process to the state of depression (Kendler, Thornton, & Gardner, 2000; Post, 1992). Recurrent episodes might lead to a change in the neuronal system (or create an increased reliance on patterns of negative information processing) in a way that the person reacts depressogenicly on minimal cues.

Further research from twin studies regarding genetic liability to major depression, specific personality traits and similar familial adverse events, proposed that some events (especially personal network events) also might be markers of more fundamental risk factors such as high neuroticism (Kessler, 2000; Van Os & Jones, 1999).

The purpose of the present study is to analyse the effects of a broad range of adverse childhood experiences and recent stressful events on first onset (incidence) and the further course of depressive disorders. The following research questions were addressed: (1) Are there differences in numbers, accumulation and patterns of adverse childhood and recent events between mentally healthy persons and individuals with an incidence, relapse or remittance of minor or major depression (mMD) in middle adulthood? (2) Are specific stressful events more important in relation to depression as the aggregated measure (accumulation) of SLEs? (3) Are recent events cause or consequence of a depressive disorder or a marker of a more fundamental risk factor like neuroticism? and (4) Do positive experiences in childhood and positive personality attributes diminish the negative impact of adverse events on mMD?

1. METHOD

1.1. Sample

The present study is based on the two examination waves 4 years apart of the younger cohort (born between 1950 and 1952) of the Interdisciplinary Longitudinal Study on Adult Development (ILSE; Martin et al., 2000). Data collection took place between September 1993 and April 1996 (T1) and between September 1997 and April 2000 (T2), respectively. At T1 the younger sample consisted of 500 participants (mean age: 44.2 years), half of the subjects were examined in East Germany (Leipzig), and half in West Germany (Heidelberg, Mannheim and Ludwigshafen). It is assumed that our sample is largely representative for the German-speaking population of Germany since it is based on local registries and compares with general populations in terms of family status, income and housing status (Martin et al., 2000). However, the sample has a somewhat higher level of educational attainment than the general population of Germany. Among the 1950/1952 birth cohort, 448 subjects participated at both measurements. The sample used in this analysis ($N = 349$) consists of all participants with a DSM III-R diagnosis of mMD up to $T2$ ($n = 122$) and all mentally healthy individuals ($n = 227$, no DSM III-R diagnosis, neither at T1 nor at T2). Participants with unclear diagnosis or pure anxiety, substance abuse, eating disorder and somatoform disorder were excluded from the study ($n = 99$). The attrition rate at T2 was at 10.4% ($n = 52$) and we lost nine persons with a lifetime MD, but dropout analysis indicated that the relative proportion of depressives was slightly lower in the dropout group (17.3%) compared to subjects still participating at T2 (27.2%).

The included depressive disorders were of moderate or high severity regarding the number of reported symptoms. The lifetime depressives at T1 ($n = 101$) reported an average of 5.7 (±1.8) symptoms. At T2 the participants with recurrence or first onset of a depressive episode reported an average of 6.7 (±1.5) symptoms.

The sample used in this analysis consists of 227 mentally healthy participants (no psychiatric diagnoses, neither at T1 nor at T2), 78 participants with a lifetime history of mMD up to T1, who stayed remitted in the catamnestic period, 23 participants with a relapse of a depressive episode between T1 and T2 and 21 participants with an incident depressive episode between T1 and T2.

1.2. Measures

Depression: Minor and major depression was assessed using the German version of the Structured Clinical Interview for DSM III-R (SCID; Wittchen et al., 1991).

Depressive mood was assessed using the self-depression rating scale (SDS; Zung, 1986).

Neuroticism: Neuroticism was assessed using the German version of the NEO-FFI of Costa and McCrae (Borkenau & Ostendorf, 1993).

Generalised perceived control: A modified version of the "Questionnaire of generalised competence and control beliefs" was used (Krampen, 1990).

Childhood adversities: Adversities were retrospectively assessed in a semi-structured interview at T1 (experience that occurred before the respondent was 16 years of age). The participants answered open-ended questions concerning their childhood and youth familial situation, health conditions, etc. Using qualitative content analysis the adverse experiences were classified into 19 categories of 4 event types: loss events (death of a parent, parental divorce and detachment from parent), parental psychopathology (mentally ill, substance abuse and suicide or suicide attempts), traumatic events (sexual abuse, familial violence and accident) and other adversities such as discord in family, chronic illness in childhood/youth, parental physical illness and poverty.

Recent SLEs: At T2 participants were asked in a semi-structured interview about the life events and life changes in the preceding 4 years. Using content analysis, recent events were classified into 34 categories of 9 life-domians (work, health, residence/housing, finances, legal problems, partnership, social network, death and others).

Protective factors: Based on a principal component analysis, 5 factors were extracted out of a pool of 20 primary variables, regarding positive experiences in childhood/youth and positive personality attributes. Factors 1–5 accounted for 63% of total variance. For purpose of comparability with the included dichotomous adverse events in logistic regression analysis we created new dichotomous variables that contain factor-based scores in a commonly used way (Hatcher, 1994). The following factors were built up: (1) *Extended and supportive parental environment* (above median supportive father/mother and experience of an expanded and opened "Lebensraum"); (2) *High self-efficacy* (lower than median neuroticism-scores and external control beliefs scores); (3) *High peer-group integration in youth* (spent leisure time with others, belonging to peer group in youth and having a lot of friends, all above the median). (4) *Positive self-esteem in youth* (high positive self-perception as teen, highly integrated in first apprenticeship/job and having a lot of friends); (5) *High cognitive ability and high positive self-esteem as pupil* (an above median total score on four subtests of the Wechsler Intelligence Scales (WAIS-R German version; Tewes, 1991): "information", "block design", "similarities" and "picture completion" and high positive self-image as a good pupil).

1.3. Statistical Analysis

In each step of the statistical analyses, the healthy participants were compared to each of the three depressive groups separately. Chi-square and t-test statistics were used to investigate group differences in the amount and accumulation of stressful events, depressive mood at time of data assessment (SDS) and neuroticism. Bivariate and multivariate logistic regression analyses were employed to compute the odds ratios (ORs) and 95% confidence intervals for the associations between single and combined adverse events and the lifetime risk for depression, for relapse and incidence.

2. RESULTS

Concerning the overall lifetime prevalence (T2) of minor and major depression, more than one-fourth of the middle-aged ILSE participants ($N = 448$) experienced a depressive episode once in their lifetime (n = 102/22.7% of all participants had suffered from at least one depressive episode and n = 20/4.5% from a sub-syndromal depressive dysfunction). In the group of 101 lifetime depressed up to T1, 78 subjects stayed remitted (77.2%; female: 71.8%), and more than one-fifth (23/22.8%) had had a relapse (female = 75%). Between T1 and T2 (female = 62.5%), 21 persons developed a first-onset depressive disorder. Regarding the total sample of 448 participants (T2), a first onset of a depressive episode (incidences) was given in 4.7%.

The three depressive groups differed significantly from the healthy controls regarding the female/male ratio (in the group of healthy controls only 38.3% were female; $\chi^2(3, N=349)=30.4, p<0.0001$), marital status ($\chi^2(9, N=349)=50.3, p<0.0001$) and employment status ($\chi^2(9, N = 349) = 17.5, p = 0.04$). Regarding marital status, 9.3% of the healthy controls, 26.9% of the remitted, 43.5% of the relapsed and 23.8% of the incident cases were divorced. Lesser proportions of the depressed subjects were employed (healthy: 82.8%, remitted: 69.2%, relapsed: 65.2% and incident: 71.4%).

2.1. *Numbers and Accumulation of Reported Adverse Events in Childhood/Adolescence and Middle Adulthood*

Nearly 46% (160) of the included 349 middle-aged participants reported no adverse childhood experience. One-third (32.4%) reported one and more than one-fifth reported two to seven events (21.8%). One or more adverse childhood events was given in 48.7% of the healthy group, in 62.8% of the remitted group, in 60.9% of the relapsed and in 71.4% of the incident group. Regarding the proximal or recent events only a minority reported none (2%) or only one adverse event (5.2 %). More than one-half experienced between two and seven (56.3%) events, and a further third reported 8–26 adverse proximal events.

Looking at the mean number of reported distal events, we found a significant increase from the mentally healthy group to the group of relapsed and incident cases (Table 1). The same was true for recent events. But in this case, also the remitted participants differed significantly in the mean number of events (Table 1).

Furthermore, the three depressive groups showed steadily increasing proportions of participants with accumulation of distal (two or more adverse childhood events and median split) and proximal events (seven or more events and median split), respectively. This proportion of "childhood-high-risk" participants increased from 18% (healthy) to 43% (incident). For "recent-high-risk" participants, we found an increase from 37% (healthy) to 76% (incident). Forty-two participants (12%) could be classified into the groups "childhood-high-risk" and "recent-high-risk". As might be expected, the proportion of "double high-risk" participants increased from the mentally healthy (7.5%) to the remitted group (16.7%), to relapsed (21.7%) and the incident cases (33.3%) ($\chi^2(3, N = 349) = 17.1, p = 0.0007$).

2.2. *Prevalences of Specific Adverse Events in Childhood/Youth*

The most prominent events in the included sample ($N = 349$) were own chronic illness ($n = 50$), discord in family ($n = 42$), aggressive father ($n = 28$), temporary detachment

Table 1. Mean number and accumulation of adverse childhood events (ACE) and recent events (RE) in healthy persons and three depressive sub-samples

	Healthy *(N = 227)*	*Remitted* *(N = 78)*	*Relapsed* *(N = 23)*	*Incident* *(N = 21)*	*F-value*
Means and standard deviations of adverse childhood and recent events					
ACE (M; SD)	0.8 (1.2)	1.0 (1.1)	1.3 (1.6)	1.4 (1.3)	2.6*
RE (M; SD)	5.9 (3.9)	8.6 (5.1)	9.7 (5.0)	9.5 (4.5)	13.8***
Accumulation of adverse childhood and recent events: High-risk proportion					
ACE ≥ 2	41 (18.1%)	19 (24.4%)	7 (30.4%)	9 (42.9%)	8.6*
RE ≥ 7	85 (37.4%)	47 (60.3%)	16 (69.6%)	16 (76.2%)	25.7***

$^{+}p \leq 0.10$; $^{*}p \leq 0.05$; $^{**}p \leq 0.01$; $^{***}p \leq 0.001$.

Note: 27.2% of the T2-ILSE-participants (N = 448) with a clear SCID-diagnoses suffered from at least one depressive episode once in their lifetime. These participants (n = 122) were classified into one of the following three depressive groups:

- Remitted: Lifetime diagnoses of mMD but stayed remitted between T1 and T2 (4 years apart);
- Relapsed: Recurrence of mMD between T1 and T2;
- Incident: A first onset of mMD between T1 and T2; and compared to
- Healthy controls: No SCID-diagnoses, neither at T1 nor at T2.

from parents ($n = 25$), accident or trauma ($n = 21$), poverty ($n = 20$) and parental psychopathology ($n = 19$).

Significant differences in prevalences between healthy participants and depressive sub-samples were found for three of the distal events. This was true for parental psychopathology (19/5.4%; $\chi^2(3, N = 349) = 10.9$, $p = 0.01$), which was most frequently found for relapse (17.4%) or incident depressives (14.3%) and it was also true for discord in family (42/12.0%; $\chi^2(3, N = 349) = 8.3$, $p = 0.03$), which we found was given two to three times more often among all depressed, especially relapsed participants. Also, parental somatic disease (17/4.9%) was given more often in the group of relapsed and incident cases ($\chi^2(3, N = 349) = 8.4$, $p = 0.04$).

2.3. *Prevalences of Specific Adverse Recent Events in the Preceding 4 Years*

The most prominent recent events in the sample ($N = 348$) were common physical health problems ($n = 209$), strained relations with children ($n = 182$), changes in work conditions ($n = 140$), strained relations with parents/parents-in-law ($n = 138$), changes in housing conditions ($n = 115$), strained housing conditions ($n = 84$), serious problems at job ($n = 82$), strained partner ($n = 75$), unemployment/job loss ($n = 69$) and surgery ($n = 64$).

Looking at differences in prevalences between healthy participants and depressive sub-samples concerning specific recent events we found a characteristic pattern of depressive disorder: All depressive groups, including the remitted, have significantly more health problems regarding common physical health problems ($\chi^2(3, N = 348) = 10.0$, $p = 0.02$), surgeries ($\chi^2(3, N = 348) = 11.1$, $p = 0.01$) and life-threatening diseases ($\chi^2(3, N = 348) = 10.8, p = 0.01$). Depressive participants experience significantly more changes in their housing situation ($\chi^2(3, N = 348) = 26.4, p =< 0.0001$), and problems with landlords, neighbours, etc. especially relapsed depressives ($\chi^2(3, N = 348) = 14.2, p = 0.01$). Incident depressives in particular are significantly more hit by job loss/unemployment (43% compared to 17% of the healthy participants; $\chi^2(3, N = 348) = 8.5, p = 0.04$), and by serious problems with their boss and colleagues (relapsed and incident cases; $\chi^2(3, N = 348) = 11.1, p = 0.01$). Interpersonal problems, including increased arguments with the spouse/partner ($\chi^2(3, N = 348) = 21.8, p = <0.0001$), separation/divorce ($\chi^2(3, N = 348) = 13.1, p = 0.004$) and strained relations with friends ($\chi^2(3, N = 348) = 18.5, p = 0.0003$), were more frequent for all depressive participants, especially for those with incidence, but there were also higher rates for remitted participants. Furthermore, all three depressive groups had been more often involved in a legal conflict ($\chi^2(3, N = 348) = 13.5, p = 0.004$), or were affected by financial problems ($\chi^2(3, N = 348) = 15.1, p = 0.002$).

2.4. Long-Term Impact of Adverse Childhood Events

In the first step, we used bivariate logistic regression followed by multivariate analyses including all relevant distal and proximal events in one model to show the interdependence of stressful distal and proximal events and the risk of belonging to one of the depressive groups. The multivariate approach showed high intercorrelations of some distal events. Therefore, we present the results of bivariate regression analysis here.

The long-term impact of adverse childhood events on the course of depression in middle adulthood is displayed in Table 2.

Table 2. Impact of adverse childhood events on depressive disorder (bivariate)

	Depressives		
	Remitted (N = 78)	*Relapsed (N = 23)*	*Incident (N = 21)*
	OR (CI 95%)	*OR (CI 95%)*	*OR (CI 95%)*
Death of father	2.0 (0.7–5.9)		
Parental psychopathology		5.1** (1.4–18.1)	4.0* (1.0–16.2)
Trauma	2.8* (1.1–7.2)		
Discord in family	1.9+ (0.9–4.1)	3.7** (1.3–10.3)	2.4 (0.7–7.9)
Accumulation of distal events	1.5 (0.8–2.7)	2.8 (0.8–5.1)	3.4* (1.3–8.6)
Combined effect of parental psychopathology and family discord	1.5 (0.3–8.1)	8.4** (1.7–40.0)	5.9* (1.0–34.1)

$^+p \leq 0.10$; $^*p \leq 0.05$; $^{**}p \leq 0.01$; $^{***}p \leq 0.001$.
Note: In each step of the bivariate logistic regression analyses the three depressive groups were compared separately to the healthy participants as reference group.

Out of 19 adverse childhood experiences only traumatic events such as accidents and injury (given in 6% of the total sample, 11.5% of the remitted cases and 9.5% of the incident cases) significantly increased the risk of a lifetime depression nearly threefold (OR: 2.8, $p \leq 0.05$). A substantial effect was also related to discord in family (OR: 1.9, $p \leq 0.10$) and death of father (OR: 2.0, $p > 0.10$). The latter reached significance only in the multivariate model, in which recent stressful events were included. Parental psychopathology and discord in family significantly heightened the risk for relapse fivefold (OR: 5.1, $p \leq 0.01$) and nearly fourfold (OR: 3.7, $p \leq 0.01$), respectively. Compared to the healthy subjects, the risk of developing a first-onset depression in middle adulthood was considerably affected by parental psychopathology (OR: 4.0, $p \leq 0.05$) and the accumulation of events (OR: 3.4, $p \leq 0.05$). The long-term negative impact through the accumulation of events on a first-onset depression in middle adulthood in particular led us to look at interaction effects. For example, the combined effect of parental psychopathology and discord in family increased the risk of a relapse eightfold and of an incidence nearly sixfold (Table 2).

2.5. Impact of Recent Stressful Life Events

The impact of recent SLEs on the course of depression in middle adulthood are displayed in Table 3.

Recent stressful events that showed a significant increase in the ORs for a lifetime depression, but staying remitted in the last 4 years, could be interpreted as a consequence or marker of the illness. This was true for the vast majority of health-related events (common physical health problems, surgeries, hospitalisation and life-threatening disease, with ORs in the range of 1.9–4.4) and interpersonal events (increased arguments with partner, separation/divorce, extremely increased or minor arguments with children, and increased arguments with parents, with ORs in the range of 1.7–3.1). Several recent stressful events heightened the risk for relapse and/or incidence, but we found varying links for the two groups. Considering proximal events which showed a significant increase for relapse, the vast majority involve interpersonal problems (problems getting along with boss/colleagues, crisis involving landlord/neighbours, separation/divorce, extremely increased arguments with children and increased arguments with other relatives, with ORs in the range of 2.6–10.2). Three events involve change and financial burden (in working conditions and removal) and two involve threat (surgery) and loss (death of a child). Six proximal events led to a significant increase in the risk of developing a first-onset depression in middle adulthood, with ORs ranging from 3.5 to 7.4. This was true for loss of job/unemployment, problems getting along with boss/colleagues, a life-threatening disease, financial burden, increased arguments with partner and separation/divorce.

The accumulation of recent events nearly fourfold the risk for relapse and fivefold the risk for first onset of a depressive disorder in middle adulthood. But there were several specific events (e.g. move, increased arguments with friends, death of a child in the case of relapse, and life-threatening disease and increased arguments with partner in the case of first onset) that showed higher impact than the aggregated measure.

Table 3. Impact of recent events on depressive disorder (bivariate)

	Depressives		
	Remitted (N = 78)	*Relapsed (N = 23)*	*Incident (N=21)*
	OR (CI 95%)	*OR (CI 95%)*	*OR (CI 95%)*
Work events			
Loss of job/unemployment			3.7** (1.5–9.4)
Problems getting along with others (boss/associates)		3.1* (1.1–8.9)	3.5* (1.2–10.0)
Changes in work conditions		2.5** (1.1–6.1)	
Health events			
Common physical health problems	2.2** (1.2–3.8)		
Life-threatening disease	4.4** (1.3–14.2)		7.4** (1.6–33.3)
Surgery	1.9* (1.0–3.7)	3.9* (1.6–9.8)	
Hospitalisation	2.8* (1.0–7.4)		
Housing			
Move	1.6* (1.1–7.2)	10.0*** (3.5–28.0)	
Having crisis involving landlords and neighbours		5.7* (2.1–16.0)	
Miscellaneous burden			
Financial burden		3.6* (1.3–10.3)	5.2** (1.9–14.2)
Interpersonal events			
Increased arguments with partner	2.8* (1.4–5.5)	2.6+(0.9–7.6)	6.9*** (2.6–18.3)
Separation/ divorce	3.0** (1.3–6.8)	3.4* (1.0–11.6)	5.1** (1.6–16.2)
Extremely increased arguments with children	3.1* (1.0–9.1)	4.7* (1.1–19.6)	
Increased arguments with children	1.9* (1.1–3.2)		
Increased arguments with parents	1.7* (1.0–2.8)		
Increased arguments with other relatives		10.2*** (2.8 36.7)	
Death of a child		21.4*** (1.9–246.3)	
Accumulation of recent events	2.5* (1.5–4.3)	3.8* (1.5–9.7)	5.3** (1.9–15.1)

$^{+}p \leq 0.10$; $^{*}p \leq 0.05$; $^{**}p \leq 0.01$; $^{***}p \leq 0.001$.

Note: In each step of the bivariate logistic regression analyses the three depressive groups were compared separately to the healthy participants as reference group.

To examine the role of adverse childhood events as stress exacerbating factors on the impact of recent events on relapse and first incidence of depression, two separated logistic regression analyses were done for participants who reported at least one adverse distal event and for participants who reported none. The analysis showed that the impact of specific recent events (especially interpersonal events) substantially increased in the first group and decreased in the second group. For example, the impact of "separation/divorce" sevenfold the risk for relapse (OR: 7.2; CI: 1.4–36.5 vs. OR: 1.5; CI: 0.2–13.2) and 13-fold the risk for incidence (OR: 13.2; CI: 3.1–57.4) if at least one distal event had occurred and dropped to insignificance in the other case. In the group of incident depressives each participant with "separation/divorce" in the preceding time since T1 reported at least one distal adverse event.

2.6. Positive Experiences in Childhood/Youth and Positive Personality Attributes (T1) as Possible Counterbalancing Factors

Including positive childhood experiences and personality attributes (assessed at T1) in the analysis, we found a significant impact of three of the five factors in reducing the risk of ever becoming depressed (remitted), of relapse or of developing a first-onset depressive disorder (Table 4). High self-efficacy reduced the risk to fall into the remitted group about 2.2 times, about 5 times for relapse and 4.5 times for incidence. Having experienced an extended and highly supportive (parental) environment reduced the risk for a first-onset depressive disorder in middle adulthood 3.3 times. Furthermore, a high positive self-esteem in youth reduced the risk of developing a lifetime depression (but staying remitted) about 1.8 times. Additionally, high peer-group integration substantially diminished the risk of suffering from lifetime depression and relapse in middle adulthood. High cognitive ability combined with a positive self-perception as a pupil showed no protective effect (Table 4).

Including these "protective" factors in a series of multivariate models, the effects of specific childhood adverse events diminished and some even lost significance. This was true for traumatic events, parental psychopathology and discord in family.

Table 4. Impact of protective factors (bivariate)

	Depressives		
	Remitted (N = 78)	*Relapsed (N = 23)*	*Incident (N = 21)*
Protective factors	*OR (CI 95%)*	*OR (CI 95%)*	*OR (CI 95%)*
Extended/high supportive family environment	0.80(0.5−1.4)	0.88(0.4−2.1)	0.30*(0.1−0.9)
High self-efficacy	0.45**(0.3−0.8)	0.20**(0.1−0.6)	0.22**(0.1−0.6)
High peer-group integration	0.63+(0.4−1.1)	0.43+(0.2−1.1)	0.70(0.3−1.8)
Positive self-esteem youth	0.57*(0.3−1.0)	0.50(0.2−1.2)	0.60(0.3−1.5)
Cognitive ability/ self-perception	1.4(0.8−1.4)	1.4(0.5−4.1)	0.90(0.2−3.1)

$^{+}p \leq 0.10$; $^{*}p \leq 0.05$; $^{**}p \leq 0.01$; $^{***}p \leq 0.001$.

Note: In each step of the bivariate logistic regression analyses the three depressive groups were compared separately to the healthy participants as reference group.

Table 5. Interactive effects of protective factors and increased arguments with partner

	Depressives		
	Remitted (N = 78)	*Relapsed (N = 23)*	*Incident (N = 21)*
	OR (CI 95%)	*OR (CI 95%)*	*OR (CI 95%)*
Increased arguments with partner	2.8* (1.4–5.5)	2.6^{+} (0.9–7.6)	6.9*** (2.6–18.3)
Increased arguments and extended/supportive family environment	2.2 (0.8–5.7)	2.8 (0.7–11.0)	3.5^{+} (0.9–14.0)
Increased arguments and high self-efficacy	2.0 (0.7–5.8)	1.1 (0.1–9.0)	2.5 (0.5–12.6)
Increased arguments and positive self-esteem youth	1.6 (0.7–3.9)	2.1 (0.6–7.9)	5.6** (1.9–16.6)

$^{+}p \leq 0.10$; $^{*}p \leq 0.05$; $^{**}p \leq 0.01$; $^{***}p \leq 0.001$.
Note: In each step of the bivariate logistic regression analyses the three depressive groups were compared separately to the healthy participants as reference group.

2.7. Increased Arguments with Partner: Provoking Agent or Marker for a More Fundamental Risk Factor

In a last step of our exploratory analyses, we combined a single recent event ("increased arguments with partner", as a significant predictor of first-onset depression in middle adulthood) with each of the above listed significant protective factors, to test for the causal role or marker function of a recent event (Table 5). "Increased arguments with partner" was given in nearly 10% of the healthy group, 23% of the remitted group, 22% of the relapsed and 43% of the incident cases.

"Increased arguments with partner" combined with an extended and highly supportive (family) environment led to a reduction in the risk of incidence to half. Considering the combination with high self-efficacy (neuroticism and external control beliefs lower than median), "increased arguments with partner" lost its negative effect for relapse and incidence. The combination with high positive self-esteem in youth also showed a reducing effect.

3. CONCLUSIONS AND DISCUSSION

More than one-fourth of the middle-aged adults in the Interdisciplinary Study of Adult Development (ILSE) had developed at least one minor or major depressive episode up to the second measurement occasion. All three depressive groups experienced significantly higher numbers of distal (with the exception of the remitted group) and proximal adverse events, with a continuous increase from healthy participants to remitted, to relapsed and to incident depressives. This was also true for the accumulation of adverse experiences (high-risk and double high-risk proportion).

As Harris (1996) points out, depressed individuals may have a biased view of their past, making them more likely to report SLEs. In our study, we found significantly higher scores of state depressive mood at T1 (SDS; Zung, 1986) in each of the three depressive groups compared to healthy controls. But there were no significant differences between the depressive groups themselves. Therefore, the different numbers of adverse childhood experiences (at T1) could not be distorted by the degree of depressive mood between the three depressive groups. Furthermore, state depressive mood at T1 and T2 did not predict the reported numbers of adverse childhood and recent events, respectively (results not presented here).

Distal events (more than 30 years ago), which strongly distinguish between the healthy subjects and the depressive sub-samples were parental psychopathology (in our study combined with parental drinking problems), discord in family, traumatic events and death of father (remitted group). Referring to parental psychopathology and discord in family, we confirmed also the findings of the Kauai study (Werner & Smith, 1992). Regarding the results of the separated logistic regression analysis (participants with and without at least one adverse event in childhood), distal events might be interpreted as vulnerability enhancing and recent stress (especially the impact of interpersonal events) exacerbating factors. Further, our findings demonstrate a differential long-term impact of the above adverse events. Death of the father and a childhood trauma only heightened the risk of a lifetime depression (but staying remitted). This finding may support the hypothesis of Kessler and Magee (1993) that the effect of some childhood adversities (early parental death) decrease over time and even might lose their depressogenic effect when young people have passed through their teenage years without becoming depressed and/or have been protected by supportive factors. Parental psychopathology and discord in family increased the risk of relapse fivefold and for a first-onset depression in middle adulthood fourfold. The effects of family mental illness and family drinking problems have been examined in a number of high-risk studies of children of depressed parents or parents with drinking problems (e.g. Fendrich, Warner, & Weissman, 1990). The evidence is consistent in these studies that family history of drinking problems and of mental illness are both strong predictors of adult depression. Our study confirmed the long-term importance of these risk factors for relapse and first onset of a depressive episode in middle adulthood. This finding could be interpreted as a high genetic load for psychiatric disorders but another plausible interpretation could be that the familial environment could have been extremely disturbed by the mental illness of a parent (Kessler, 2000).

By also considering protective factors (i.e. extended/supportive parental environment, high self-efficacy and social integration), the effects of specific childhood adverse events diminished and some even lost their significance. The finding supports the idea that a long-term depressogenic effect of some childhood adversities is only given in combination with unfavourable attributes such as high neuroticism and/or high external control beliefs (Kessler, 2000).

Comparing lifetime depressives (remitted), depressives with relapse and first-onset cases allowed us to analyse the role of recent SLEs as cause, marker or consequence of a depressive disorder. The findings demonstrated differential short-term impact of events. A trigger or provoking effect could be seen in the impact of unemployment (only incident cases), in the impact of a life-threatening disease (remitted and incident cases) and death of a child (relapsed). Health events were most prominent in the remitted group and could be seen (partly) as consequence of a depressive disorder. Compared to the mentally healthy controls, interpersonal problems (increased arguments with spouse and other family members) were much more pronounced in the depressive groups and showed a higher risk of falling within one of the three depressive groups. The findings are consistent with previous epidemiological and clinical studies examining the role of recent events as predictors for incident depressive disorders (e.g. the Netherlands Mental Health and Incidence Study; de Graaf, Bijl, Ravelli, Smit, & Vollebergh, 2002) or comparing remitted patients with current depressives (Bodenmann, Schwerzman, & Cina, 2000) or examining the risk for relapse in former patient samples (Keller, 1997).

A moderate association between the aggregated measure of the number of recent events (accumulation) and depression has been observed, but specific events have been shown to be more important in relation to depression (move, increased arguments with friends, death of a child in the case of relapse, and life-threatening disease and increased arguments with partner in the case of first onset). This finding supports the assumption of Brown and Harris (1989) that one severe event (in a cluster of related events) is sufficient enough to provoke a depressive episode.

Including positive factors, especially high self-efficacy, displayed a protective role in all three depressive groups. Combining the interpersonal event "increased arguments with partner" with high self-efficacy decreased the risk of developing a first-onset depression and the risk of relapse in middle adulthood to insignificance. This finding supports the hypothesis that interpersonal events especially might be a marker for a more fundamental risk factor such as high neuroticism (Kendler, Gardner, & Prescott, 2003; Kessler, 2000).

The findings demonstrate the differential long-term (more than 30 years ago) and short-term impacts of several adverse recent events. The results underline the urgent need for a greater awareness of adverse events in childhood and the early diagnosis of minor and major types of depression (looking at consequential health events and disturbed social relationships).

As a first step to demonstrate the separate long-term effects of a broad range of adverse distal and recent events on relapse and first onset of a depressive disorder in middle adulthood the results of bivariate logistic regression analyses are described here. The multivariate analyses, in which all relevant distal and proximal events (OR > 1.5) as well as the group specific relevant positive factors were included (three separated models, one model for lifetime depression, one for relapse and one for incidence), and showed an overlapping of effects and increasing importance of adult risk factors (the recent events) that dilute the effects of the early adversities as well as the effects of the positive factors in the case of relapse and incidence. These results are part of the dissertation work of the first author of this report. Furthermore, no distinctions are made among parental losses that occurred in the respondent's infancy, early childhood or adolescence. Neither do we distinguish between parental drinking problems and mental health problems, even though there is interest in these distinctions in the literature (Kessler & Magee, 1993). The results need to be interpreted with these limitations in mind.

AFFILIATIONS

[1]*The German Centre for Research on Ageing at the University of Heidelberg*

[2]*Section of Geriatric Psychiatry at the University of Heidelberg*

REFERENCES

Angst, J. (1988). Clinical course of affective disorders. In T. Helgasen & R. J. Daily (Eds.), *Depressive illness: Prediction of course and outcome* (pp. 1–45). Berlin: Springer.

Blum, R. W. (2002). *Risk and resilience: A model for public health interventions for adolescents* [Online]. Retrieved from: www.asca-caahca/Ang/documents/riskandresilience. Pdf.

Bodenmann, G., Schwerzman, S., & Cina, A. (2000). Kritische Lebensereignisse und Alltagsstress bei Depressiven und Remittierten. *Zeitschrift für Klinische Psychologie, Psychiatrie und Psychotherapie, 48*, 1–17.

Borkenau, P., & Ostendorf, F. (1993). *NEO-Fünf-Faktoren-Inventar (NEO-FFI)*. Göttingen: Hogrefe.

Brilman, E. I., & Ormel, J. (2001). Life events, difficulties and onset of depressive episodes in later life. *Psychological Medicine, 31*, 859–869.

Brown, G. W., & Harris, T. (1978). *Social origins of depression: A study of psychiatric disorder in women.* London: Tavistock Press.

Brown, G. W., & Harris, T. (1989). *Life events and illness.* London: Unwin Hyman, Guilford Press.

De Graaf, R., Bijl, R. V., Ravelli, A., Smit, F., & Vollebergh, A. M. (2002). Predictors of first incidence of DSM-III-R psychiatric disorders in the general population: Findings from the Netherlands Mental Health Survey and Incidence Study. *Acta Psychiatrica Scandinavica, 106*, 303–313.

Farmer, A., & McGuffin, P. (2003). Humiliation, loss and other types of life events and difficulties: A comparison of depressed subjects, healthy controls and their siblings. *Psychological Medicine, 33*, 1169–1175.

Fendrich, M., Warner, V., & Weissman, M. M. (1990). Family risk factors, parental depression, and psychopathology in offspring. *Developmental Psychology, 26*, 40–50.

Harris, T. (1996). Life events and health. In A. Baum (Ed.), *Cambridge handbook of psychology, health and medicine* (pp. 136–139). Cambridge: Cambridge University Press.

Harris, T., Brown, G. W., & Bifulco, A. (1990). Loss of parent in childhood and adult psychiatric disorder: A tentive overall model. *Development and Psychopathology, 2*, 311–328.

Hatcher, L. (1994). *A step-by-step approach to using the SAS system for factor analysis and structural equation modelling.* Cary: SAS Institute Inc.

Keller, F. (1997). *Belastende Lebensereignisse und der Verlauf von Depressionen.* Münster: Waxmann.

Kendler, K. S., Gardner, C. O., & Prescott, C. A. (2003). Personality and the experience of environmental adversity. *Psychological Medicine, 33*, 1193–1202.

Kendler, K. S., Thornton, L. M., & Gardner, C. O. (2000). Stressful life events and previous episodes in the etiology of major depression in women: An evaluation of the "Kindling" hypothesis. *The American Journal of Psychiatry, 157*, 1243–1251.

Kessing, L. V., Agerbo, E., & Mortensen, P. B. (2003). Does the impact of major stressful life events on the risk of developing depression change throughout life? *Psychological Medicine, 33*, 1177–1184.

Kessler, R. C. (2000). The long-term effects of childhood adversities on depression and other psychiatric disorders. In T. O. Harris (Ed.), *Where inner and outer worlds meet* (pp. 111–126). London: Routledge Ltd.

Kessler, R. C., & Magee, W. J. (1993). Childhood adversities and adult depression: Basic patterns of association in a US national survey. *Psychological Medicine, 23*, 679–690.

Klerman, G. L., & Weisman, M. M. (1992). The course, morbidity, and cost of depression. *Archives of General Psychiatry, 49*, 831–834.

Krampen, G. (1990). *Fragebogen zu Kompetenz- und Kontrollüberzeugungen.* Göttingen, Hogrefe.

Lepine, J. P., Gastpar, M., Mendlewicz, J., & Tylee, A. (1997). Depression in the community: The first pan-European study DEPRES (Depression Research in European Society). *International Clinical Psychopharmacology, 12*(1), 19–29.

Martin, P., Martin, M., Schmitt, M., Sperling, U., Ettrich, K. U., Fischer-Cyrulies, A., Roether, D. & Lehr, U. (2000). Interdisziplinäre Längsschnittstudie des Erwachsenenalters (ILSE). Abschlussbericht über den 2. Untersuchungsdurchgang. Forschungsberichte aus dem DZFA, Nr. 8.

Murray, C. J., & Lopez, A. D. (1996). Evidence-based health policy-lessons from the Global Burden of Disease Study. *Science, 274*(5288), 740–743.

Paykel, E. (2003). Life events: Effects and genesis. *Psychological Medicine, 33*, 1145–1148.

Post, R. M. (1992). Transduction of psychosocial stress into the neurobiology of recurrent affective disorder. *American Journal of Psychiatry, 149*, 999–1010.

Rutter, M. (1989). Pathways from childhood to adult life. *Journal of Child Psychology and Psychiatry and Allied Disciplines, 38*, 23–51.

Tewes, U. (1991). *HAWIE-R. Hamburg-Wechsler Intelligenztest für Erwachsene/Revision 1991* (2nd ed.). Bern: Huber.

Van Os, J., & Jones, P. B. (1999). Early risk factors and adult person–environment relationships in affective disorder. *Psychological Medicine, 29*, 1055–1067.

Werner, E. E., & Smith, R. S. (1992). *Overcoming the odds. High risk children from birth to adulthood.* Ithaca: Cornell University Press.

WHO. (2002). *The World Health Report 2002: Reducing risks, promoting healthy life.* World Health Organization (Murray, C. & Lopez, A.) Geneva, Switzerland.

Wittchen, H. U., Müller, N., Schmidtkunz, B., Winter, S., & Pfister, H. (2000). Erscheinungsformen, Häufigkeit und Versorgung von Depressionen. Ergebnisse des bundesweiten Gesundheitssurveys "Psychische Störungen". *Fortschritte der Medizin, 118*, 4–10.

Wittchen, H. U., Zaudig, M., Spengler, P., Mombour, W., Klug, J., & Horn, R. (1991). S*KID: Strukturiertes klinisches Interview für DSM III-R* (2. Aufl.). Weinheim: Beltz Test.

Zung, W. W. K. (1986). Self-rating depression scale. In Collegium Internationale Psychiatrie (Hrsg), *Internationale Skalen für Psychiatrie.* Göttingen: Beltz-Test.

ELAINE WETHINGTON

COMMENTARY: STRESSFUL LIFE EVENTS AND DEPRESSIVE DISORDERS: THE PARADIGM SHIFT

The author acknowledges the support of the Cornell Institute for Translational Research on Aging (5 P30 AG22845, P. I. Karl Pillemer) in writing this commentary.

In the last 15 years there has been a major change in the way researchers have investigated the role of adverse events and other experiences in triggering or provoking onsets of depression and other disorders in adulthood. Innovations in data collection and research methods such as those developed for the U.S. National Comorbidity Survey (e.g. Kessler et al. 2004) have spurred these long-needed revisions. Among the agents of this revision—which in fact could be termed a paradigm shift—are three critical and converging findings.

First, the majority of onsets of depression observed in cross-sectional studies of adults are recurrent, rather than first onsets of depression (e.g. Kendler, Thornton, & Gardner, 2000). Second, exposure to severely stressful events and situations in childhood may produce a life-long liability toward depressive onset among genetically and socially vulnerable people (e.g. Kessler, Berglund, Demler, Jin, & Walters, 2005). Third, proximal or recent stressful life events, even very severe, are less likely to provoke a depression episode in those who do not have a recurrent depressive disorder (Kendler et al., 2000). Conversely, those who have a severe recurrent depressive disorder may not require a major or severe event to experience an onset of depression. (Monroe & Harkness, 2005; Post, Rubinow, & Ballenger, 1992).

The chapter by Voss, Stegmann, and Schroeder makes sophisticated use of the literature emerging from this paradigm shift. The authors take an important step in this paper by also exploring protective factors from childhood that may mitigate the impact of distal and proximate stressors in middle age. In this commentary, I will emphasize the authors' most important conclusions, and suggest some ways to expand the current research.

First, the chapter confirms that discord in the childhood family, traumatic childhood events, loss of father and parental psychopathology are associated with onset of depression in adulthood, but that the risk of onset and recurrence varies according to history of depressive disorder. Parental psychopathology appears to exacerbate the risk of first onset in adulthood, in the presence of a severe proximal event. Thus the chapter contributes to accumulating evidence that childhood adversities may in some cases continue to affect vulnerability to events into middle age (Caspi et al., 2002; Repetti, Taylor, & Seeman, 2002). The data suggest in turn that difficulties in adult primary relationships, such as arguments with spouses, neuroticism (which could be a trigger

H.-W. Wahl et al. (eds.), The Many Faces of Health, Competence and Well-Being in Old Age, 115–118.

for interpersonal difficulties), and a less robust self-image are the mediating factors that produce the vulnerabilities.

Second, Voss and her colleagues find that stressful events are more frequent among all three sub-types of participants (remitted from a previous depression episode, relapsed into a depression episode and new incidents/first onsets) who report depressive disorder. Taken in tandem with the finding that mood at the time of the interview does not have an impact on the recall of adverse childhood experiences and proximate events (Schraedley, Turner, & Gotlib, 2002), this suggests that the relationship between stressful experiences and depressive onset is a dynamic one. Major stressful experiences can both provoke a recurrent episode and trigger a first onset in middle age.

The chapter shows, moreover, that many more types of stressful experiences are associated with onset of depression among relapsed subjects than first onset (incident) subjects. The authors emphasize the interesting difference in the pattern of events: interpersonal events are more frequently associated with onset among the relapsed than the first onset subjects. Such a pattern may be indicative of subjects suffering from a recurrent disorder that provokes arguments and difficulties with others. This is consistent with the well-known work of Brown and Harris (1978) on the sequelae of affective disorder and also with the possibility that disorder provokes life difficulties (see also Monroe & Harkness, 2005). Recurrent disorders, moreover, are more likely to be severe and comorbid with other types of mental disorders and substance use (e.g. Kessler, Chiu, Demler, & Walters, 2005), which in combination might be more likely to provoke more severe or chronic interpersonal difficulties.

A weakness of the paper by Voss and colleagues is that the number of cases of each course of depression is relatively small. Even in this large sample there are only 23 relapsed subjects and 21 first onset subjects, which reduces the number of people in each category who experience a particular type of stressful event that may trigger an episode. It would therefore be useful to classify the stressful events into more generic categories. These categories would include a rating of the probability of "independence" of the event from an underlying disorder, and probable long-term threat, using the category systems developed by other investigators (e.g. Brown & Harris, 1978, 1989; Dohrenwend, Raphael, Schwartz, Stueve, & Skodol, 1993; Kendler, Hettema, Butera, Gardner, & Prescott, 2003), such as loss, danger, humiliation, entrapment or fatefullness. Categorizing stressful events into smaller groups based on previous theoretical reasons would clarify these important findings. It is also possible that such classification analyses will confirm that first onsets are associated only with the most objectively severe events, while recurrent depressions are provoked by less severe agents (Post et al., 1992; but see also Coyne, Thompson, & Pepper, 2004).

Third, there is a small but growing accumulation of research on the role of social status, gender and age on the relationship of accumulating stressors, both distal and proximate, on onset of depression in adulthood. Adverse childhood experiences are more frequent among those who were raised in lower income households (McLeod & Kaiser, 2004). This raises the possibility that the great majority of depression episodes in adulthood for those of lower social status are recurrent episodes. Counterbalancing this supposition is that being female or growing older may be associated with a higher probability of exposure to severely threatening events that may provoke first onset throughout adulthood, such as job loss (Turner, Wheaton, & Lloyd, 1995).

I urge the authors to expand their life course approach to examine the progression of exposure to adversity across life and how that differs by starting point in life (George, 2003). They have already taken the very important step of investigating the role of protective factors in preventing first onset or relapse of depression. Researchers might learn the most by focussing on the unusual cases: for example, how those at risk from a disadvantaged childhood accumulate the resources to avoid further exposure to risks in adulthood (George, 2003; Repetti et al., 2002; Wethington, 2005). An exclusive focus on adversity, at the expense of protective factors, leads to overly deterministic conclusions about the relationship between life stressors and mental disorder. Thus the most important step that the Voss paper takes is to consider the interplay of risk and resilience over time.

AFFILIATION

Department of Human Development and Department of Sociology, Cornell University

REFERENCES

Brown, G. W., & Harris, T. O. (1978). *Social origins of depression.* New York: The Free Press.

Brown, G. W., & Harris, T. O. (1989). *Life events and illness.* New York: Guildford Press.

Caspi, A., McClay, J., Moffitt, T., Mill, J., Martin, J., Craig, I., et al. (2002). Role of genotype in cycle of violence in maltreated children. *Science, 297*, 851–853.

Coyne, J. C., Thompson, R., & Pepper, C. M. (2004). The role of life events in depression in primary medical care versus psychiatric settings. *Journal of Affective Disorders, 82*, 353–361.

Dohrenwend, B. P., Raphael, K. G., Schwartz, S., Stueve, A., & Skodol, A. (1993). The structured event probe and narrative rating method for measuring stressful life events. In I. Goldberger & S. Breznitz (Eds.), *Handbook of stress: Theoretical and clinical aspects* (pp. 174–199). New York: The Free Press.

George, L. K. (2003). Life course research: Achievements and potential. In J. Mortimer & M. Shanahan (Eds.), *Handbook of the life course* (pp. 671–680). New York: Kluwer Academic/Plenum Publishers.

Kendler, K., Hettema, J., Butera, F., Gardner, C. O., & Prescott, C. (2003). Event dimensions of loss, humiliation, entrapment, and danger in the prediction of onsets of major depression and generalized anxiety. *Archives of General Psychiatry, 60*, 789–796.

Kendler, K. S., Thornton, L. M., & Gardner, C. O. (2000). Stressful life events and previous episodes in the etiology of major depression in women: An evaluation of the "kindling" hypothesis. *American Journal of Psychiatry, 157*, 1243–1251.

Kessler, R. C., Berglund, P., Chiu, W. T., Demler, O., Heeringa, S., Hirip, E., et al. (2004). The U.S. National Comorbidity Survey Replication (NCS-R): Design and field procedures. *International Journal of Methods in Psychiatric Research, 13*, 69–78.

Kessler, R. C., Berglund, P., Demler, O., Jin, R., & Walters, E. (2005). Lifetime prevalence and age-of-onset distributions of DSM-IV disorders in the National Comorbidity Survey Replication. *Archives of General Psychiatry, 62*, 593–602.

Kessler, R. C., Chiu, W. T., Demler, O., & Walters, E. (2005). Prevalence, severity, and comorbidity of 12-month DSM-IV disorders in the National Comorbidity Survey Replication. *Archives of General Psychiatry, 62*, 617–627.

McLeod, J. D., & Kaiser, K. (2004). Childhood emotional and behavioral problems and educational attainment. *American Sociological Review, 69*, 636–658.

Monroe, S. M., & Harkenss, K. L. (2005). Life stress, the "kindling" hypothesis, and the recurrence of depression: Considerations from a life stress perspective. *Psychological Review, 112*, 417–445.

Post, R., Rubinow, D. R., & Ballenger, J. C. (1992). Conditioning and sensitization in the longitudinal course of affective illness. *British Journal of Psychiatry, 149*, 191–201.

Repetti, R. Taylor, S. E., & Seeman, T. (2002). Risky families: Childhood social environments and the mental and physical health of offspring. *Psychological Bulletin, 128*, 330–366.

Schraedley, P. K., Turner, R. J., & Gotlib, I. H. (2002). Stability of retrospective reports in depression: Traumatic events, past depressive episodes, and parental psychopathology. *Journal of Health and Social Behavior, 43*, 307–316.

Turner, R. J., Wheaton, B., & Lloyd, D. A. (1995). The epidemiology of social stress. *American Sociological Review, 60*, 104–125.

Wethington, E. (2005). The life course perspective on health: Implications for health and nutrition. *Journal of Nutritional Education and Behavior, 37*, 115–120.

CHRISTOPH ROTT, DANIELA JOPP, VERA D'HEUREUSE and GABRIELE BECKER

PREDICTORS OF WELL-BEING IN VERY OLD AGE

Research on oldest old and centenarians has demonstrated that very old age is associated with enormous negative changes in various domains of functioning. The Berlin Aging Study (Baltes & Mayer, 1999), the Danish Longitudinal Centenarian Study (Andersen-Ranberg, Schroll, & Jeune, 2001) and also the Heidelberg Centenarian Study (Becker, Rott, d'Heureuse, Kliegel, & Schönemann-Gieck, 2003; Rott, d'Heureuse, Kliegel, Schönemann, & Becker, 2001) have revealed that physical frailty and chronic conditions are very common at the age of 100 years and above (cf. Jeune, 2002). There is also converging evidence that the prevalence rate of dementia is at least 50% beyond the age of 95 years (Hagberg, Alfredson, Poon, & Homma, 2001; Kliegel, Moor, & Rott, 2004). In addition to the losses in physical and cognitive functioning the social network is substantially reduced (Antonucci, 2001; Rook & Schuster, 1996). The Georgia Centenarian Study showed that being widowed and having lost a child is the fate of the majority of centenarians (Martin et al., 1992). Although older individuals seem to be characterised by high levels of resilience allowing positive adaptation under adverse circumstances (Staudinger & Fleeson, 1996), the accumulating negative conditions in very old age represent a serious challenge to mental health and subjective well-being (SWB). Applying a diathesis–stress model to examine the prevalence of psychopathology in later life, Gatz (1998) hypothesised that age-related stressful life circumstances such as loss of social partners or chronic illness deplete the individual's affective reserve capacity (i.e. plasticity in affect resulting from regulatory competence) which endangers the individual to develop depressive symptoms or a manifest depression. In line with this assumption, even the highly positively selected participants of the Georgia Centenarian Study revealed more depressive symptoms than representative samples of sexagenarians and octogenarians (Martin, Rott, Kerns, Poon, & Johnson, 2000). Staudinger and Fleesen (1996) posited that, especially, extreme physical constraints appear to limit resilience. Some authors even suspect that the individual's capacity for adaptation would break down in extremely old age, resulting in a phenomenon called "psychological mortality" which is characterised by loss of intentionality, personal identity and psychological control over one's future as well as the chance to live and die in dignity (Baltes & Smith, 2003).

This pessimistic view about SWB and quality of life (QOL) in old age seems to stand in contrast to several empirical studies. For instance, many studies found that indicators of subjective well-being are surprisingly stable far into very old age (e.g. Smith, Fleeson, Geiselmann, Settersten, & Kunzmann, 1999), which would speak

H.-W. Wahl et al. (eds.), The Many Faces of Health, Competence and Well-Being in Old Age, 119–129.

against the assumption that the adaptational system would be no longer available or have lost some of its functioning. Moreover, authors such as Lawton (1999, 2000) have pointed out that much of the research on QOL conducted with older individuals would have a much too strong focus on health-related quality of life (HRQOL), which could lead to a biased perspective on the QOL in advanced age. Although health and physical integrity are important throughout the whole life span, a concentration on HRQOL bears three basic problems (Lawton, 2000). First, positive features in non-health-related areas such as affectional ties, leisure time pursuits or self-growth effort are often excluded. There is simply more that gives life meaning than physical health and functioning. Second, the HRQOL research is characterised by a decrement model of QOL. Illness, pain and disability erode QOL, but excellent and ordinary health just reflect "no pathology". Lawton hypothesised that anticipating positive affect may compensate or override the poor aspects of life engendered by pain and disability. Thus, knowledge of both positive and negative considerations is necessary to draw conclusions about the individual's subjective QOL or the wish to live. The third problem of HRQOL lies in the assumption that the meaning of different health states is the same across all ages. It is ignored or even denied that the adaptive potential of human beings can, and in most cases, will lead to a rearrangement of preferences when one's own health is changing. This adaptive process is assumed to be associated with the maintenance of SWB. Thus, the existing concepts of QOL, especially HRQOL do not sufficiently address and cannot completely explain end-of-life-phenomena such as wish for life, life-extending treatments and how life should end.

To overcome these shortcomings and especially to address SWB at the end of life, Lawton and colleagues developed the concept of valuation of life (VOL) (Lawton et al., 1999, 2001). The basic idea was to examine the factors that may influence a person's wishes to continue to live and that may affect his or her end-of-life attitudes and behaviours. Many factors are expected to have an impact on these judgements, negative as well as positive ones, and people integrate the many sources of positive and negative features of life in order to define their attitudes regarding longevity in terms of the number of years older people wish to live (years of desired life). But positive aspects of mental health have not received the same attention in research as has been the case for indicators of poor mental health, such as depressive symptoms or anxiety. Thus VOL represents a new era in QOL research by focussing on the intervening psychological mechanism, the dynamic cognitive–affective thought process, operating between the total of good and bad conditions of life and the wish to live.

VOL is understood as a complex of judgments, emotions and projections into the future and reflects the subjectively experienced worth of and the active attachment to one's present life. In a very general sense, VOL is greater when one anticipates a future in positive terms and should be influenced at least to the same degree by positive factors in one's life as by poor health and low functioning. Furthermore, Lawton et al. (2001) suggested that VOL included that individuals positively anticipate and plan for the future (futurity) and believe that the future is positive (hope), that individuals feel competent (self-efficacy) and believe in their competence to solve problems (persistence), and pursue goals that guide their lives (purpose). Thus, in Lawton's model, VOL acts as a mediator between background characteristics such as health, QOL and mental health and the years that an individual desires to live (Lawton et al., 1999). Although a number of indicators of QOL are related to VOL, they influence the years of desired life only indirectly to the extent that they affect VOL. Years of desired life is one possible outcome of VOL.

Because VOL is primarily conceptualised as a positive affective state, it can be assumed that the determinants of positive affect could also be effective for VOL. More specifically, according to Lawton's "dual-channel" model of psychological well-being externally engaging phenomena are hypothesised to enhance positive affect but not to influence negative affect. In contrast, intrapersonal factors including personality factors such as neuroticism contribute to negative affect but do not influence positive affect (Lawton, Parmelee, Katz, & Nesselroade, 1996; Lawton, Winter, Kleban, & Ruckdeschel, 1999). Usually, higher scores of extraversion are connected with more activities, thus this personality trait should emerge as a predictor of VOL while neuroticism should not exert a substantial influence.

The questionnaire developed to operationalise VOL mirrors the above described structure and includes no direct expression of life expectancy, wish for longevity, reference to physical and mental pathology or death. The construct validity of VOL was demonstrated in several studies with older people (Lawton et al., 1999, 2001). However, VOL has never been investigated in extremely old individuals such as centenarians. Because centenarians represent a highly constrained group of individuals in terms of cognitive functioning, health and social network and because they are very close to their end of life, exploring the levels of VOL and its predictors at this extremely old age can be considered as especially meaningful for testing the central assumptions of Lawton's concept.

The present study pursued three aims. First, we wanted to find out whether the concept of VOL is theoretically and psychometrically applicable to extremely old individuals with severe functional limitations whose remaining life expectancy is very limited. We hypothesised that VOL can be reliably assessed within a representative sample of centenarians who possess sufficient cognitive capacity to answer questions about themselves. Second, we wanted to evaluate the level of VOL in centenarians by comparing this age group with younger persons. In line with Lawton's theoretical framework (Lawton, 1996), we hypothesised that the level of VOL will be not substantially lower than that of younger individuals. Third, we tried to predict interindividual differences in VOL by using personal resources such as extraversion as well as risk factors such as neuroticism. Following Lawton's assumptions (Lawton et al., 1996, 1999, 2001; Lawton, Winter et al., 1999), we hypothesised that physical and cognitive functioning as well as neuroticism should have only a minor or no influence on VOL while extraversion as a positive intrapersonal resource should emerge as a major predictor of VOL.

1. METHODS

1.1. Participants

The subjects for this study ($N = 56$) are a sub-sample of the Heidelberg Centenarian Study (Rott et al., 2001) because investigating issues of subjective well-being was only possible with those very old individuals who are able to give self-reports. In order to better understand the probable selectivity of this sample, the recruitment process will be described in the following in some detail. All inhabitants of a defined geographical region approximately 60 km around Heidelberg, Germany (comprising 172 communities and 2.6 million inhabitants) who were aged between 100 years and 1 month and 100 years and 11 months between January 1, 2000 and April 30, 2001, as well as all individuals who were aged 99 years and 4 months to 99 years and 11 months between February 15, 2001 and April 30, 2001 were potential participants. Based on the records provided by the city registries (in Germany, registration is compulsory), 156 centenarians or persons close to their 100th birthday were eligible and identified. Out of these 156 potential subjects 91 individuals (58%) were assessed in a face-to-face interview. The main reasons not to participate were dementia, health problems or psychiatric disorders. Other reasons for refusal were a lack of interest in the study or fear especially expressed by the proxies that the interview would be too stressful. As indicated in Table 1 (column "face-to-face interview"), most of these individuals were women, very frequently widowed and in about three out of four cases had received an

Table 1. Basic characteristics of the participants of the face-to-face interview, the drop-outs and the participants of the present study

	Face-to-face interview		*Drop-out*		*Present study*	
	(N = 91)		*(N = 35)*		*(N = 56)*	
Variable	*%*	*M (SD)*	*%*	*M (SD)*	*%*	*M (SD)*
Gender (% women)	89		97		84	
Widowed	80		77		82	
Married	4		6		4	
Never married	12		9		14	
Divorced	3		9		0	
Elementary school	71		89		59	
Intermediate school	26		11		35	
High school	3		0		6	
Institutionalised	48		66		37	
ADL		7.0 (4.44)		3.6 (3.50)		9.2 (3.55)
IADL		3.1 (3.42)		0.9 (1.55)		4.6 (3.53)
SMMSE		10.0 (7.32)		3.7 (5.96)		13.8 (5.12)
GDS		4.0 (2.09)		5.7 (1.70)		3.0 (1.59)

ADL, activities of daily living; IADL, instrumental activities of daily living; SMMSE, Shortened Mini Mental State Examination; GDS, Global Deterioration Scale elementary school education. Roughly half of them lived in institutions (e.g. a nursing home). The average age was 100.2 years ($SD = 0.41$). On scales evaluating the activities of daily living (ADL) and the instrumental activities of daily living (IADL) the face-to-face-interview subjects reached scores of 7.0 and 3.1, respectively. With respect to cognitive status, participants reached a score of 10.0 on a shortened version of the Mini Mental State Examination (SMMSE) and a score of 4.0 on the Global Deterioration Scale (GDS; see measures section for more details on these instruments).

Given that reduced cognitive functioning represents a risk to the reliability and validity of self-reports, information about VOL was only assessed if the individual was not affected by severe cognitive impairment. Taking into account cut-offs that had been utilised in earlier studies (e.g. Kliegel et al., 2004), we determined a score of 4 or higher on the SMMSE to indicate the necessary cognitive capacity for answering self-report questions. Based on this cut-off, 35 individuals were excluded (drop-outs) resulting in the final sample of 56 centenarians for the present study (Table 1).

Because drop-outs are usually worse off we investigated differences between this group ($n = 35$, i.e. persons unable to contributing valid self-reports) and the full participants ($n = 56$, present sample) in basic sociodemographic variables and the three domains of functioning, ADL, IADL and cognitive status. Fisher's exact tests showed significant differences for education ($p < 0.01$) and living arrangement ($p < 0.05$), but not for gender ($p = 0.08$) and marital status ($p = 0.12$). Thus, the drop-outs were less educated and were more likely to live in a care-providing institution than the full participants. With respect to physical and cognitive functioning, drop-outs scored significantly lower (ADL: $t(88) = -7.27$, $p < 0.001$; IADL: $t(73.66) = -6.59$, $p < 0.001$; SMMSE: $t(88) = -8.51$, $p < 0.001$; GDS: $t(88) = 7.61$, $p < 0.001$). Consequently, the sample for this study only represents a selected range of physical and cognitive functioning within centenarians. Results cannot be generalised to the entire centenarian population but are only valid for those very old individuals who are able to give self-reports.

1.2. *Measures*

To assess VOL as well as personal resources, we administered established instruments. The individual level of VOL was obtained with the Positive Valuation of Life Scale (PosVOL), a 13-item instrument (Lawton et al., 1999, 2001). Three sample items shall provide an impression about the content of the PosVOL Scale. The scale reads like "I have a strong will to live right now", "Life has meaning for me" or "I intend to make the most of my life". Compared to the original version the presentation format was changed. We used questions instead of statements, like "Does life have meaning for you?". In order to further reduce cognitive load, the answering format was reduced from 5 to 3 categories: "yes", "in between", "no" were the alternatives. Cronbach's alpha in this study was 0.85, demonstrating high reliability of the scale within this sample of extremely old individuals.

The ADL and the IADL were assessed with the Duke Older Americans Resources and Services Procedures (OARS; Fillenbaum, 1988). With the exception of five cases, the evaluation was based on proxy reports. The scales range from 0 (completely dependent) to 14 (fully independent). Cognitive status was assessed with a shortened version of the Mini Mental State Examination (MMSE; Folstein, Folstein, & McHugh, 1975) with a maximum score of 21 points instead of 30. More specifically, the Language section was not administered because many centenarians suffered from sensory–motor constraints that would have biased the results (Kliegel et al., 2004). In addition, the Global Deterioration Scale (GDS; Reisberg, Ferris, de Leon, & Crook, 1982) was used. Low scores of this instrument indicate good performance. The scores of the SMMSE and the GDS were highly correlated ($r = -0.92$, $p < 0.01$).

As additional determinants, extraversion as personal resource and neuroticism as risk factor were chosen. These personality traits were assessed with the NEO-FFI (Costa & McCrae, 1989; German version by Borkenau & Ostendorf, 1993). Again, the presentation format was changed from statements to questions and the number of answer categories was reduced to three ("yes", "in between", "no"). Cronbach's alpha was 0.55 for extraversion and 0.71 for neuroticism.

2. RESULTS

The results are presented along the three hypotheses underlying this study. First, we report the degree of endorsement of each item of the PosVOL scale. Next, the mean level of the centenarians' PosVOL scores is compared with that of individuals in their 70s by using data published by Lawton et al. (Lawton et al., 1999). Finally, the results of a hierarchical regression analysis are reported that evaluate the impact of personal resources and risk factors on PosVOL.

Table 2 shows the rank ordering of endorsement of the 13 PosVOL items. The question with the highest agreement was "Do you intend to make the most of your

Table 2. Centenarians' endorsements of items establishing positive valuation of life

Rank	*Item*	*M (SD)*
1	Make most of life	2.82 (0.43)
2	Maintain hopeful attitude	2.66 (0.58)
3	Religious and ethical beliefs	2.61 (0.71)
4	Meet goals set for oneself	2.59 (0.63)
4	Life has meaning	2.59 (0.76)
6	Much to look forward to	2.57 (0.71)
7	Strong will to life	2.54 (0.76)
7	Hopeful right now	2.54 (0.66)
9	Able to accomplish life goals	2.32 (0.69)
10	Many ways to get out of a jam	2.27 (0.80)
11	Way to solve the problem	2.23 (0.71)
12	Useful life	2.20 (0.86)
13	Get important things in life	2.14 (0.70)

life?" Eighty-four percent of the centenarians answered with "yes". Next followed the statement that the centenarians' personal beliefs allowed them to maintain a hopeful attitude. In contrast, the items "Is your life these days a useful life?" and "Do you think of many ways to get the things in life that are most important to you?" ranked lowest.

In order to determine whether the level of VOL is stable in very old age or subject to decline, we compared the PosVOL level of our centenarian sample to the PosVOL level of 600 septuagenarians (mean age 77 years) reported by Lawton et al. (1999). Of course, a difference could also reflect a cohort effect rather than an age effect, because of the cross-sectional nature of the comparison. First we adjusted for the different answering format used in both studies (5 point scale in the Lawton et al. study, 3 point scale in our study). More specifically, a score of 1 (no agreement) in our study was set to the average disagreement (1 disagree very strongly, 2 disagree strongly) in Lawton's study. Our score 3 (agreement) indicated the average agreement (4 agree strongly, 5 agree very strongly) of Lawton's original scale. Our medium category of 2 was set equivalent to Lawton's middle category 3. We then compared the resulting mean levels with that obtained in Lawton's study (Lawton et al., 1999). While the centenarians reached a mean score of 48.1 points ($SD = 8.20$), Lawton's septuagenarians depicted a mean score of 50.2 points ($SD = 6.35$) (Figure 1). Although the two mean scores were significantly different from each other (t (136.25) = 2.24, $p < 0.05$, adjusted degrees of freedom because of heterogeneous variances), this age effect has to be considered as small ($d = 0.31$).

Subsequently, we conducted a series of hierarchical regression analyses to evaluate the impact of health, cognitive status, personal resources and risk factors on PosVOL.

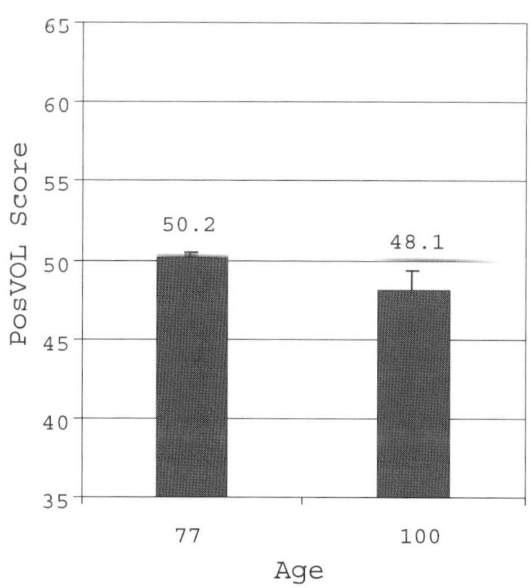

Figure 1. Age differences in positive valuation of life between septuagenarians and centenarians. Note: Bars indicate standard errors.

Table 3. *Hierarchical regression analyses predicting positive valuation of life from personal resources*

Predictors	Standardised coefficients *Model 1*	*Model 2*	*Model 3*
ADL competence	0.03	−0.16	−0.12
Cognitive impairment	−0.14	−0.02	0.10
IADL competence		0.34	0.38*
Extraversion			0.42**
Neuroticism			−0.15
R^2	0.02	0.07	0.29**
R^2 change	0.02	0.05	0.22**
Adjusted R^2	−0.02	0.01	0.22

*$p < 0.05$.
**$p < 0.01$.

In the first model, we only included basic components of functioning, ADL competence and cognitive impairment (represented by the GDS scores) as predictors, which resulted in a non-significant overall model explaining 2% of the variance (Table 3). In the second model, we added IADL competence to the above reported predictors what explained additional 5% of the variance of PosVOL. The β for this predictor was 0.34 but failed to reach statistical significance like the total model. In the third model, the two personality dimensions extraversion and neuroticism were included in a separate step to the predictors tested before. With these predictors, 29% of the variance of PosVOL was explained, resulting in a significant overall model. This model thus explained 22% more than the previous model. Having a closer look at the predictive pattern, extraversion but not neuroticism was significantly related to PosVOL ($\beta = 0.42$). Moreover, IADL competence had a β of 0.38 and passed the 5% level of significance in this final model. In sum, the regression results confirm our hypotheses: Extraversion predicts interindividual differences in VOL, whereas ADL competence, cognitive constraints and neuroticism are without predictive value. Why IADL emerged as positive predictor has to be discussed.

3. DISCUSSION

According to Lawton's theoretical framework, the concept of VOL should be of high relevance for individuals approaching their end of life. Given that this is certainly the case for very old individuals who have already outlived most of their cohort, we assumed that VOL is of key relevance for centenarians. Knowing how severely restricted centenarians usually are with respect to their physical functioning, we expected that evaluating VOL with centenarians represents a strong empirical test of Lawton's assumptions that positive features of mental health and well-being included in VOL should be maintained despite adverse life circumstances. Given that our results are in convergence with his central hypotheses, namely that individuals would be able to keep high levels of VOL, our results provide important evidence supporting the VOL concept. Additionally, our results may be helpful for developing future directions of VOL research, since the VOL construct is not only another conceptualisation of SWB, but has the potential to predict why, how and how long people wish to live under the adverse circumstances characterising the end of the life span.

More specifically, the results clearly confirmed the three hypotheses addressed in this study. First, although very old individuals may reveal some decrement in orientation and short-term memory, the items of the PosVOL scale had meaning for them and the centenarians were able to answer properly. Thus, the present study demonstrates that there is no reason to restrict the administration of the instrument only to fully functioning individuals who do not reveal any sign of cognitive impairment if age-related constraints are accommodated by minor changes to the PosVOL items (i.e. using questions instead of statements and restricting the answering format to three options). The psychometric properties obtained confirmed that reliable and valid data on this facet of SWB for rather low functioning persons can be collected. Thus, the findings are noteworthy and encouraging, since the collection of self-report on extremely long-lived individuals such as centenarians is challenging due to their multiple sensory, literacy and cognitive limitations.

Second, the centenarians revealed a high degree of VOL. Their level of VOL was almost comparable to that of septuagenarians. This result is intriguing because our participants faced a tremendous amount of especially physical limitations and losses in multiple domains of functioning. In fact, high levels of VOL seem not to support the assumption that psychological resilience is depleted in extremely old age, as Staudinger and Fleesen (1996) assumed. Since high levels of VOL also speak against a break down of the adaptational system, we also found no support for an increase in the prevalence of psychological mortality in extremely old age as suspected by Baltes and Smith (2003).

Third, when having a specific look at the predictors of VOL, the central assumptions related to the VOL concept were replicated in this sample of extremely old individuals. More specifically, physical functioning, cognitive status and neuroticism made no independent contribution to VOL as expected by Lawton and colleagues (Lawton et al., 1996, 1999, 2001; Lawton, Winter et al., 1999). The strongest predictor was the personality trait extraversion which is in line with the theoretical framework. Thus, it seems to be the case that living a socially active life and enjoying social contacts remains an essential factor even in very old age, speaking for a life-long positive impact of extraversion on well-being. The absence of a negative association between neuroticism and VOL is also in line with previous studies that found links of neuroticism to well-being indicators only when negative well-being facets were used as outcomes. For instance, Isaacowitz and Smith (2003) reported that neuroticism was only associated with negative affect, but not with positive affect in old and very old participants of the Berlin Aging Study.

Interestingly, IADL showed a significant positive association to VOL. It could be the case that centenarians with high engagement in IADL activities, such as preparing one's own meal, profit from the emotional uplifts associated with mastery experiences related to these activities and the feeling of not being completely dependent on other persons. Thus, we interpret the emerging impact of IADL competence on VOL as the continuing motivation of the individual to remain proactive and influence one's environment by behaviour.

One limitation of this study is that our sample is positively selected as shown by the selectivity analyses. Nevertheless, although one could have expected that the individuals who dropped out were much more restricted compared to the individuals who participated in the study, the selectivity effects were found to be only of moderate size. However, when evaluating the results, one has to keep in mind that the findings should only be generalised to very old individuals who are still able to give valid information about themselves.

Moreover, it can also be seen as a limitation of the study that we did not include the target variable that Lawton's concept considered as essential for this research, namely the years of desired life. It would be very interesting to know how long the centenarians wanted to live under their specific personal circumstances. Nevertheless, according to our results we have good reasons to conclude that even after a very long life and with the presence of substantial limitations, these individuals want to live and not to die. To them, life seems to have meaning and appears worth living until the very end of the life span.

AFFILIATION

German Centre for Research on Ageing at the University of Heidelberg

REFERENCES

Andersen-Ranberg, K., Schroll, M., & Jeune, B. (2001). Healthy centenarians do not exist, but autonomous do: A population-based study of morbidity among Danish centenarians. *Journal of the American Geriatrics Society, 49*, 900–908.

Antonucci, T. C. (2001). Social relations: An examination of social networks, social support, and sense of control. In J. E. Birren & K. W. Schaie (Eds.), *Handbook of the psychology of aging* (5th ed., pp. 427–453). San Diego, CA: Academic Press.

Baltes, P. B., & Mayer, K. U. (Eds.). (1999). *The Berlin aging study: Aging from 70 to 100*. New York: Cambridge University Press.

Baltes, P. B., & Smith, J. (2003). New frontiers in the future of aging: From successful aging of the young old to the dilemmas of the fourth age. *Gerontology, 49*, 123–135.

Becker, G., Rott, C., d'Heureuse, V., Kliegel, M., & Schönemann-Gieck, P. (2003). Funktionale Kompetenz und Pflegebedürftigkeit nach SGB XI bei Hundertjährigen. Die besondere Bedeutung des kognitiven Status. *Zeitschrift für Gerontologie und Geriatrie, 36*, 437–446.

Borkenau, P., & Ostendorf, F. (1993). *NEO-Fünf-Faktoren Inventar (NEO-FFI)*. Göttingen: Hogrefe.

Costa, P. T., & McCrae, R. R. (1989). *The NEO PI/FFI manual supplement*. Odessa, FL.: Psychological Assessment Resources.

Fillenbaum, G. G. (1988). *Multidimensional functional assessment of older adults: The Duke Older Americans Resources and Services Procedures*. Hillsdale: Lawrence Erlbaum Associates.

Folstein, M., Folstein, S. E., & McHugh, P. R. (1975). "Mini-Mental State": A practical method for grading the cognitive state of patients for the clinician. *Journal of Psychiatric Research, 12*, 189–198.

Gatz, M. (1998). Towards a developmentally informed theory of mental disorder in older adults. In J. Lomranz (Ed.), *Handbook of aging and mental health: An integrative approach.* (pp. 101–120). New York: Plenum Press.

Hagberg, B., Alfredson, B. B., Poon, L. W., & Homma, A. (2001). Cognitive functioning in centenarians: A coordinated analysis of results from three countries. *Journal of Gerontology: Psychological Sciences, 56B*, P141–P151.

Isaacowitz, D. M., & Smith, J. (2003). Positive and negative affect in very old age. *Journal of Gerontology: Psychological Sciences, 58B*, P143–P152.

Jeune, B. (2002). Living longer—but better? *Aging Clinical and Experimental Research, 14*, 72–93.

Kliegel, M., Moor, C., & Rott, C. (2004). Cognitive status and development in the very oldest old: A longitudinal analysis from the Heidelberg Centenarian Study. *Archives of Gerontology and Geriatrics, 39*, 143–156.

Lawton, M. P. (1996). Quality of life and affect in later life. In C. Magai & S. McFadden (Eds.), *Handbook of emotion, adult development and aging.* (pp. 327–348). Orlando, FL: Academic Press.

Lawton, M. P. (1999). Quality of life in chronic illness. *Gerontology, 45*, 181–183.

Lawton, M. P. (2000). Quality of life, depression and end-of-life attitudes and behaviors. In G. M. Williamson, D. R. Shaffer, & P. A. Parmelee (Eds.), *Physical illness and depression in older adults: A handbook of theory, research, and practice* (pp. 147–171). New York: Kluwer Academic/Plenum Publishers.

Lawton, M. P., Moss, M., Hoffmann, C., Grant, R., Have, T. T., & Kleban, M. H. (1999). Health, valuation of life, and the wish to live. *The Gerontologist, 39*, 406–416.

Lawton, M. P., Moss, M., Hoffmann, C., Kleban, M. H., Ruckdeschel, K., & Winter, L. (2001). Valuation of life: A concept and a scale. *Journal of Aging and Health, 13*, 3–31.

Lawton, M. P., Parmelee, P., Katz, I., & Nesselroade, J. R. (1996). Affective states in normal and depressed older people. *Journal of Gerontology: Psychological Sciences, 51B*, P309–P316.

Lawton, M. P., Winter, L., Kleban, M. H., & Ruckdeschel, K. (1999). Affect and quality of life: Objective and subjective. *Journal of Aging and Health, 11*, 169–198.

Martin, P., Poon, L. W., Clayton, G. M., Lee, H. S., Fulks, J. S., & Johnson, M. A. (1992). Personality, life events, and coping in the oldest-old. *International Journal of Aging and Human Development, 34*, 19–30.

Martin, P., Rott, C., Kerns, M. D., Poon, L. W., & Johnson, M. A. (2000). Predictors of depressive symptoms in centenarians. In P. Martin, C. Rott, B. Hagberg, & K. Morgan (Eds.), *Centenarians: Autonomy versus dependence in the oldest old.* (pp. 91–104). Paris: Serdi.

Reisberg, B., Ferris, S. H., de Leon, M. J., & Crook, T. (1982). The Global Deterioration Scale for assessment of primary degenerative dementia. *American Journal of Psychiatry, 139*, 1136–1139.

Rook, K. S., & Schuster, T. L. (1996). Compensatory processes in the social networks of older adults. In G. R. Pierce, B. R. Sarason, & I. G. Sarason (Eds.), *Handbook of social support and the family* (pp. 219–248). New York: Plenum.

Rott, C., d'Heureuse, V., Kliegel, M., Schönemann, P., & Becker, G. (2001). Die Heidelberger Hundertjährigen-Studie. Theoretische und methodische Grundlagen zur sozialwissenschaftlichen Hochaltrigkeitsforschung (The Heidelberg Centenarian Study: Theoretical and methodological foundations of psychosocial research in the oldest old). *Zeitschrift für Gerontologie und Geriatrie, 34*, 356–364.

Smith, J., Fleeson, W., Geiselmann, B., Settersten, R. A., & Kunzmann, U. (1999). Sources of well-being in very old age. In P. B. Baltes & K. U. Mayer (Eds.), *The Berlin Aging Study: Aging from 70 to 100* (pp. 450–471). New York: Cambridge University Press.

Staudinger, U. M., & Fleeson, W. (1996). Self and personality in old and very old age: A sample case of resilience. *Development and Psychopathology, 8*, 867–885.

BO HAGBERG

COMMENTARY: WELL-BEING IN VERY OLD AGE: OLD AND NEW ISSUES

Well-being, the good life, perceived quality of life, healthy ageing, active ageing, ageing well and successful ageing are all, in one way or another, expressions for the quality aspect of ageing. What is meant by the various concepts is, however, rather seldom explicated and few have been properly defined. There are at least two definitions which seem to have gained wider acceptance. Lawton (1991) offers the following definition: "Quality of life is the multi-dimensional evaluation, by both intrapersonal and social normative criteria of the person environment system of an individual in time past, current and anticipated." This definition is meant to subsume the full spectrum of quality of life in its most inclusive meaning. The major characteristic is its anchorage in various domains. In particular, psycholcgical well-being, behavioural competence, perceived quality of life and objective environment are considered in this definition. As we see, the multi-dimensionality and the integration of perspectives come from a broad area of experiences that the individual accumulates during the life span. Coverage of as many of these aspects as possible is both necessary and important to understand the essence of the concept as it applies to old age.

Furthermore, conceptual clarity in the target variable significantly effects the selection of predictors for well-being. Going even further, the point in time from which prediction is made, together with the choice of predictor variables, brings further obscurity to the challenge of predicting well-being in very old age. With this in mind and by also taking the excellent paper of Dr. Rott et al. into consideration, a number of old and new questions and issues related to research on well-being in very old adults can be raised.

1 A SELECTION OF FUNDAMENTAL QUESTIONS AND ISSUES

Here is a selection of the most fundamental questions and issues, most of them representing now classic but still not fully resolved questions in the field: Do general models of ageing well apply in the very old? From which age do we predict, what is the baseline, and does it matter for the outcome? What about structural invariance of well-being? What kind of mechanism do we envisage to obtain well-being? What are the well-being areas of interest in the very old? What are the special predictors of well-being in the very old? What are the major threats to well-being in the very old?

With these questions in the background, the study of well-being in the oldest old should take into account the specificity and uniqueness of these persons who have lived a very long life. In addition, a focus may also be directed to aspects that eventually come as a consequence of such a long life.

H.-W. Wahl et al. (eds.), The Many Faces of Health, Competence and Well-Being in Old Age, 131–134.

First of all, as Dr. Rott and colleagues pointed out in their paper, that negative changes that come with extreme ageing put subjective well-being (SWB) at risk. According to the authors, maintenance of personal and social resources is of great importance for coping with these negative changes, a statement that holds for the young old as well.

Second, long living persons have accumulated a large number of experiences during their lives, experiences that could be considered an additional resource in dealing with ageing changes at a very high age.

Third, Dr. Rott et al. also point to existential and meaning related life issues as particularly critical in very old age. Such a reflective attitude often found in the very old can well become a natural way of applying autobiographical review, which has been found in many studies to promote SWB (Birren & Deutchman, 1991).

Fourth, for comparative studies of well-being in younger age groups, there is always the question of structural invariance of the concept. The question whether SWB should be equally defined for young-old as compared to the oldest old is hard to tackle. It seems, however, highly likely that physical and social activity have different value in the subjective experience of SWB in different age groups.

Fifth, not only does defining SWB in different age groups imply difficulties, but it is also difficult to identify predictors valid for different ages. This also relates to the problem that predictors may change, driven by their location at different points in time, as seen from the target variable as the subject of prediction. Factors that are positively predictive in younger age groups might be negatively related to SWB in very old age or vice versa. One example is blood pressure (BP), which is used as a predictor for health: High BP is a negative predictor in young age groups for both survival and well-being, but has been found to be a positive predictor in centenarians.

Sixth, there are also different ways to conceive of how SWB is experienced. One suggestion has been the distinction between the additive approach, the key issue approach and the dynamic approach (Hagberg, 2003). The *additive* approach follows the guideline "the more the better," which means that experiences can be added in linear fashion to increase the quality of life. The *key issue* approach means that if one important quality is lost—for instance health or the experience of a good marriage—other experiences also lose their quality value. The *dynamic* approach considers changes in life quality over time in a life span perspective and implies that as life goes on, valuable experiences are exchanged for other equally valuable ones.

2. LIFE QUALITY FROM QUALITATIVE RESEARCH

Another way of looking at life quality can be found in recent qualitative research. Hagberg (2002) has strived to understand life quality through a phenomenological perspective. As was found, the meaning of quality of life can be reduced to a number of basic constituents. This pattern contains one component which is central and called *commitment*, added by two components coined *balance* and *continuity*. Finally, there are two complementary functions of a more expressive nature, i.e., to be *creative* and to be *transcending*.

3. OTHER DOMAINS

In addition to the dimensions and aspects of life quality presented above and in Dr. Rott et al.'s paper, we should be aware of the fact that there are still numerous aspects to be considered for a full coverage of the concept. Below are a few examples that add further qualities to the concept.

Life satisfaction, studied extensively by Neugarten et al. (1961), is the most frequently investigated marker of well-being at large. Major components included are mood, zest, congruency, resolution, and fortitude.

Self esteem, confidence, and self-acceptance have been studied by Ryff (1995) and others. Included in these components are having a positive attitude towards oneself, acknowledging and accepting one's good and bad sides, as well as feeling positive about one's past life.

Adaptive capacity, studied by Lazarus and Folkman (1984), Smith et al. (1999) and others, has been understood as a dynamic concept that constantly changes during ageing.

Life values, introduced by Allport (1937), address central life values as crucial to purposeful development, particular in old age. Life values might be insight and truth, usefulness, material benefits, beauty and harmony, relations and belongingness, power and influence and transcendence to other realities than the material.

Additional concepts put forward by Ryff (1995) include autonomy, that is, the perception of the degree to which one is self-determining and independent, resistance to social pressure to think and act in certain ways, and regulation of behaviour from within as well as the ability to evaluate one's self from personal standards. Environmental mastery means a sense of mastery and competence in managing the environment, being in control of a complex array of external activities, making effective use of surrounding opportunities, and being able to choose or create a context suitable to personal needs and values. Personal growth involves the feeling of continued development, seeing one's self as growing and expanding, being open to new experiences, having the sense that one's potential is being realised, seeing improvement in self and behaviour over time and being able to change in a way that reflect more self-knowledge and effectiveness. Positive relations with others cover warm, satisfying and trusting relationships, showing concern for the welfare of others, being capable of strong empathy, affection, and intimacy and understanding the give and take in human relations. Finally, purpose in life means having goals in life and a sense of directedness, being driven by feelings that there is meaning in one's present and past life, holding beliefs that give life purpose, and having aims and objectives for living (see also Reker, 1977).

4. CONCLUSION

There are a number of conclusion that can be drawn from Dr. Rott et al.'s paper and the questions that it has raised. General models of well-being and quality of life might apply to very old age, but only selectively. Predictors may differ depending on distance to outcome. Well-being may differ in meaning at different ages. Different mechanisms for well-being might be assumed at different ages; critical domains might differ at different ages. Individual resources seem to increase in importance with age. Aspects of well-being might increase, decrease or remain stable with age. Life span predictors seem to be important for determining well-being also in the oldest old. Different correlates at different ages can be expected to predict well-being in young old, old and the oldest old. Threats to well-being increase by age. The majority of the oldest old seem to find ways to accommodate to ageing decline and thereby preserve acceptable levels of well-being.

In sum, it seems that even in a classic field of gerontology and life span research such as well-being, addressed in many studies and theoretical writings, the major challenges are still ahead of us.

AFFILIATION

Lund University

REFERENCES

Allport, G. (1937). *Personality*. New York: Holt.

Birren, J. E., & Deutchman, D. E. (1991). *Guiding autobiography groups for older adults. Exploring the fabric of life*. London: John Hopkins Press Ltd.

Hagberg, B. (2003). How can gerontological knowledge contribute to well-being in old age? In K. Eisfeld, U. Wiesmann, H.-J. Hannich & P. Hirtz (Eds.). *Gesund und bewegt im Alter. Interdisziplinäre Ansätze für eine Community Medicine.* Butzbach-Greidel: Afra-Verlag.

Hagberg, M. (2002). *To become a coherent whole. Shaping meaning and worth in older life. Thesis*. Lund: Dept of Psychology at Lund University.

Lawton M. P. (1991). A multidimensional view of quality of life in frail elders. In J. E. Birren, J. Lubben, J. W. Rowe, D. E. Deutchman (Eds.). *The concept and measurement of quality of life in the frail elderly* (pp. 3–27). New York: Springer Press.

Lazarus, R. S., & Folkman, S. (1984). *Stress, appraisal and coping*. New York: Springer Publishing.

Neugarten, B. L., Havighurst, R. J., & Tobin S. S. (1961). The measurement of life satisfaction. *Journal of Gerontology, 16*, 134–143.

Reker, G.T. (1977). The purpose-in-life test in an inmate population: An empirical investigation. *Journal of Clinical Psychology, 33*, 688–693.

Ryff, C. D. (1995). The structure of psychological wellbeing revisited. *Journal of Personality and Social Psychology, 69*, 719–727.

Smith, J., Fleeson, W., Geiselmann, B., Settersten Jr. R. A., & Kunzmann, U. (1999). Sources of well-being in very old age. In P. B. Baltes & K. U. Mayer (Eds.). *The Berlin Aging Study. Aging from 70 to 100* (pp. 450–471). Cambridge: Cambridge University Press.

PART III

FOCUSING ON EPIDEMIOLOGICAL RESEARCH—CONTRIBUTION TO HEALTH, COMPETENCE, AND WELL-BEING

HERMANN BRENNER

INTRODUCTION: EPIDEMIOLOGICAL PERSPECTIVES IN AGEING RESEARCH

Until very recently, epidemiology and gerontology, both of which are relatively young disciplines in the academic spectrum of many countries, including Germany, have had their own separate and specific development. Only in recent years have expertise from both fields been brought together to extend and strengthen the spectrum of ageing research.

It is clear from its definition, as "the study of the distribution and determinants of health-related states in specific populations, and the application of this study to control of health problems" (Last, 2001) that epidemiology is central to ageing research given the prominent role of health in the lives of older adults.

Until about the middle of the 20th century, epidemiology dealt mainly with infectious diseases, which were then the leading causes of morbidity and mortality in most parts of the world. In the understanding of the lay public, it is still often exclusively linked to the study of communicable diseases. However, with the profound demographic changes in the past decades and the emergence of "epidemics" in rapidly ageing societies of chronic, non-communicable diseases, such as cardiovascular disease, cancer and rheumatic diseases, the rise of a new epidemiology, starting after World War II, focused on distribution, determinants and possibilities of prevention and control of those diseases.

Up to the middle of the 1960s, basic designs and approaches to analysis were developed for studying the causes of chronic, non-communicable diseases; the two most important prototypes include cohort and case-control studies. By the early 1980s, a theoretical framework for epidemiologic methods, including clarification of concepts such as confounding and interaction, was constructed to specifically address the complex etiologies of chronic diseases (Greenland, 1987). Further methodological and conceptual developments during the last two decades were strongly influenced by the revolutionary developments in computer technology on one hand, and in techniques of molecular biology on the other.

Whereas a central and integrating role of epidemiology in modern ageing research is not in question, there are at least three conceptually different approaches to epidemiology in ageing research (Brenner & Arndt, 2004). The oldest concept considers epidemiology in ageing research as the epidemiology in old age (e.g. Ebrahim & Kalache, 1996; Wallace & Woolson, 1992) or geriatric epidemiology. The focus of this approach lies on the study of the determinants of longevity, on the evaluation of health care and on studies addressing the frequency and natural history of diseases common in old age, such as diabetes, coronary heart disease, cancer, or dementia, as well as

H.-W. Wahl et al. (eds.), The Many Faces of Health, Competence and Well-Being in Old Age, 137–138.

their functional sequelae (Ebrahim, 1996). The restriction of the exclusive focus on old age was overcome by Miettinen (1991), who declared epidemiology of aging as the epidemiologic study of the biologic aging process across the entire life span. However, even that approach appears to be overly restrictive by the focus on biologic aging, which is difficult to measure in the individual. A more comprehensive view is taken in the life course approach (Kuh & Ben-Shlomo, 1997), which follows the notion that the risk of most non-communicable diseases accumulates with age and is influenced by factors acting at all stages of the life span. This view also implies that preventive measures often have to be taken well before old age, which is now widely accepted.

The following two chapters provide examples of recent contributions of epidemiology to the study of cancer and cardiovascular diseases, which are two of the major groups of chronic non-communicable diseases in older adults. The life course view taken in these contributions enables the identification of possibilities for prevention well before old age. Despite their focus on specific common diseases, particular emphasis is placed on aspects of co- and multimorbidity, which are the rule rather than the exception among older patients. Functional aspects and aspects of quality of life are often more important than the mere medical features for the lives of the affected patients.

A third contribution provides an example of application of epidemiologic methods to the study of medical care, which focuses on the rapidly growing population of nursing home residents in particular.

AFFILIATION

German Centre for Research on Ageing at the University of Heidelberg

REFERENCES

Brenner, H., & Arndt, V. (2004). Epidemiology in ageing research. *Experimental Gerontology, 39*, 679–686.

Ebrahim, S. (1996). Principles of epidemiology in old age. In S. Ebrahim, & A. Kalache (Eds.). *Epidemiology in old age* (pp. 12–21). London: BMJ Publishing Group.

Ebrahim, S., & Kalache, A. (1996). *Epidemiology in old age*. London: BMJ Publishing Group.

Greenland, S. (1987). *Evolution of Epidemiologic Ideas*. Newton Lower Falls, MA: Epidemiology Resources Inc.

Kuh, D., & Ben-Shlomo, Y. (1997). *Life course approach to chronic disease epidemiology*. Oxford: Oxford University Press.

Last, J. M. (2001). *A dictionary of epidemiology* (4th ed.). New York: Oxford University Press.

Miettenen, O. S. (1991). Epidemiological research on ageing: an orientation. *International Journal Epidemiology, 20*(Suppl. 1), 2–7.

Wallace, R. B., & Woolson, R. F. (1992). *The epidemiologic study of the elderly*. New York, Oxford: Oxford University Press.

HERMANN BRENNER and VOLKER ARNDT

CANCER AMONG OLDER ADULTS: INCIDENCE, PROGNOSIS AND NEW AVENUES OF PREVENTION

More than one-third of people living in Germany are expected to develop cancer during their lives. Most cancers occur in older adulthood. In Germany, about 75% of male cancer patients and about 71% of female cancer patients are 60 years or older at the time of diagnosis (Arbeitsgemeinschaft Bevölkerungsbezogener Krebsregister in Deutschland, 2004). The proportion of elderly persons has increased in Germany as in many other countries during the last few decades, and will increase further in the coming years (Pötzsch & Sommer, 2003). Hence, both the absolute number and the proportions of older cancer patients are expected to increase strongly in the years to come. Furthermore, given the steady improvement in survival for many forms of cancer, the proportion of older adults living with some form of cancer, i.e. the cancer prevalence among older adults, will continue to rise.

However, most previous epidemiological and clinical studies have focused on younger cancer patients, and patients above age 75 or 80 have often been excluded entirely from pertinent studies. Therefore, evidence regarding risk factors, the impact of preventive and therapeutic measures, or regarding major outcomes (including survival and quality of life) is quite limited for these age groups. Preliminary evidence indicates that older patients often tend to be undertreated, have poorer prognosis and benefited less from recent improvements in effective cancer management than younger cancer patients. Much age bias is based on misinformation by the attending physician (Muss & Longo, 2004). The median life expectancy of older patients is often underestimated. A person in average health surviving to age 80 can now expect to live on average another 8 years (Pötzsch & Sommer, 2003). This number exceeds the average survival durations of most untreated cancers. Still, older people remain at risk of having their lives shortened by cancer and, conversely, stand to have their lives extended by successful treatment. Extension of clinical and epidemiological studies to older cancer patients is badly needed to explore new avenues of prevention and to provide adequate care to older cancer patients.

1. CANCER INCIDENCE

Cancer is a major health problem in developed countries, in many of which it is the second most common cause of death behind cardiovascular disease for all ages combined (WHO, 1998). In Europe, the number of new cancer cases diagnosed annually has been increasing steadily in recent decades (Muir et al., 1987; Parkin et al., 1992, 1997). All the major malignancies primarily affect the elderly. The incidence of most

H.-W. Wahl et al. (eds.), The Many Faces of Health, Competence and Well-Being in Old Age, 139–151.

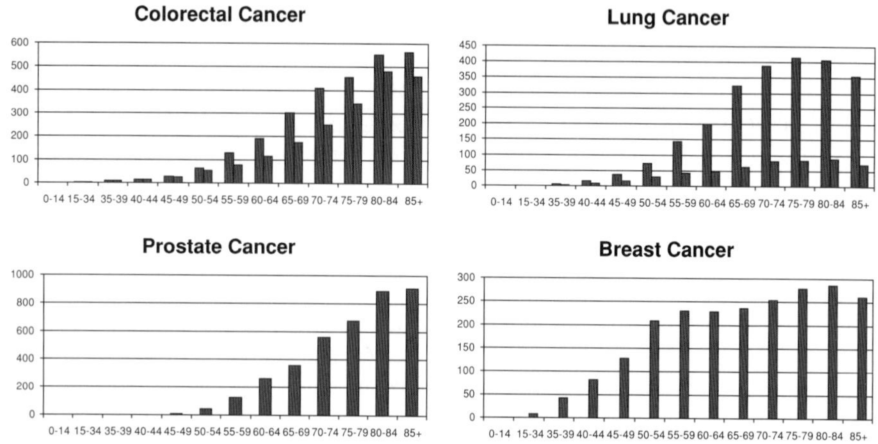

The vertical bars reflect the number of new cases per 100 000 (blue for men, red for females).

Figure 1. Cancer incidence for major tumour sites by age and gender, Germany 2000 (Arbeitsgemeinschaft Bevölkerungsbezogener Krebsregister in Deutschland, 2004)

common cancer cases as well as of all tumours combined increases with age. Rates are generally higher for men than for women, except for persons below the age of 50, where women have slightly higher cancer incidence rates. Persons aged 65 or older have a risk of cancer 7–11 times greater than that of persons under the age of 65 (Hansen, 1998; Yancik & Ries, 2004). However, large variations exist between different cancer sites with respect to the pattern of age specific rates (Figure 1).

Contrary to the pattern in younger age groups, in which annual cancer rates are almost equally distributed among the two genders, elderly men have an almost double cancer incidence rate compared with elderly women. For all major specific cancer sites except testicular cancer, the incidence rate is significantly higher among the elderly than among any groups of younger and middle-aged persons. Among elderly men, cancer of the prostate, the lung and the colon make up around half of all diagnosed cancers. Prostate cancer is around 22 times more frequent among elderly men than among younger men. The most frequent cancers among elderly women are breast, colon, stomach and lung cancer (Arbeitsgemeinschaft Bevölkerungsbezogener Krebsregister in Deutschland, 2004; Hansen, 1998).

For the four most common cancers (breast, prostate, lung and colorectal), the percentage of persons aged 65 years and older ranges from nearly 50% to more than 70%. Although the median age for the incidence of all cancers combined is currently around 68 years, the median age range at diagnosis varies widely for specific cancers (Data from the US, 1995–1999, cited in Edwards et al., 2002).

Although old age is associated with cancer disease, age itself is not considered a causal risk factor (Peto & Doll, 1997). Rather, the age distribution of cancer is thought to reflect a multi-stage process involving several consecutive genetic changes, with the rate of progression of a partially altered cell from one stage to another being largely unaffected by age (Armitage & Doll, 2004). In addition, age-related biological changes such as reduced DNA repairing ability and decreased carcinogen catabolism are discussed to play an important role in the promotion of the carcinogenic process in the elderly (Denduluri & Ershler, 2004).

There is no uniform picture regarding the issue, whether tumours observed in late age are more aggressive and are diagnosed more often at a late stage. According to Goodwin et al. (1986) cancers of the bladder, breast, cervix, ovary, thyroid, and uterus, and for melanoma tend to be diagnosed at more advanced stages in older patients, whereas cancers of the lung, pancreas, rectum and stomach are more likely to be diagnosed at an earlier stage in older patients. No association between age and stage at diagnoses seems to exist for cancers of the colon, kidney, liver and prostate. The situation becomes even more complex as tumour stage and tumour aggressiveness are not necessarily in parallel, as could be demonstrated within a large population-based study in the case of breast cancer. While our group found that older women are more likely to be diagnosed at more advanced stages of breast cancer (Arndt et al., 2001) and tend to delay the initiation of diagnostic work-up more often than younger women (Arndt et al., 2002), malign breast tumours in older women appear to be less aggressive, indicated by results from our group showing that the prognosis of women diagnosed with breast cancer at old age is better than the prognosis of women with breast cancer at younger age (Brenner & Arndt, 2004a).

2. CANCER MORTALITY

2.1. *Trends in Cancer Mortality*

In contrast to other major causes of death among the elderly (such as heart disease which declined among older adults in the United States during the second half of the 20th century by over 30%), cancer mortality has not in general declined over the past decades (Edwards et al., 2002). Indeed, there has been a significant increase in cancer mortality by over 20% during the period between 1950 and 1990, mainly attributable to the dramatic rise in death due to cancers of the respiratory system (Fried, 2000). Similar figures are reported for Europe. No more than a decade ago, cancer mortality started to decline (Levi, Lucchini, Negri, Boyle, & La Vecchia, 2003, 2004). This very recent favourable development in cancer mortality is largely driven by the decline of tobacco-related cancer mortality in men. Other significant components of the trend are the persistent substantial fall in gastric cancer mortality, the recent decline in intestinal cancer mortality in both sexes and of breast cancer mortality in women, together with the long-term falls in mortality from uterine cancer, leukaemias, Hodgkin's disease and other neoplasms amenable to advancements in diagnosis and treatment. Trends in cancer mortality have long been unfavourable in the case of the elderly (Levi, Lucchini, Negri, Boyle, & La Vecchia, 2001; Office of Cancer Communications, 1997), but are on the decline in both males and females (with the exception of lung cancer mortality in females) in Germany as in other parts of Central and Western Europe since the late 1980s. In contrast, cancer mortality has continued to rise for both sexes in Eastern Europe throughout the 1990s.

2.2. *Cancer Mortality Rates by Age at the End of the 20th Century*

Eighty-two percent of all cancer deaths occur in the age segment of the population 60 years and older in Germany (Arbeitsgemeinschaft Bevölkerungsbezogener Krebsregister in Deutschland, 2004). Persons in this age group bear the brunt of the cancer burden. As in case of cancer incidence, cancer mortality rates increase with age and males have a much higher mortality rate. This is explained in part by higher rates of tobacco-related tumours in males (e.g. lung cancer) and the different types of tumours that affect each sex. For the cancers common to both sexes, women have lower death rates.

3. CANCER SURVIVAL

The survival of cancer patients among all ages combined is well described (e.g. Sant et al., 2003) and shows quite different survival rates for different types of cancer. Obviously, when assessing survival among elderly cancer patients one has to take the relatively high prevalence of other potentially fatal diseases (comorbidity) into account. Therefore, it is particularly important when comparing survival of cancer among the elderly or between older and younger patients to use relative survival rates which are calculated as the ratios of absolute (observed) and expected survival rates (i.e. survival rates expected in a group of people of similar age without cancer). These relative survival rates reflect "net survival" after adjustment for deaths from other causes.

A major limitation of previous cancer survival studies is that they referred to patients diagnosed over a decade ago and dismissed potential progress in prognosis during the last decade, mostly due to the limitations of previously available statistical methods of survival analysis. During the past few years, we developed an entirely new approach to population-based survival analysis, denoted as period analysis, which allows to disclose trends in long-term cancer patient survival in a much more timely fashion (Brenner, Gefeller, & Hakulinen, 2004). After careful empirical evaluation (Brenner and Hakulinen, 2002a,b; Brenner, Söderman, & Hakulinen, 2002), this method has been successfully applied to disclose recent improvements and up-to-date estimates of long-term cancer survival in various countries (Brenner, 2002; Brenner, Stegmaier, & Ziegler, 2005). Pertinent analyses showed, that, overall, long-term prognosis has substantially improved for many (though not all) forms of cancer in recent years. For example, 10-year relative survival rates achieved in Germany by the beginning of the 21st century were shown to be close to 100% for patients with testis and thyroid cancer, >85% for patients with melanomas of the skin, about 80% for patients with endometrial cancer and prostate cancer, close to 70% for patients with breast cancer and kidney cancer, and close to 60% for patients with colon cancer and lymphomas (Brenner, Stegmaier, Ziegler, 2005).

The literature on cancer survival among the elderly is relatively sparse. Earlier studies from the United States (Kant, Glover, Horm, Schatzkin, & Harris, 1992) and Europe (Sant et al., 2003; Vercelli et al., 1998, 2000) reported a decrease in 5-year relative survival with advancing patient age for all cancers combined and the major tumour sites. We recently were able to demonstrate that for many forms of cancer

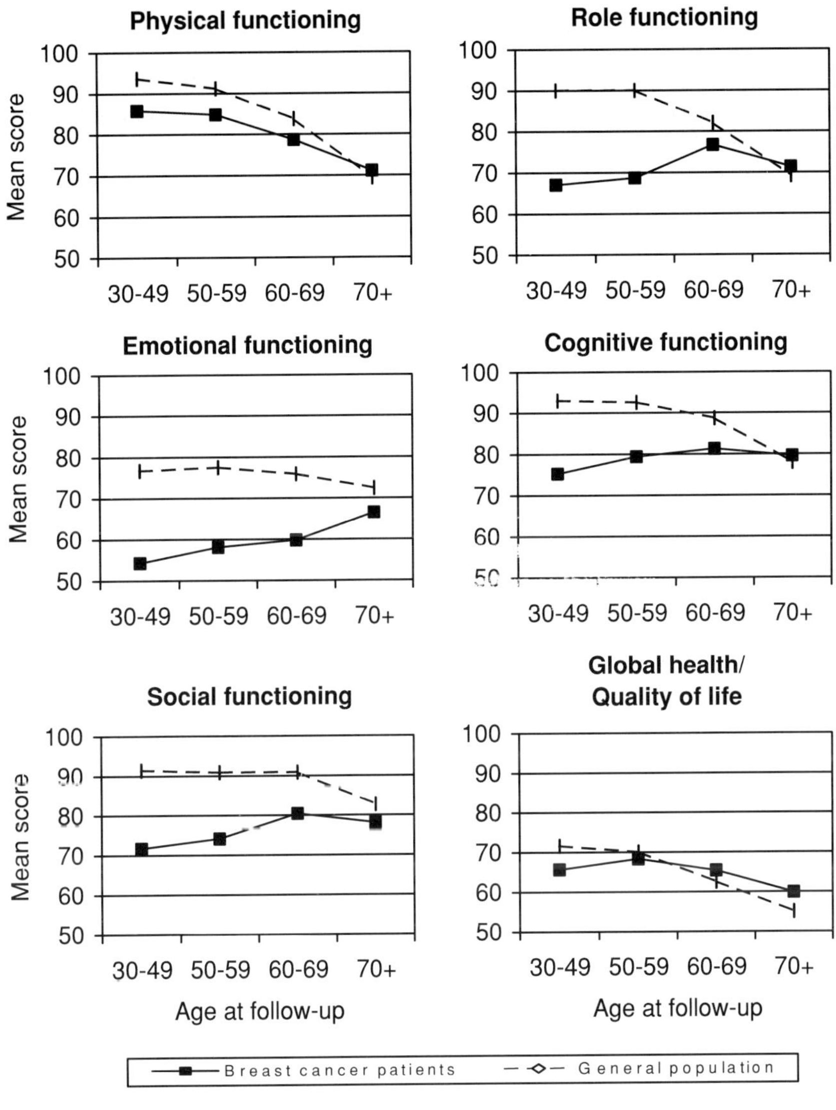

Figure 2. Recent progress in survival for all cancer sites and both sexes combined indicated by contrasting age-specific 10-year relative survival curves for the 1986–1990 cohort (left panel) and for the 1996–2000 period (right panel) (Brenner and Arndt, 2004a).

long-term survival expectations of patients have increased throughout the 1990s at all ages but that relative survival rates in older patients continue to be lower than in younger patients (Brenner and Arndt, 2004a). Indeed, our results show that the increase in survival throughout the 1990s was generally less pronounced in older than in younger patients (Figure 2).

With increasing survival rates, both the absolute numbers and the proportions of elderly people who have had a diagnosis of cancer at some time in their life is increasing. Fortunately, for most forms of cancer, patients who have survived their cancer for more than 10 years usually can be considered as cured and do not have any excess mortality compared to people without cancer any longer. Unfortunately, this does not hold for breast cancer, the most common form of cancer among women. In a recent study from our group, it was shown that older women who have had breast cancer at relatively young age, continue to have an excess risk of death even decades after diagnosis (Brenner & Hakulinen, 2004). Further research should address the reasons for and ways to overcome this continued excess mortality.

On the other hand, there are very good news for patients with prostate cancer, by far the most common form of cancer in high age among men, which were disclosed in another recent study from our group: In populations where screening by a test for prostate specific antigen in blood is common, such as the United States, the vast majority of patients diagnosed with prostate cancer no longer have excess mortality compared to men of the same age from the general population (Brenner & Arndt, 2005). Thus, with the available options in therapy, which include surgery, radiotherapy, hormone therapy and watchful waiting, the diagnosis of prostate cancer should become much less frightening than it was before, and optimising quality of life rather than prolongation of life might become the most important challenge in management of this disease and for further research.

4. CANCER PREVALENCE AND QUALITY OF LIFE

Cancer incidence, mortality and survival do not fully reflect the magnitude of the cancer burden. For the evaluation of the cancer burden in a population, measuring the prevalence is also relevant. The prevalence of a disease is the number of patients diagnosed with that disease, present in the population at a given time.

Before the publication of the EUROPREVAL study (Lutz et al., 2003), information on cancer prevalence had been largely unavailable for central European countries. The EUROPREVAL data show that within central Europe overall cancer prevalence is highest in Germany and Switzerland, with breast cancer as the most frequent malignancy among women and prostate cancer as the leading malignancy among men. For all tumours combined and for all major tumours sites (with the exception of Hodgkin's disease), prevalence sharply increases with age. For all tumours combined, prevalence was estimated to be 11.3% and 11.2% among women and men, respectively, in the age group 65+ in Germany. The prevalence is 3–4 times higher than those in the age group 45–64 years and 25–30 times higher than those in the age group up to 44 years. The age gradient is particularly high for tumours of the prostate, stomach, colon, rectum, lung and corpus uteri.

In terms of absolute numbers, people aged ≥65 years account for 68% of all prevalent cases in Germany. Compared to other countries from central Europe, this is the second highest proportion next to Switzerland (72%). The proportion of older persons

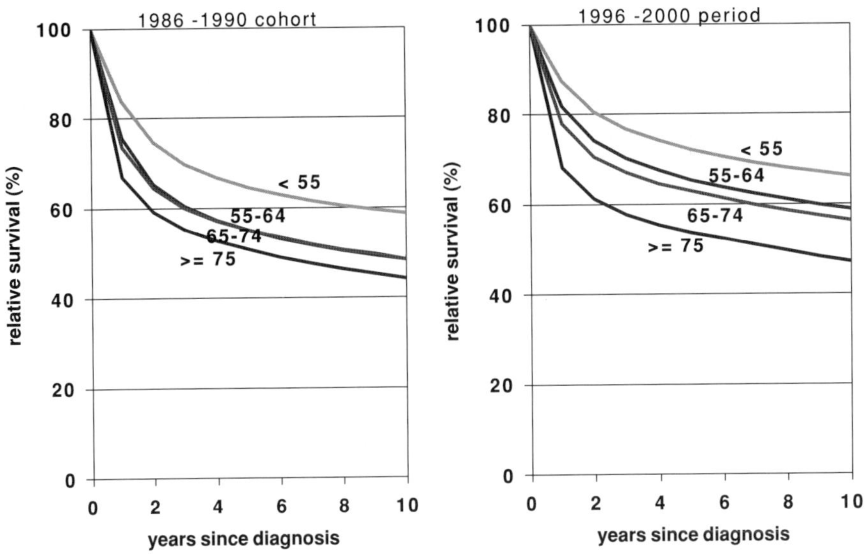

Figure 3. Age-specific health-related quality of life in women with breast cancer in comparison to women from the general population (Arndt et al., 2004a).

was highest for stomach, colon, rectum, prostate and endometrial cancer. In all these tumour entities over 75% of all cancer patients were older than 75 years. In contrast, the proportion of older patients was lowest for Hodgkin's disease and leukaemia.

Even more important than the mere prevalence of a previous diagnosis of cancer is the health-related quality of life associated with the prevalence. However, data regarding this major outcome are even sparser on the population level. In two recent population-based studies from Germany, we found health-related quality of life among patients with breast and colorectal cancer one year after diagnosis not too different from levels found in the general population of comparable age (Arndt et al., 2004; Arndt, Merx, Stegmaier, Ziegler, & Brenner, 2004). Nevertheless, deficits in emotional, cognitive, social and—in case of breast cancer—role functioning were observed. Although older persons, in general, report poorer quality of life in many dimensions, the deficits of cancer patients in contrast to healthy controls were less pronounced among the elderly (Figure 3). Furthermore, while quality of life among younger patients was primarily hampered by psychosocial deficits and financial difficulties, older cancer patients reported poorer physical functioning and poorer overall quality of life than younger patients. Apparently older persons consider their physical health in a different reference frame and tend to assess their health in terms of their age peers, whereas young cancer patients view cancer as a greater threat to their lives and manifest poorer mental health than older patients. Further follow-up of this cohort shall explore whether these deficits in quality of life continue to persist over a longer period or whether patients start to recover from the psychosocial and physical sequelae of cancer.

5. PROJECTIONS

Because of complex factors that affect changes in cancer incidence, it is difficult to anticipate what the rates will be over the next 50 years. However, if current cancer incidence rates are assumed to be constant for the next five decades, the number of cancer patients in developed countries is expected to double between 2000 and 2050 due to population growth and aging (Edwards et al., 2002). In particular, the number of cancer patients aged 85 years and older is expected to increase by more than fourfold between 2000 and 2050.

6. RISK FACTORS AND AVENUES FOR PREVENTION

Major risk factors and protective factors have meanwhile been identified for many common forms of cancer by epidemiological studies. Most of these studies have excluded older patients, however, mainly for logistic reasons. Therefore, it is often unknown to what extent findings about risk factors of cancer at younger ages can be generalized to older ages. Although there is usually no reason to assume that risk factors that increase (decrease) cancer risks at younger ages should have qualitatively different effects (i.e. opposite effects or no effect at all) at older ages, the relative importance of various risk factors and protective factors may vary substantially. For example, genetic factors, which may be major cancer risk factors at younger ages, often only play a minor role at higher ages. Vice versa, the role of certain lifestyle factors may often become increasingly important at older ages, partly reflecting very long induction periods. For example, the now well-established association between smoking and colorectal cancer emerged only with the accrual of sufficient numbers of men and women who had been smoking at least 40 years in the past, and who would typically be 60 years and older at the time of diagnosis (Giovannucci & Martinez, 1996).

These long induction periods and the major role of lifetime lifestyle factors at the same time imply that prevention of cancer among older adults could and should be aimed for at throughout the life span (Brenner & Arndt, 2004b). For example, our group has identified potential barriers to the promotion of smoking cessation and consequently initiated a cluster-randomized intervention study assessing new strategies for smoking cessation promotion in general practices in the Heidelberg-Mannheim area (Twardella & Brenner, 2005).

Besides modifications of lifestyle factors, with prevention of smoking uptake, promotion of smoking cessation, prevention of excessive alcohol consumption, promotion of a diet rich in fruits and vegetables and of physical activity being the key elements, there has recently been much interest in possibilities of chemoprevention. For example, aspirin, folate, vitamin D and calcium supplementation are now considered promising candidates for reducing the risk of colorectal cancer (Chia & Newcomb, 2004; Peters et al., 2004). However, as lessons from failed previous attempts of chemoprevention of lung cancer have shown, avenues of chemoprevention suggested by observational studies have to be confirmed by large-scale intervention trials which are yet to be completed. Finally, recent progress in disclosing the key role of infections for some forms of cancer, such as stomach cancer (e.g. Brenner, Arndt, Stegmaier, Ziegler, & Rothenbacher, 2004a; Rothenbacher & Brenner, 2003), may open new avenues of prevention by anti-infective therapy, preventive or therapeutic vaccination in the future.

Other new avenues for prevention and early detection of cancer and its precursors might be paved by breakthroughs in medical technology and molecular biology. For example, colonoscopy with removal of precancerous lesions appears to have the potential to prevent between 60% and 90% of colorectal cancers (Brenner, Arndt, Stegmaier, Ziegler & Stürmer, 2005; Brenner et al., 2001). Although colonoscopy has now been implemented in cancer screening programs in some countries including Germany, compliance with this offer remains questionable, given the invasiveness of the procedure. The effectiveness of screening colonoscopy in Germany is currently evaluated in two large-scale epidemiologic studies carried out in collaboration with various partners by our group. The first study is a case-control study conducted in the Rhine-Neckar area, the second study is a population-based cohort study conducted in Saarland.

Possibly, invasiveness of examinations can soon be overcome by new technical developments, such as virtual colonoscopy (Pickhardt et al., 2003). Similarly, detection of new molecular markers of cancer, e.g. in urine, stool, sputum or blood, may strongly enhance new opportunities for early detection of cancer (Garcea et al., 2003; Haug & Brenner, 2005b). In particular, the combination of new stool tests with colonoscopic follow-up of positive results may be a promising approach to reduce incidence and mortality from colorectal cancer (Haug & Brenner, 2005a).

7. TREATMENT AND OUTCOMES

Progress in therapy has meanwhile increased perspectives of survival and quality of life for many forms of cancer. Most likely, however, older cancer patients have benefited less from these developments for several reasons.

Firstly, older patients have often been excluded from pertinent clinical trials (Hutchins, Unger, Crowley, Coltman, & Albain, 1999). As a result, evidence regarding safety and efficacy of various therapeutic regimens in this group is much poorer than for younger cancer patients. It is therefore not surprising that treatment recommendations are often quite inconsistent for elderly cancer patients.

Secondly, even where pertinent evidence of the efficacy of treatment is available, elderly cancer patients often tend to remain undertreated. Although the consequences of therapeutic disparities, and more particularly of undertreatment of the elderly, have been poorly assessed to date, there is evidence that the consequences of such undertreatment may be substantial. For example, a recent study from Switzerland found half of the patients with breast cancer aged 80 or older were undertreated, resulting in a large excess of preventable breast cancer mortality (Bouchardy et al., 2003). There could though be major differences between various countries. Although more than 70% of breast cancer patients above 80 years of age suffered from severe comorbidity compared to 6% of those aged 40–49 years, treatment was not influenced by severity of comorbidity (Houterman et al., 2004). However, as consistently reported from other studies (e.g. Yancik et al., 1998, 2001) comorbidity was associated with a much worse prognosis.

Given the increasing prevalence of comorbidity with age, it is not surprising that studies from population-based cancer registries have consistently shown decreasing relative survival with increasing age for almost all cancer sites (Vercelli et al., 2000). However, the widening gap in relative survival in recent years described above (Brenner & Arndt, 2004a) may reflect that older cancer patients have had the least benefit even from the more recent improvements in cancer care.

8. CONCLUSION

Although the vast majority of cancer patients are older than 65 years in developed countries, and although the numbers and proportions of older cancer patients will further increase strongly in the years to come, older patients with cancer continue to be underrepresented in epidemiological and clinical studies, which severely limits empirical evidence regarding optimal prevention and treatment strategies. Uncertainty regarding optimal prevention and treatment strategies has been shown to go along with underuse of such strategies in many instances, thereby unduly withholding effective measures of cancer control from older patients. Major efforts are needed both in cancer research and clinical care to overcome this specific and severe form of "ageism."

AFFILIATION

German Centre for Research on Ageing at the University of Heidelberg

REFERENCES

Arbeitsgemeinschaft Bevölkerungsbezogener Krebsregister in Deutschland (2004). Krebs in Deutschland [Cancer in Germany] (4th ed.). Saarbrücken. Available at http://www.rki.de/cln_006/nn_403600/DE/Content/GBE/DachdokKrebs/Broschuere/brosc-huere_node.html_nnn=true (Accessed 15.06.2005).

Armitage, P., & Doll, R. (2004). The age distribution of cancer and a multi-stage theory of carcinogenesis (reprint of the classical work published in *British Journal of Cancer* 1954; 8:1–12). *British Journal of Cancer, 91*, 1983–1989.

Arndt, V., Stürmer, T., Stegmaier, C., Ziegler, H., Dhom, G., & Brenner, H. (2001). Socio-demographic factors, health behavior and late-stage diagnosis of breast cancer in Germany: A population-based study. *Journal of Clinical Epidemiology, 54*, 719–727.

Arndt, V., Stürmer, T., Stegmaier, C., Ziegler, H., Dhom, G., & Brenner, H. (2002). Patient delay and stage of diagnosis among breast cancer patients in Germany—a population based study. *British Journal of Cancer, 86*, 1034–1040.

Arndt, V., Merx, H., Stürmer, T., Stegmaier, C., Ziegler, H., & Brenner, H. (2004) Age specific detriments to quality of life among breast cancer patients one year after diagnosis. *European Journal of Cancer, 40*, 673–680.

Arndt, V., Merx, H., Stegmaier, C., Ziegler, H., & Brenner, H. (2004). Quality of life in patients with colorectal cancer 1 year after diagnosis compared with the general population: A population-based study. *Journal of Clinical Oncology, 22*, 4829–4836.

Bouchardy, C., Rapiti, E., Fioretta, G., Laissue, P., Neyroud-Caspar, I., Schafer, P., Kurtz, J., Sappino, AP., & Vlastos, G. (2003). Undertreatment strongly decreases prognosis of breast cancer in elderly women. *Journal of Clinical Oncology, 21*, 3580–3587.

Brenner, H. (2002). Long-term survival rates of cancer patients achieved by the end of the 20th century: A period analysis. *Lancet, 360*, 1131–1135.

Brenner, H., & Arndt, V. (2005). Long-term survival rates of patients with prostate cancer in the PSA screening era: Population-based estimates for the year 2000 by period analysis. *Journal of Clinical Oncology, 23*, 441–447.

Brenner, H., & Arndt, V. (2004a). Recent increase in cancer survival according to age: Increase in all age groups, but widening age gradient. *Cancer Causes Control, 15*, 903–910.

Brenner, H., & Arndt, V. (2004b). Epidemiology in aging research. *Experimental Gerontology, 39*, 679–686.

Brenner, H., Arndt, V., Stegmaier, C., Ziegler, H., & Rothenbacher, D. (2004a). Is *Helicobacter pylori* a necessary condition of noncardia gastric cancer? *American Journal of Epidemiology, 159*, 252–258.

Brenner, H., Arndt, V., Stürmer, T., Stegmaier, C., Ziegler, H., & Dhom, G. (2001). Long lasting reduction of the risk of colorectal cancer following screening endoscopy. *British Journal of Cancer, 85*, 972–976.

Brenner, H., Arndt, V., Stegmaier, C., Ziegler, H., & Stürmer, T. (2005a). Reduction of clinically manifest colorectal cancer by endoscopic screening: Empirical evaluation and comparison of screening at various ages. *European Journal of Cancer Prevention, 14*, 231–237.

Brenner, H., Gefeller, O., & Hakulinen, T. (2004). Period analysis for up-to-date cancer survival data: Theory, empirical evaluation, computational realization and applications. *European Journal of Cancer, 40*, 326–335.

Brenner, H., & Hakulinen, T. (2004). Are patients diagnosed with breast cancer below age 50 ever cured? *Journal of Clinical Oncology, 22*, 432–438.

Brenner, H., & Hakulinen, T. (2002a). Up-to-date long-term survival curves of patients with cancer by period analysis. *Journal of Clinical Oncology, 20*, 826–832.

Brenner, H., & Hakulinen, T. (2002b). Advanced detection of time trends in long-term cancer patient survival: Experience from 50 years of cancer registration in Finland. *American Journal of Epidemiology, 156*, 566–577.

Brenner, H., Söderman, B., & Hakulinen, T. (2002). Use of period analysis for providing more up-to-date estimates of long-term survival rates: Empirical evaluation among 370,000 cancer patients in Finland. *International Journal of Epidemiology, 31*, 456–462.

Brenner, H., Stegmaier, C., & Ziegler, H. (2005). Long-term survival of cancer patients in Germany achieved by the beginning of the 3rd millennium. *Annals of Oncology, 16*, 981–986.

Chia, V., & Newcomb, P. A. (2004). Calcium and colorectal cancer: Some questions remain. *Nutrition Review, 62*, 115–124.

Denduluri, N., & Ershler, W. B. (2004). Aging Biology and Cancer. *Seminar in Oncology, 31*, 137–148.

Edwards, B. K., Howe, H. L., Ries, L. A., Thun, M. J., Rosenberg, H. M., Yancik, R., Wingo, P. A., Jemal, A., & Feigal, E. G. (2002). Annual report to the nation on the status of cancer, 1973–1999, Featuring implications of age and aging on U.S. cancer burden. *Cancer, 94*, 2766–2792.

Fried, L. P. (2000). Epidemiology of ageing. *Epidemiological Review, 22*, 95–106.

Garcea, G., Sharma, R. A., Dennison, A., Steward, W. P., Gescher, A., & Berry, D. P. (2003). Molecular biomarkers of colorectal carcinogenesis and their role in surveillance and early intervention. *European Journal of Cancer, 39*, 1041–1052.

Giovannucci, E., Martinez, M. E. (1996). Tobacco, colorectal cancer, and adenomas: A review of the evidence. *Journal of the National Cancer Institute, 88*, 1717–1730.

Goodwin, J. S., Samet, J. M., Key, C. R., Humble, C., Kutvirt, D., & Hunt, C. (1986). Stage at diagnosis of cancer varies with the age of the patient. *Journal of American Geriatric Society, 34*, 20–26.

Hansen, J. (1998). Common cancers in the elderly. *Drugs Aging, 13*, 467–478.

Haug, U., & Brenner, H. (2005a). A simulation model for colorectal cancer screening: Potential of stool tests with various performance characteristics compared to screening colonoscopy. *Cancer Epidemiology, Biomarkers & Prevention, 14*, 422–428.

Haug, U., & Brenner, H. (2005b). New stool tests for colorectal cancer screening: A systematic review focusing on performance characteristics and practicalness. *International Journal of Cancer* doi:10.1002/ijc.21016 (published online 4 May 2005).

Houterman, S., Janssen-Heijnen, M. L., Verheij, C. D., Louwman, W. J., Vreugdenhil, G., van der Sangen, M. J. et al. (2004). Comorbidity has negligible impact on treatment and complications but influences survival in breast cancer patients. *Br J Cancer, 90*, 2332–2337.

Hutchins, L. F., Unger, J. M., Crowley, J. J., Coltman, C. A. Jr., & Albain, K. S. (1999). Underrepresentation of patients 65 years of age or older in cancer-treatment trials. *New England Journal of Medicine, 341*, 2061–2067.

Kant, A. K., Glover, C., Horm, J., Schatzkin, A., & Harris, T. B. (1992). Does cancer survival differ for older patients? *Cancer, 70*, 2734–2740.

Levi, F., Lucchini, F., Negri, E., Boyle, P., & La Vecchia, C. (2004). Cancer mortality in Europe, 1995–1999, and an overview of trends since 1960. *International Journal of Cancer, 110*, 155–169.

Levi, F., Lucchini, F., Negri, E., Boyle, P., & La Vecchia, C. (2003) Mortality from major cancer sites in the European Union, 1955–1998. *Annals of Oncology, 14*, 490–495.

Levi, F., Lucchini, F., Negri, E., Boyle, P., & La Vecchia, C. (2001). Changed trends of cancer mortality in the elderly. *Annals of Oncology, 12*, 1467–1477.

Lutz, J. M., Francisci, S., Mugno, E., Usel, M., Pompe-Kirn, V., Coebergh, J. W., Bieslka-Lasota, M.; EUROPREVAL Working Group (2003). Cancer prevalence in Central Europe: The EUROPREVAL Study. *Annals of Oncology, 14*, 313–322.

Muir, C. S., Waterhouse, J., Mack, T., Powell, J., & Whelan, S. (1987). Cancer Incidence in Five Continents, Vol. V. IARC Scientific Publications No. 88. *International Agency for Research on Cancer*, Lyon, France.

Muss, H. B., & Longo, D. L. (2004). Introduction: Cancer in the elderly. *Seminar in Oncology, 31*, 125–127.

Office of Cancer Communications, National Cancer Institute (1997). Questions and Answers on Trends in Cancer Mortality. Available at: http://rex.nci.nih.gov/massmedia/backgrounders/cancermortality. HTM (accessed 15.06.2005).

Parkin, D. M., Muir, C. S., Whelan, S. L., Gao, Y. T., Ferlay, J., & Powell, J. (1992). Cancer Incidence in Five Continents, Vol VI. IARC Scientific Publications No. 120. International Agency for Research on Cancer, Lyon, France.

Parkin, D. M., Whelan, S., Ferlay, J., Raymond, L., & Young, J. (1997). Cancer Incidence in Five Continents, Vol. VII. IARC Scientific Publications No. 143. International Agency for Research on Cancer, Lyon, France.

Peters, U., Hayes, R. B., Chatterjee, N., Shao, W., Schoen, R. E., Pinsky, P., Hollis, B. W., & McGlynn, K. A.; Prostate, Lung, Colorectal and Ovarian Cancer Screening Project Team (2004). Circulating vitamin D metabolites, polymorphisms in vitamin D receptor, and colorectal adenoma risk. *Cancer Epidemiology Biomarkers & Prevention, 13*, 546–552.

Peto, R., & Doll, R. (1997). There is no such thing as aging. *BMJ, 315*, 1030–1032.

Pickhardt, P. J., Choi, J. R., Hwang, I., Butler, J. A., Puckett, M. L., Hildebrandt, H. A., Wong, R. K., Nugent, P. A., Mysliwiec, P. A., & Schindler, W. R. (2003). Computed tomographic virtual colonoscopy to screen for colorectal neoplasia in asymptomatic adults. *The New England Journal of Medicine, 349*, 2191–2200.

Polednak, A. P. (1997). Estimating the prevalence of cancer in the United States. *Cancer, 80*, 136–141.

Pötzsch, O., & Sommer, B. (2003). Bevölkerung Deutschlands bis 2050. Ergebnisse der 10. koordinierten Bevölkerungsvorausberechnung [German population by the year 2050. Results of the 10th coordinated population projection]. Statistisches Bundesamt, Wiesbaden. Available at http://www.destatis.de/presse/deutsch/pk/2003/ Bevoelkerung_2050.pdf (Accessed 15.06.2005).

Rothenbacher, D., & Brenner, H. (2003). Burden of *Helicobacter pylori* and *H. pylori* related diseases in developed countries: Recent developments and future implications. *Microbes & Infection, 5*, 693–703.

Sant, M., Aareleid, T., Berrino, F., Bielska Lasota, M., Carli, P.M., Faivre, J., Grosclaude, P., Hedelin, G., Matsuda, T., Moller, H., Moller, T., Verdecchia, A., Capocaccia, R., Gatta, G., Micheli, A., Santaquilani, M., Roazzi, P., & Lisi, D. The EUROCARE Working Group (2003). EUROCARE-3: Survival of cancer patients diagnosed 1990–94—results and commentary. *Annals of Oncology, 14* (Suppl. 5), V61–V118.

Twardella, D., & Brenner, H. (2005). Lack of training as a central barrier to the promotion of smoking cessation: A survey among general practitioners in Germany. *European Journal of Public Health, 15*, 140–145.

Vercelli, M., Quaglia, A., Casella, C., Parodi, S., Capocaccia, R., & Martinez Garcia, C., EUROCARE Working Group (1998) Relative survival in elderly cancer patients in Europe. *European Journal of Cancer, 34*, 2264–2270.

Vercelli, M., Capocaccia, R., Quaglia, A., Casella, C., Puppo, A., & Coebergh, J. W. W., EUROCARE Working Group (2000). Relative survival in elderly European cancer patients: Evidence for health care inequalities. *Critical Review on Oncology and Hematology, 35*, 161–179.

WHO. (1998). Health for all (CD-Rom). World Health Organization, Geneva.

Yancik, R. M., Ries, L. A. G. (2004). Cancer in Older Persons: An international issue in an aging world. *Seminar in Oncology, 31*, 128–136.

Yancik, R., Wesley, M. N., Ries, L. A., Havlik, R. J., Edwards, B. K., & Yates, J. W. (2001). Effect of age and Comorbidity in postmenopausal breast cancer patients aged 55 years and older. *Jama, 285*, 885–892.

Yancik, R., Wesley, M. N., Ries, L. A., Havlik, R. J., Long, S., Edwards, B. K., & Yates, J. W. (1998). Comorbidity and age as predictors of risk for early mortality of male and female colon carcinoma patients. A population-based study. *Cancer, 82*, 2123–2134.

JAN WILLEM COEBERGH

COMMENTARY: CANCER IN THE ELDERLY: PREVENTION AND BETTER CARE NEEDED

The contribution of Brenner and Arndt (in press) deals with a range of issues in relation to cancer occurring at older age, especially over age 70: For the more frequent tumours, incidence rises usually up to age 80 and at older age survival decreases, even after adjustment for dying from other causes. Because of increasing opportunities for (hope of) effective treatment and decreasing fatalism, an intriguing set of dilemmas emerges from a basic clinical question: What is the right treatment, can over- or undertreatment be estimated or even predicted, and what type of studies are needed within the framework of a population-based setting that cover the whole spectre of patients? According to clinical researchers in cancer centres, more randomised trials should be carried out, but they often focus on a selection of patients without co-morbidity, which in old age is, of course, a minority. Moreover, if indeed the heterogeneity of the patients that clinicians observe increases with age, resulting from combinations of co-morbid conditions and diversity in social condition and coping strategy, then what can be done to learn from experience? Let us realise that despite the large and increasing numbers of newly diagnosed older patients, the numbers per hospital of such patients, even with frequent tumours, become low at old age (Table 1).

As cancer survival has been increasing in the last decade, also in the elderly, e.g. for ovarian, breast and colorectal cancer, the proposed survival estimation using most recent survival data seems warranted. But for tumours amenable to early detection and even screening like prostate or breast cancer, an impression of overtreatment as an indicator of side effects (up to fivefold in the case of prostate cancer) should also be given. From a strategic point of view, the major question seems whether and when primary or secondary prevention can work in the elderly without too many side effects on quality of life. A more general question is how to avoid too great of an inequity, or which socio-conditions are required for large scale early detection and adequate oncological treatment?

Given the fact that a high and increasing proportion of newly diagnosed patients is over 70 (between 30% and 50%), the resources available for health services appear to be a determinant of outcome across Europe as suggested by a recent paper of Quaglia et al. (2005). On the other hand, social support also mattered. The variation across Europe at least was (and probably still is) so large that the European Union would be wise in providing more resources for the framework to study the social and medical determinants of this variation. Of major interest is also to estimate the rapidly rising demand for future care. (Coebergh, 2001)

H.-W. Wahl et al. (eds.), The Many Faces of Health, Competence and Well-Being in Old Age, 153–158.

Table 1. Estimation of number of new elderly cancer patients according to age in a general hospital in the Netherlands in 2000: range according to hospital size

Tumour	*75+ years*	*80+ years*	*85+ years*	*90+ years*
Lung	20–40	6–12	1–4	0–1
Prostate	8–24	3–12	2–6	0–2
Breast	12–35	10–20	4–7	0–2
Digestive tract	25–75	20–40	5–15	2–4
Haemopoietic system	3–15	1–6	0–3	0–1
All sites	115–260	60–120	25–50	6–18
(% of total)	(26%)	(12%)	(5%)	(1.2%)

Source: Netherlands Cancer Registry.

For those who ultimately die from cancer, a large proportion is older than 60 years, even 80% in Germany, but adequate palliative care can nowadays increasingly be given due to specific training, better drugs, etc. Based on experience in the Netherlands, it seems increasingly relevant to have regional organisations for coordination of the many medical and nursing disciplines involved, including also geriatricians, because of the complexities and interactions of co-morbidities with medical care at old age. Such organisations (called Integraal Kankercentrum) do not need to cost more than 1 euro per inhabitant, to which one should add almost 0.5 euro for the cancer registry, 50% for collection of data and 50% for research with the registry. This registry is an essential element for studies of adequacy of care. (Brewster, Coebergh, & Storm, 2005)

Some specific comments will be given on primary and secondary prevention and on the role of co-morbidity, also based on current experience and plans.

1. PRIMARY PREVENTION

For most tumours incidence increases, more or less exponentially, with the rise of age, especially when lifestyle played a role, usually at young and middle age. Based on current knowledge, primary prevention of cancer in the elderly would have to be based on avoiding (or stopping) excessive exposures to UV-radiation (mortality rates of skin melanoma are rapidly rising in elderly men across Europe with a possible flattening in males born after the 1950s). Larger effects would be attained by a lower intake of tobacco, alcohol and calories (Doll, 1999); together with regular physical exercise and intake of enough fruits and vegetables, a large proportion of cancers, up to 50% in most countries, would be avoidable. Scandinavian researchers have realistically estimated the proportion of avoidable cancers (mostly relevant at older age) to be about 25% (Olsen et al., 1997), but their incidence rates are generally lower.

In a starting project within the EU 6th framework (www.eurocadet.org), a group of European researchers will estimate the feasibility and potential of healthy lifestyle interventions to substantially lower the future incidence of cancer across Europe.

A time axis will be chosen up to 2040, since it takes decades to implement major interventions and also show their effects.

2. SECONDARY PREVENTION

Most mass screening programmes indirectly focus on the elderly. Even if their upper age limit is at middle age, the effects hold on for another 5–15 years, at least because of lead-time (an earlier detection and a better treatment option). Cervical cancer screening usually stops at age 60 and breast cancer screening at age 70 (in Holland at 75); PSA-prostate cancer screening, still tested in the ERSPC (European Randomised Study of Screening for Prostate Cancer)—trial usually stops at age 70 and endoscopic colorectal cancer screening at mass scale has nowhere been implemented with substantial compliance; it would have protective value for 10–15 years, if not longer. In America (like in Germany), much more so called opportunistic screening occurs for most of these tumours, also resulting in substantial overtreatment. On every death avoided, up to 10 patients might also be overtreated and, depending on the tumour type and other characteristics, between 500 and 2500 persons need to be screened to avoid one death. An individual policy for screening has also been developed if healthy persons (no symptomatic patients of course) demand screening tests (Coebergh, 2004; Walter & Covinski, 2001): their life expectancy would need to be at least 5 years, based on a classification of candidates for screening (in fact symptom-free persons) according to life expectancy in three to four groups, from favourable to unfavourable. But not only are the side effects of screening considerable, as has been eloquently delineated by Welch (2005), also are the forces of fear and commerce, often by organisations. Candidates for screening should be more aware of this and help their caregiver out of the dilemma by asking questions as to why, what if and for what. This should rather evolve in a high risk strategy, because for low risk persons screening has in fact too many side effects, albeit remaining invisible to the public. Considering complexity and logistics, I also tend to favour a risk based approach from high risk screening, gradually moving to standard screening, and avoiding as much as possible screening of low risk persons (Coebergh, 2004).

3. ADEQUACY OF CARE IN THE ELDERLY

Many studies show that adherence to guidelines decreases with age, in fact more than warranted. But few studies on complications of treatment in elderly have been carried out on those not caused by overtreatment. The presence of co-morbidity seems rather crucial, which was studied during the past 12 years in our registry (Janssen-Heijnen & Coebergh, 2003) using the score of Charlson. A summary of these studies (Janssen-Heijnen, et al., 2005) shows that co-morbidity plays a role when sufficiently severe and especially for tumours with a relatively good prognosis. But the major impact of these studies is to create awareness for better multi-disciplinary care. In particular, this would be necessary for cancer patients that also suffer from diabetes, because their hazard ratio seems unnecessarily almost 2-fold increased.

An overview of our studies of breast cancer (Tables 2–4) clearly shows the impact (Louwman et al., 2005; Houterman et al., 2004).

Table 2. Age-specific prevalence of co-morbidity in newly diagnosed patients with cancer

Co-morbidity	*50–59(%)*	*Age (years) 60–74(%)*	*75+ (%)*
None	55	35	26
Previous cancer	7	12	16
COPD	8	15	16
Heart diseases	6	15	19
Vascular diseases peripheral	2	5	6
Hypertension	9	16	16
Diabetes mellitus	4	8	10
CVA/hemiplegia	1	4	6

Source: Eindhoven Cancer Registry (Janssen-Heijnen et al., in press).

Table 3. Breast cancer: Prevalence of co-morbidity (%) in the south of the Netherlands during 1995–2001: according to age

	<50 (N = 2308)	*50–69 (N = 4186)*	*70–79 (N = 1665)*	*80+ (N = 800)*
Co-morbidity number (%)				
0	79	67	50	35
1	8	16	27	34
2+	1	4	14	22
Unknown	13	12	9	9
Co-morbidity type (%)				
Previous cancer	2	5	8	12
Cardiovascular	1	5	14	21
Cerebrovascular	0	1	5	8
COPD	2	4	7	7
Diabetes	1	6	14	17
Dementia	0	0	1	5
Digestive tract	1	1	2	4

Source: Eindhoven Cancer registry (Louwman et al., 2005)

Table 4. Breast Cancer, 1995–2001: Age-specific crude and relative 5-year survival by age and presence of co-morbidity at diagnosis

	Age 50–69 % (se)	*Age 70+ % (se)*	*Relative % (se)*
None	84 (1)	68 (2)	93 (2.1)
Previous cancer	73 (4)	59 (5)	78 (6)
Cardiovascular	83 (5)	56 (4)	77 (6)
COPD	84 (4)	62 (7)	88 (8)
Diabetes	84 (4)	53 (4)	69 (6)
Cerebrovascular	72 (10)	48 (7)	75 (10)
Dementia	—	27 (9)	—
>1 co-morbidity	65 (4)	35 (2)	53 (3)

Source: Eindhoven Cancer registry (Louwman et al., 2005)

Table 5. Multivariate analysis of hazard ratio of co-morbidity in breast cancer (N = 8000) diagnosed in the south of the Netherlands, 1995–2001

Co-morbidity	*Hazard ratio*	*95% CI*
Cardiovascular	1.8	1.6–2.1
COPD	1.5	1.2–1.8
Diabetes	1.65	1.4–1.9
Cerebrovascular	2.0	1.8–2.4
Dementia	3.2	2.4–4.3

Source: Eindhoven Cancer Registry (Louwman et al., 2005)

To conclude, given the growing proportion of older adults in most European populations, management, and prevention of cancer is a major challenge that will put the health system in general and specialised oncologists and nurses to the test. Regional coordinating organizations are needed that are comprehensive and attain the ideal of adequate multi-disciplinary care for the elderly.

AFFILIATIONS

Erasmus University, Medical Centre Rotterdam

Comprehensive Cancer Centre South (IK2), Eindhoven

REFERENCES

Brenner, H., & Arndt, V. (2005). Cancer among older adults: Incidence, prognosis and new avenues of prevention. In H.-W. Wahl, H. Brenner, H. Mollenkopf, D. Rothenbacher, & C. Rott (Eds.), *The many faces of health, competence and well-being in old age: Integrating epidemiological, psychological and social perspectives*. Amsterdam: Springer.

Brewster, D. H., Coebergh, J. W., & Storm, H. H. (2005). Population-based cancer registries: the invisible key to cancer control. *The Lancet Oncology, 6*, 193–195.

Coebergh, J. W. W. (2004). Colorectal cancer screening in Europe: first things first. *European Journal of Cancer, 40*, 638–642.

Coebergh, J. W. W. (2001). Cancer in the elderly: epidemiology in Europe. *European Journal of Cancer, 37*, s217–s228.

Doll, R. (1999). The Pierre Denoix Memorial Lecture: nature and nurture in the control of cancer. *European Journal of Cancer, 35*, 16–23.

Houterman, S., Janssen-Heijnen, M. L. G., Verhey, K., Louwman, W. J., Vreugdenhil, G., van der Sangen, M., et al. Co-morbidity has negligible impact on treatment and complications, but influences survival from breast cancer in the first year. *British Journal of Cancer, 90*, 2332–2337.

Janssen-Heijnen, M. L. G., Coebergh, J. W. W. (2003). Co-morbidity. In: R. Sankila, J. W. W. Coebergh, E. Demaret, R. Black, D. Forman, G. Gatta, et al. (Eds.). *Evaluation of clinical care utilizing cancer registries* (pp. 27–33). Lyon: IARC Technical Publications No. 37.

Janssen-Heijnen, M. L. G., Houterman, S., Louwman, W. J., Lemmens, V. E., Coebergh, J. W. W. (2005). Prognostic impact of increasing age and co-morbidity in cancer patients: A population-based approach. *Critical Reviews in Oncology/Hematology*.

Louwman, W. J., Janssen-Heijnen, M. L. G., Houterman, S., Voogd, A. C., van der Sangen, M. J. C., Nieuwenhuijzen, G. A. P., et al. (2005). Less extensive treatment and inferior prognosis for breast cancer patients with co-morbidity: a population-based study. *European Journal of Cancer, 41*, 779–785.

Olsen, J. H., Andersen, A., Dreyer, L., Pukkala, E., Trygvadottir, L., Gerhardsson de Verdier, M. et al. (1997) Avoidable cancers in the Nordic countries. APMIS;105(suppl 76). 1–146.

Quaglia, A., Vercelli, M., Lilini, R., Mugnos, E., Coebergh, J. W. W., Quinn, M., et al. (2005). Socio-economic factors and health care system characteristics related to cancer survival in the elderly. A population-based analysis in 16 European countries (ELDCARE project).*Critical Reviews in Oncology/Hematology, 54*, 117–128.

Schroder, F., Roobol, M., Damhuis, R., de Koning, H., Bleyenberg, W., van der Kwast Th, et al. (2005) Rotterdam randomized pilot studies of screening for prostate cancer—an overview after 10 years. *Journal of National Cancer Institute. 97*, 696.

Walter, L. C., & Covinsky, K. E. (2001). Cancer screening in elderly patients: a framework for individualized decision making. *JAMA, 285*, 2776–2278.

Welch, H. G. (2005). Should I be tested for cancer? Maybe not and here's why. University of California Press, 2004. (also: Search and destroy—the right cancer strategy for Europeans? *European Journal of Cancer, 41*, 660–663.

DIETRICH ROTHENBACHER and HERMANN BRENNER

CARDIOVASCULAR DISEASES AMONG OLDER ADULTS: INCIDENCE, PROGNOSIS AND NEW AVENUES FOR PREVENTION

The demographic transition that we are currently observing in the Western countries leads to a considerable increase in the proportion of elderly members of the society, whereas the proportion of younger subjects decreases mainly due to a decrease in birth rates. The increase in the group of subjects 80 years and older will be most emphasized and, according to estimates from Germany, this group will triple within the next 50 years (Statistisches Bundesamt, 2000). By the year 2050, over 9 million of subjects will be in the age group 80 years and older and this age segment will comprise 12% of the total population. Currently about 3.2 million subjects or 4% of the total population are in this age segment. This demographic transition will also lead to a considerable increase and shift in the burden of the respective diseases these societies will have to cope with in future decades. The increase in the prevalence of chronic diseases in the elderly, in particular, will present a major challenge for our society in upcoming decades. This increase will also pose a special challenge to epidemiologists and other researchers working in this field (Brenner & Arndt, 2004). In the following, the specific situation and the future developments of coronary heart diseases will be outlined in order to lay the ground for a discussion of the urgency and specific possibilities of preventive measures in order to cope with these challenges. Thereby, the situation in the elderly will be emphasized. In addition, two examples will be used to exemplify own research results and their implication for prevention of coronary heart disease in the general population, both for the sake of the individual and society.

1. INCIDENCE AND PREVALENCE OF CARDIOVASCULAR DISEASES

Cardiovascular diseases are still the leading cause of disability and death in Western countries. According to the official cause of death statistics, they are responsible for about 50% of all deaths per year in Germany (see Figure 1) and half of all these cases are directly attributable to coronary heart disease (Statistisches Bundesamt, 1999). The incidence of cardiovascular diseases increases with increasing age. Age specific incidence rates are three to four times higher in men compared to women.

A World Health Organization Working Group has developed a major international collaborative study with the objective of measuring over 10 years the trends in, and determinants of, cardiovascular disease. The MONICA (Monitoring Trends and Determinants in Cardiovascular Disease)-study was conducted in various regions of the world. The study recorded morbidity and mortality of acute myocardial infarctions

H.-W. Wahl et al. (eds.), The Many Faces of Health, Competence and Well-Being in Old Age, 159–168.

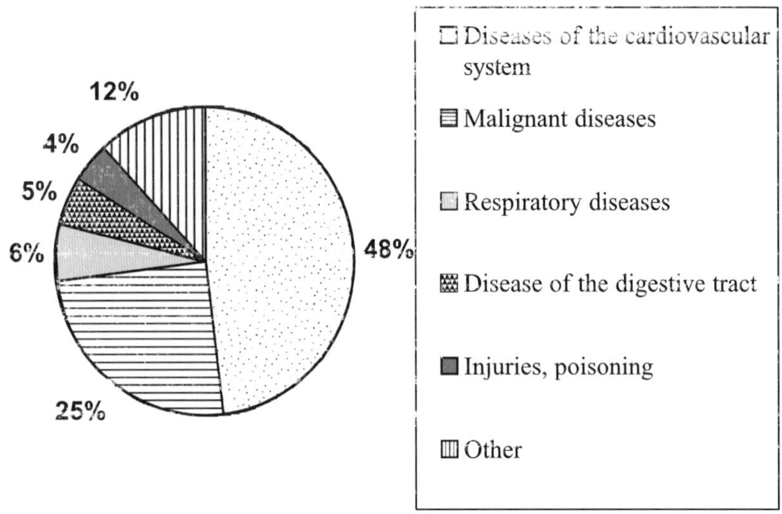

Figure 1. Main causes of death in Germany. Source: National Death Statistics (Statistisches Bundesamt, 1999).

(which is an acute manifestation of an ischaemic heart disease) on a population based level between the years 1984 and 1995. According to data from the population based KORA/MONICA-registry in Augsburg (Germany), the incidence of an acute myocardial infarction varied in men between 78 cases per 100,000 in the age category of 35–44 years and 1,648 cases per 100,000 in the age category 65–74 years, and it was 14 cases and 645 cases in women in the respective categories (Löwel et al., 2002). From 1985 to 1998, morbidity from myocardial infarction declined from 560 to 397 cases per 100,000 in men and from 161 to 145 cases in women; the mortality decreased from 317 to 232 in men and from 101 to 96 in women (Löwel et al., 2002). The decline in men was mainly due to the decrease in incident and recurrent myocardial infarction, and the decline in women was mainly due to a reduction of recurrent myocardial cases. This general trend to a decrease of age specific death rates during the last years was seen in almost all participating MONICA centres; the exact reasons, however, are still unclear (Tunstall-Pedoe et al., 1999).

Although over the past years and decades we could observe a steady decrease of coronary heart disease lethality (Tunstall-Pedoe et al., 1999), the prognosis is still severe. Mortality of an acute coronary syndrome which results in a myocardial infarction is highest during the pre- and early hospital phase. Within the pre-hospital phase and within the early hospital phase (first day in hospital) almost 32% and 24% of men, and 39% and 31% of women died, respectively. After the first month of an acute myocardial infarction only 54% of men and only 36% of women were still alive (Löwel et al., 1993; Löwel et al., 2002). Thereafter mortality is relatively low. Because of the dramatic change of the age composition in our society with an increase of the elderly population in addition to an increasing life expectancy, the prevalence of coronary heart disease will increase within the next years. This will occur despite the observed age and gender standardized decrease of incident cases and will be further furnished by the decrease of case-fatality rates with an increasing proportion of patients who will survive an acute manifestation. It is estimated that coronary heart disease will be the number one cause of disability and death by the year 2020 worldwide (Murray & Lopez, 1997).

In a recently started large cohort study (ESTHER-study) initiated from our department in the Saarland (Germany) which was especially designed for epidemiological investigations of the chances of preventing, recognizing and optimally treating chronic diseases in an elderly population, already 77% of the subjects aged 50–74 years had at least one cardiovascular risk factor (hypertension, hyperlipidaemia, diabetes, adiposity or cigarette smoking) at baseline, underlining the high priority that cardiovascular diseases will have in the future (Löw, Stegmaier, Ziegler, Rothenbacher, & Brenner, 2004). In line with observations from other countries, this study also showed that cardiovascular diseases in elderly subjects often occur simultaneously with other chronic diseases. The resulting multimorbidity often requires the use of multiple drugs which poses the risk of drug interactions with potential side effects (Bergk et al., 2004). According to recent data from the US, although octogenarians comprised currently about 5% of the population, they represent 20% of all hospitalisations from myocardial infarction and 30% of all myocardial infarction related hospitals deaths (Wenger, 1999).

Therefore, both new avenues and concepts of primary and secondary prevention are urgently needed to face these developments and the special situation in the elderly patients with the aim to reduce the burden of disease for the individual as well as to compensate for the burden of the disease for the society.

2. PATHOPHYSIOLOGY OF CORONARY HEART DISEASE

Coronary heart disease is basically the clinical manifestation of an atherosclerosis of the coronary vessels, which itself is the result of many pathophysiologic changes in these vessels over decades until finally a plaque has grown and becomes clinically manifest. Atherosclerotic changes involve the following steps: firstly, an endothelial dysfunction with monocyte adhesion to endothelial cells by expression of adhesion molecules, secondly, oxidized LDL-uptake of macrophages and thirdly, proliferation of migrated smooth muscle cells by activation of platelet derived growth factors.

Meanwhile, convincing evidence suggests that coronary heart disease is an inflammatory process, and a variety of inflammatory and other biochemical markers potentially related to atherogenesis have been identified (Danesh, Collins, Appleby, & Peto, 1998; Hoffmeister et al., 2001; Ross, 1999). After a vessel stenosis has developed over time, the rupture of a plaque is often a very acute event which occludes the coronary vessel and leads to an acute myocardial infarction. This process is both initiated and aggravated by established risk factors such as hypertension, smoking, obesity, diabetes, physical inactivity and of special importance, hyperlipidaemia (Hoffmeister et al., 2001; Imhof et al., 2003; Rothenbacher, Hoffmeister, Brenner, & Koenig, 2003; Twardella et al., 2004).

3. STRATEGIES FOR PREVENTION OF CORONARY HEART DISEASE

Strategies for primary as well as secondary prevention of coronary heart disease are very similar. Both are mainly targeted at the elimination or alleviation of coronary heart disease risk factors as they initiate or accelerate the disease process. Current knowledge about risk factors for atherosclerosis is immense. Landmark observational studies such as the Framingham study have established a number of determinants and risk factors (Dawber, 1980). However, the results have to be adapted for the German population as otherwise the risk for coronary heart diseases is overestimated to some degree (Hense, Schulte, Löwel, Assmann, & Keil, 2003). Male sex and a positive family history of cardiovascular diseases are important determinants of coronary heart disease. Among the well-established modifiable risk factors are hypertension, obesity, cigarette smoking, physical inactivity, hyperlipidaemia and diabetes (Assmann, Cullen, & Schulte, 2002; Hense et al. 2003).

After an individual risk assessment has been conducted, a concept for therapeutic interventions should be elaborated. The preventive potential of pharmacological treatment of even moderate levels of hypertension and hyperlipidaemia and of low-dose aspirin is now beyond controversy in order to reduce the risk for coronary heart disease or improve its prognosis (Wood et al., 1998).

However, results of recent studies suggest that a large risk reduction could also be achieved by lifestyle changes such as adoption of a Mediterranean diet pattern, moderate alcohol consumption or even modest increase in physical activity (Wood, 2001). At least in primary prevention of coronary heart disease, changes in lifestyle should precede drug treatment. This should also be a key component in secondary prevention of coronary heart disease. However, an effectively managed lifestyle change in patients with already manifest coronary heart disease cannot substitute an appropriate drug therapy in order to avoid secondary coronary heart disease events and improve prognosis (Wood et al., 1998).

4. STRATEGIES OF PREVENTION IN THE ELDERLY

The aims and targets of preventive programs in patients with coronary heart disease are quite well formulated and consensus exists for how these principles should be applied in clinical practice (Wood et al., 1998). Unfortunately, very few data exist about the benefit of the various preventive strategies in elderly patients.

One reason is that elderly patients are mostly excluded both from clinical trials and population based-studies (Williams et al., 2002) because an upper age limit of 70 or 75 years is often used as a pre-formulated exclusion criteria of these studies. A second important point is that many older patients who would benefit from cardiac intervention programs do not participate in such programs because of lack of referral or a variety of societal and other barriers (Ades, Waldmann, McCann, & Weaver, 1992). As a consequence, the results of these studies can only hardly be applied to elderly subjects. Having the aforementioned demographic transition in mind, future studies should urgently include elderly subjects as they will especially compromise the future burden of coronary heart disease.

Although most of the practice guidelines are based on clinical trials or observational studies conducted in middle-aged men, more and more evidence is accumulating that the recommendations are also valid for older subjects, both in primary and secondary prevention (Williams et al., 2002). The strategies commonly used for primary and secondary reduction of coronary heart disease risk in middle-aged subjects seem also to be effective strategies in the elderly, as several large scale randomised trials and observational studies have recently suggested (Dornbrook-Lavender, Pieper, & Roth, 2003; Mayou et al., 2000).

However, in elderly patients the concepts of prevention are meeting special challenges as the patients often are suffering not only a coronary heart disease, but simultaneously have other chronic diseases present that may require pharmacological treatment with the possibility of multiple side effects and drug interactions (Bergk et al., 2004). In particular, cognitive impairment and vascular forms of dementia which become more prevalent with increasing age and may also be the result of a cerebrovascular manifestation of atherosclerosis, are other aggravating factors that limit the applicability of preventive programs which are based on self-organization and motivation.

Furthermore, as chronic diseases are also often accompanied by depression and other mood disorders, the presence of depressive symptoms and symptoms of anxiety in elderly should more often be taken into consideration. They are both primary risk factors for coronary heart disease and adverse prognostic factors in patients with already existing coronary heart disease (Blumenthal et al., 2003; Frasure-Smith et al., 2000; Mayou et al., 2000). As simple validated questionnaires exist (Herrmann, 1997), these symptoms might be evaluated on a routine basis in clinical practice. Respective treatment may be initiated if indicated, for which effective pharmacological as well as psychotherapeutic interventions exist. If not treated adequately, these symptoms are clearly associated with a worse prognosis in patients with coronary heart disease and they also lead to non-adherence to recommended health behaviour.

Yet, despite present evidence that statin therapy after myocardial infarction, in particular, reduces the risk for secondary cardiovascular events and total mortality, irrespective of age and gender (Heart Protection Study Collaborative Group, 2002), younger patients are still more likely to get these drugs prescribed in primary care compared to elderly patients (Dalal, Evans, & Campbell, 2004). Another problem is the lack of adherence to treatment regimens in the elderly. According to a recent report, up to 60% of elderly patients did not take their medication 2 years after an acute myocardial infarction had occurred (Jackevicius, Mamdani, & Tu, 2002). A study from Germany conducted in patients undergoing in-patient rehabilitation because of a coronary heart disease demonstrated that patients with increased cardiovascular risk factors showed a significant improvement in most of the risk factors (Küpper-Nybelen, Rothenbacher, Hahmann, Wusten, & Brenner, 2003). However, these improvements were only partly sustained in the long-term. Therefore, mainly factors associated with patient compliance and difficulties to implement the health related behaviour chances into the daily life are critical components of successful prevention programs. These issues may be of even more importance in elderly patients.

Beside the benefits of pharmacological treatment in the elderly, benefits of lifestyle changes such as an increase in leisure time physical activity are also evident in elderly subjects (Wannamethee et al., 2002). It is, however, not necessary to limit physical activity to structured and strenuous exercise programs that are usually conducted by younger people. Especially in elderly patients, physical activity should also include a broader interpretation, as even simple activities such as low intensity walking may lead to considerable reductions in mortality (Hakim et al., 1998).

Therefore, more and more evidence is accumulating that prevention or postponement of cardiovascular events in elderly may be achieved by the same risk factor modifications which are already established targets for intervention in younger and middle-aged subjects. However, the living environment of elderly subjects has to be taken into consideration if these strategies are to be implemented on a routine basis.

Furthermore, although the relative risk associated with the respective risk factor may decrease with increasing age, the increasing incidence of coronary heart disease with increasing age and thus the large number of affected elderly patients may compensate for this apparent loss of effectiveness on the population level and prevent a large number of otherwise occurring coronary heart disease cases.

4.1. First Example: Physical Activity and Prevention of Primary Coronary Heart Diseases

Meanwhile, the beneficial effect of physical activity on cardiovascular morbidity and mortality, and all cause mortality, is widely acknowledged (Department of Health and Human Services, 1996). As suggested in various studies (Bijnen et al., 1998; Lee, Rexrode, Cook, Manson, & Burig, 2001; Wannamethee, Shaper, & Alberti, 2000; Wannamethee, Shaper, & Walker, 1998), the beneficial effects for a reduction of coronary heart disease risk are seen already with moderate engagement in leisure time physical activities. We analysed data of a case-control study in patients with stable coronary heart disease in order to estimate the risk for coronary heart disease associated with leisure time physical activity and work related physical strain after careful adjustment for other established risk factors (Rothenbacher et al., 2003).

In this large case-control study including 312 patients with angiographically confirmed and stable coronary heart disease and 472 age- and gender-matched controls, we found a strong and independent inverse association between leisure time physical activity and risk of coronary heart disease, already effective at moderate levels. Compared to subjects who reported no summer leisure time physical activity the odds ratio (OR) for coronary heart disease was 0.85 [95% confidence interval (CI) 0.47–1.53) in the category with <1 h/week, 0.60 [95% CI 0.38–0.95] in the category with 1–2 h/week and 0.39 [95% CI 0.26–0.59] in the category with >2 h/week of leisure time physical activity after full adjustment for covariates. Similar results were obtained for winter leisure time physical activity.

In contrast, an increased risk for coronary heart disease associated with work related physical strain was seen. Furthermore, we could demonstrate that leisure time physical activity is inversely and independently associated with several acute phase proteins, pro-inflammatory cytokines, and circulating adhesion molecules, suggesting a direct role of leisure time physical activity in triggering the immune response which is characteristic for atherogenesis. Sedentary subjects had a higher inflammatory activity when compared to physically active subjects. In addition, markers of endothelial function seem to be inversely and independently associated with leisure time physical activity, indicating that several pathomechanistic pathways are involved. These data therefore strongly support the recommendation of leisure time physical activity in the general population for the prevention of primary coronary heart disease.

4.2. Second Example: Smoking Essation and Prevention of Secondary Coronary Heart Diseases

The deleterious effects of smoking on cardiovascular health and the increased risk of coronary heart disease due to smoking have been consistently demonstrated (Doll, 2000; Fagerström, 2002). Furthermore, there appears to be a clear beneficial effect of smoking cessation on prognosis and occurrence of coronary heart disease due to a decreased risk for subsequent secondary cardiovascular events (U.S. Department, 1990, Critchley & Capewell, 2003). Thus smoking is an accepted and major component of cardiac rehabilitations concepts (Ades, 2001). We addressed the impact of smoking and smoking cessation measured by self-report and by serum cotinine level (the latter is a biologic marker of cigarette smoking) on the risk of secondary cardiovascular disease events during a one year follow-up period in a cohort of patients with coronary heart disease recruited when undergoing a 3-week in-patients rehabilitation program in two rehabilitation clinics in Germany (Twardella et al., 2004).

During the 1-year follow-up, 139 of the 967 patients experienced a secondary cardiovascular disease event. Both self-reported smoking status and smoking classification according to serum cotinine measurements were associated with the occurrence of a secondary cardiovascular disease event. After reclassification of all cotinine-positive subjects to continued smokers and cotinine-negative self-reported smokers to recent quitters, this association became even stronger. The OR for a secondary cardiovascular disease event then was 0.71 (95% CI 0.38–1.33) for recent quitters, 0.64 (95% CI 0.36–1.11) for former smokers and 0.44 (0.24–0.81) for never smokers compared to continued smokers (p-value for trend = 0.009).

This study therefore suggested that the benefits of smoking cessation in cardiac patients might even be stronger than suggested by previous studies which so far exclusively relied on self-reported smoking status. The results furthermore underline the importance of efforts to support smoking cessation and to prevent relapse during and after in-patient rehabilitation of patients with coronary heart disease.

5. CONCLUSION AND FUTURE REQUIREMENTS

The prevalence of coronary heart disease will increase strongly within the next years. Prevention or postponement of cardiovascular events may also prevent or postpone disability and the necessity of nursing care in old age and therefore be important constituents of primary and secondary prevention in the elderly. However, clearly more studies are needed which investigate the effectiveness of various preventive measures on the community level and they should specifically include elderly people (Löw et al., 2004) as prevention in this group faces special challenges such as the frequent multimorbidity of the patients, and the special environmental and social context of elderly subjects.

Major efforts are needed to close the gap between current knowledge with respect to issues of primary and secondary prevention which has been elaborated mostly in middle-aged adults and the future burden of coronary heart disease, which mainly consists of patients who are of older age and possibly have multiple chronic diseases. Research efforts specifically aiming to close this gap may be the best way to cope with the future requirements and enables us to make the necessary decision on an evidence-based ground.

AFFILIATION

The German Centre for Research on Ageing at the University of Heidelberg

REFERENCES

Ades, P. A. (2001). Cardiac rehabilitation and secondary prevention of coronary heart disease. *The New England Journal of Medicine, 345*, 892–902.

Ades, P. A., Waldmann, M. L., McCann, W. J., & Weaver, S. O. (1992). Predictors of cardiac rehabilitation participation in older coronary patients. *Archives of Internal Medicine, 152*, 1033–1035.

Assmann, G., Cullen, P., & Schulte, H. (2002). Simple scoring scheme for calculating the risk of acute coronary events based on the 10-year follow-up of the prospective cardiovascular Munster (PROCAM) study. *Circulation, 105*, 310–315.

Bergk, V., Gasse, C., Rothenbacher, D., Loew, M., Brenner, H., & Haefeli, W. E. (2004). Drug interactions in primary care: impact of a new algorithm on risk determination. *Clinical Pharmacology and Therapeutics, 76*, 85–96.

Bijnen, F. C. H., Caspersen, C. J., Feskens, E. J. M., Saris, W. H. M., Mosterd, W. L., et al. (1998). Physical activity and 10-year mortality from cardiovascular diseases and all causes. The Zutphen Elderly Study. *Archives of Internal Medicine, 158*, 1499–1505.

Blumenthal, J. A., Lett, H. S., Babyak, M. A., White, W., Smith, P. K., et al. (2003). Depression as a risk factor for mortality after coronary artery bypass surgery. *Lancet, 362*, 604–609.

Brenner, H., & Arndt, V. (2004). Epidemiology in aging research. *Experimental Gerontology, 39*, 679–686.

Critchley, J. A., & Capewell, S. (2003). Mortality risk reduction associated with smoking cessation in patients with coronary heart disease: a systematic review. *The Journal of the American Medical Association, 290*, 86–97.

Dalal, H., Evans, P. H., & Campbell, J. L. (2004). Recent developments in secondary prevention and cardiac rehabilitation after acute myocardial infarction. *British Medical Journal, 328*, 693–697.

Danesh, J., Collins, R., Appleby, P., & Peto, R. (1998). Association of fibrinogen, C-reactive protein, albumin, or leukocyte count with coronary heart disease: meta-analyses of prospective studies. *The Journal of the American Medical Association, 279*, 1477–1482.

Dawber, T. R. (1980). *The Framingham study: the epidemiology of atherosclerotic disease*. Cambridge, Massachusetts, USA: Harvard University Press.

Department of Health and Human Services. (1996). *Physical activity and health: a report of the Surgeon General*. Atlanta (GA), USA: National Center for Chronic Diseases Prevention and Health Promotion.

Doll, R. (2000). Fifty years of research on tobacco. *Journal of Epidemiology and Biostatistics, 5*, 321–329.

Dornbrook-Lavender, K. A., Pieper, J. A., & Roth, M. T. (2003). Primary prevention of coronary heart disease in the elderly. *The Annals of Pharmacotherapy, 37*, 1654–1663.

Fagerström, K. (2002). The epidemiology of smoking: health consequences and benefits of cessation. *Drugs, 62*(Suppl 2), 1–9.

Frasure-Smith, N., Lesperance, F., Gravel, G., Masson, A., Juneau, M., et al. (2000). Social support, depression, and mortality during the first year after myocardial infarction. *Circulation, 101*, 1919–1924.

Hakim, A. A., Petrovitch, H., Burchfiel, C. M., Ross, G. W., Rodriguez, B. L., et al. (1998). Effects of walking on mortality among nonsmoking retired men. *The New England Journal of Medicine, 338*, 94–99.

Heart Protection Study Collaborative Group (2002). MRC/BHF heart protection study of cholesterol lowering with simvastin in 20,536 high-risk individuals: a randomized placebo-controlled trial. *Lancet, 360*, 7–22.

Hense, H.-W., Schulte, H., Löwel, H., Assmann, G., & Keil, U. (2003). Framingham risk function overestimates risk of coronary heart disease in men and women from Germany—results from the MONICA Augsburg and the PROCAM cohorts. *European Heart Journal, 24*, 937–945.

Herrmann, C. (1997). International experiences with the Hospital Anxiety and Depression Scale – a review of validation data and clinical results. *Journal of Psychosomatic Research, 42*, 17–41.

Hoffmeister, A., Rothenbacher, D., Bazner, U., Frohlich, M., Brenner, H., Hombach, V., et al. (2001). Role of novel markers of inflammation in patients with stable coronary heart disease. *The American Journal of Cardiology, 87*, 262–266.

Imhof, A., Rothenbacher, D., Khuseyinova, N., Hoffmeister, A., Maerz, W., et al. (2003). Plasma Lipoprotein Lp(a) and risk of coronary heart disease: what are the mechanisms involved? *Journal of Cardiovascular Risk 10*, 362–370.

Jackevicius, C. A., Mamdani, M., & Tu, J. V. (2002). Adherence with statin therapy in elderly patients with and without acute coronary syndromes. *The journal of the American Medical Association, 288*, 462–467.

Küpper-Nybelen, J., Rothenbacher, D., Hahmann, H., Wusten, B., & Brenner, H. (2003). Changes of risk factors in patients with coronary heart disease after in-patient rehabilitation. *Deutsche Medizinische Wochenschrift, 128*, 1525–1530.

Lee, I.-M., Rexrode, K. M., Cook, N. R., Manson, J. A., & Burig, J. E. (2001). Physical activity and coronary heart disease in women. *The Journal of the American Medical Association, 285*, 1447–1454.

Löw, M., Stegmaier, C., Ziegler, H., Rothenbacher, D., & Brenner, H. (2004). [Epidemiological investigations of the chances of preventing, recognizing early and optimally treating chronic diseases in an elderly population (ESTHER study)] (article in German). *Deutsche Medizinische Wochenschrift, 129*, 2643–2647.

Löwel, H., Dobson, A. M., Keil, U., Herman, B., Hobbs, M. S., et al. (1993). Coronary heart disease case fatality in four countries. *Circulation, 88*, 2524–2531.

Löwel, H., Meisinger, C., Heier, M., Hörmann, A., Kuch, B., et al. (2002). Sex specific trends of sudden cardiac death and acute myocardial infarction: result of the population-based KORA/MONICA-Augsburg register 1985 to 1998. *Münchner Medizinische Wochenschrift, 127*, 2311–2316.

Mayou, R. A., Gill, D., Thompson, D. R., Day, A., Hicks, N., et al. (2000). Depression and anxiety as predictors of outcome after myocardial infarction. *Psychosomatic Medicine, 62*, 212–219.

Murray, C. J., & Lopez, A. D. (1997). Mortality by cause for eight regions of the world: Global Burden of Diseases Study. *Lancet, 349*, 1269–1276.

Ross, R. (1999). Atherosclerosis—an inflammatory disease. *The New England Journal of Medicine, 340*, 115–126.

Rothenbacher, D., Hoffmeister, A., Brenner, H., & Koenig, W. (2003). Physical activity, coronary heart disease, and inflammatory response. *Archives of Internal Medicine, 163*, 1200–1205.

Statistisches Bundesamt (1999). *ed. Reihe 4 Todesursachen*, Fachserie 12: Gesundheitswesen. Wiesbaden: Metzler and Poeschel.

Statistisches Bundesamt (2000). 1. Bevölkerungsentwicklung Deutschlands bis zum Jahr 2050. Ergebnisse der 9. koordinierten Bevölkerungsvorausberechnung. Wiesbaden. at http://www.destatis.de/download/veroe/bevoe.pdf (last accessed October 10, 2005).

Tunstall-Pedoe, H., Kuulasmaa, K., Mahonen, M., Tolonen, H., Ruokokoski, E., et al. (1999). Contribution of trends in survival and coronary-event rates to changes in coronary heart disease mortality: 10-year results from 37 WHO MONICA project populations. Monitoring trends and determinants in cardiovascular disease. *Lancet, 353*, 1547–1557.

Twardella, D., Kupper-Nybelen, J., Rothenbacher, D., Hahmann, H., Wusten, B., et al. (2004). Short-term benefit of smoking cessation in patients with coronary heart disease: estimates based on self-reported smoking data and serum cotinine measurements. *European Heart Journal, 25*, 2101–2108.

U.S. Department of Health and Human Services (1990). *The health benefits of smoking cessation.* U.S. Department of Health and Human Services, Public Health Service, Centers for Disease Control, Center for Chronic Diseases Prevention and Health Promotion, Office on Smoking and Health. DHHS Publication No. (CDC) 90–8416.

Wannamethee, S. G., Lowe, G. D., Whincup, P. H., Rumley, A., Walker, M., et al. (2002). Physical activity and hemostatic and inflammatory variables in elderly men. *Circulation, 105*, 1785–1790.

Wannamethee, S. G., Shaper, A. G., & Alberti, K. G. (2000). Physical activity, metabolic factors, and the incidence of coronary heart disease and type 2 diabetes. *Archives of Internal Medicine, 160*, 2108–2116.

Wannamethee, S. G., Shaper, A. G., & Walker, M. (1998). Changes in physical activity, mortality, and incidence of coronary heart disease in older men. *Lancet, 351*, 1603–1608.

Wenger, N. K. (1999). Cardiovascular Diseases in the Octogenarian and Beyond. London: Martin Dunitz, Ltd.

Williams, M. A., Fleg, J. L., Ades, P. A., Chaitman, B. R., Miller, N. H., et al., (2002). Secondary prevention of coronary heart disease in the elderly (with emphasis on patients > or = 75 years of age): an American Heart Association scientific statement from the Council on Clinical Cardiology Subcommittee on Exercise, Cardiac Rehabilitation, and Prevention. *Circulation, 105*, 1735–1743.

Wood, D. (2001). Established and emerging cardiovascular risk factors. *American Heart Journal, 141*(2 Suppl), S49–S57.

Wood, D., DeBaker, G., Faergeman, O., Graham, I., Mancia, G., et al. (1998). Prevention of coronary heart disease in clinical practice. *European Heart Journal, 19*, 1434–1503.

S. GOYA WANNAMETHEE

COMMENTARY: CARDIOVASCULAR DISEASES AMONG OLDER ADULTS: INCIDENCE, PROGNOSIS AND NEW AVENUES FOR PREVENTION

1. BACKGROUND

Cardiovascular disease (CVD) remains a major preventable cause of morbidity and mortality in Western countries. Despite the decline in mortality rates, which has occurred since the late 1970s, CVD is still responsible for 40–50% of all deaths before the age of 74 in western societies (Petersen, Peto, & Rayner, 2004; Rayner & Petersen, 2005). The incidence of major CVD rise strongly with age by more than fivefold between 50 and 70 years. In the UK, nearly 90% of all deaths from CVD occur after the age of 65 years and almost 70% after 75 years (Rayner & Petersen, 2005) while in the US comparable figures are reported with over 85% of CVD deaths occurring in persons aged ≥65 years (American Heart Association, 2005). There is also a substantial burden of morbidity associated with CVD at older ages. CVD is one of the leading causes of physical disability, accounting for more than a third of physical disability at older ages (Hiranic & Malbut, 2002). With increasing life expectancy, this raises serious issues for CVD prevention and management.

About half of all deaths from CVD are due to coronary heart disease (CHD; Petersen et al., 2004). The identification and management of modifiable risk factors have been major contributors to the reduction in CHD deaths over the past 25 years. Several major risk factors for CHD are clearly established at the individual levels, including dietary fat-blood cholesterol, cigarette smoking, high blood pressure, physical inactivity, overweight and diabetes/insulin resistance (Grundy, Pasternak, Greenland, Smith, & Fuster, 1999; Law, Wald, & Thompson, 1994; Lewington, Clarke, Qizilbash, Peto, & Collins, 2002). Most of these classical risk factors remain predictive in older people (Dornbrook-Lavender, Pieper, & Toth, 2003; Houterman et al., 2002) although the relationship between CVD risk factors and CHD is weaker in older adults compared to middle-aged adults (Manolio et al., 1992; Selmer, 1992). In general, relative risks decrease with increasing age but absolute risk of CHD increase. There is now very strong evidence that effective control of major risk factors (particularly blood cholesterol, blood pressure and cigarette smoking) can reduce risk both in subjects without CHD (primary prevention) and with established CHD (secondary prevention) (Progress Collaborative Group, 2001; Wald & Law, 2003) and that the benefits of prevention apply among older people (Heart Protection Study Collaborative Group, 2002; Shepherd et al., 2002).

H.-W. Wahl et al. (eds.), The Many Faces of Health, Competence and Well-Being in Old Age, 169–174.

2. PRIMARY AND SECONDARY PREVENTION OF CVD

The current recommendations for prevention of CHD focus on management of blood pressure and lipids as well as aspirin therapy and targeting smoking cessation, dietary intake, physical activity, weight management and diabetes management (Pearson et al., 2002). The recommendations for primary and secondary prevention are generally similar. The paper presented by Rothenbacher and Brenner provides an overview of the current standing in primary and secondary prevention of CHD in older subjects. Although most of the practice guidelines are based on clinical trials or observational trials in middle-aged men, there is accumulating evidence that the recommendations are also valid for older subjects both in primary and secondary prevention. In older subjects absolute risks for CVD are high therefore even a small decrease in risk causes a substantial reduction in the number of CVD events.

Recommendations for the use of pharmacologic agents are based primarily on findings from large clinical trials in middle-aged populations. Although trials in older adults are still limited there is increasing evidence that antihypertensives, lipid lowering agents such as statins and aspirin therapy prevent initial coronary events in older subjects (>65 years old), people who are at very high risk (Dornbrook-Lavender et al., 2003). Much less is know about the efficacy of pharmacotherapy for prevention in subjects >75 as the oldest patients have generally been excluded from trials and clinical trials are needed to determine the magnitude of benefit in this population.

3. LIFESTYLE MODIFICATION IN THE PREVENTION OF CVD

Besides the benefits of pharmacological treatment in the elderly, Rothenbacher and Brenner points out that that prevention or postponement of CVD events in the elderly may also be achieved by lifestyle modification such as an increase in physical activity and smoking cessation which are already established targets for intervention in younger and middle-aged subjects. There is evidence that remaining active and taking up physical activity in later life is beneficial in older men with and without established CHD (Wannamethee & Shaper, 2001; Williams et al., 2002) and that light to moderate levels of activity are sufficient to achieve such benefit, levels readily attainable in an older population (Wannamethee & Shaper, 2001). This has significant implications particularly with the increase in sedentary lifestyles. Smoking cessation among older men with and without established CHD is clearly beneficial although the speed and extent of risk reduction in this group remain uncertain (Williams et al., 2002; Critchley & Capewell, 2003). The case control study data presented by Rothenbacher and Brenner provides further evidence that taking up physical activity and smoking cessation in elderly men with established CHD is beneficial and illustrates the importance of these factors for secondary prevention of CVD in the elderly. Light to moderate alcohol intake has been shown to be associated with lower risk of CHD (Corrao, Rubbiati, Bagnardi, Zambon, & Poikolainen, 2000). There has been much debate about whether subjects at high risk should be encouraged to take alcohol (Wilson, 2003) but the evidence at present is inconclusive (Muntwyler, Hennekens,

Buring, & Gaziano, 1998; Shaper & Wannamethee, 2000; Wannamethee & Shaper, 2002).

4. OBESITY AND CVD

An issue of growing concern not mentioned in the overview is the rising tide of obesity in most western societies with a dramatic increase of overweight and obesity, also seen in the elderly population (Rossner, 2001; WHO, 1998). Overweight and obesity are associated with an increased burden of CVD and disability in the elderly (Wannamethee, Shaper, & Whincup, 2004). However, the effects of weight reduction on CVD risk remains controversial. Although weight reduction is widely recommended, evidence to support benefit is lacking particularly in the elderly (Rossner, 2001). Weight loss has been associated with a significant reduction in risk of diabetes but has been associated with no benefit or even increased risk of CVD despite improvement in CV risk factors (Rossner, 2001). Recent evidence suggests that the benefit of weight reduction may be seen in overweight younger men (<50 years) but not in older men (Wannamethee, Shaper, & Walker, 2005). Duration and severity of obesity may limit the benefits of weight reduction on CVD in older men emphasising the importance of weight reduction in middle-age before CVD is well established. Thus prevention of overweight/obesity remains a key objective in reducing the burden of CVD. Although benefit for CVD risk is lacking, evidence indicates that weight reduction is associated with benefit overall with a reduction in non-cardiovascular mortality (Wannamethee, Shaper, & Lennon, 2005).

5. TYPE 2 DIABETES AND CVD

Type 2 diabetes, like obesity, is also increasing markedly in prevalence and has important implications for CVD trends as it is associated with increased risk of CVD (Zimmet, Alberti, & Shaw, 2001). It is suggested that risk among diabetic subjects is equivalent to those of pre-existing CHD and that all diabetics should be treated as if they have had a heart attack (Haffner, Lehto, Ronnemaa, Pyorala, & Laakso, 1998). Others suggest that the increase in CVD risk is smaller, although the co-existence of diabetes and CHD has been widely shown to have an exceptionally poor prognosis (Wannamethee, Shaper, & Lennon, 2004). Despite the controversy regarding attributable risk in diabetic patients, it is well established that vigorous control of established CVD risk factors particularly blood cholesterol and blood pressure reduces cardiovascular risk in these patients (Collins, Armitage, Parish, Sleight, & Peto, 2003; Turner et al., 1998).

6. DISABILITY

Moreover, increasing life expectancy has brought public health concern about the growing prevalence of disability. Physical disability whether defined as the inability to perform tasks (e.g. walking) or more specific daily living activities leads to loss of independence and is itself associated with increased mortality (Ebrahim, Wannamethee,

Whincup, Walker, & Shaper, 2000). CVD is one of the major causes of disability and in older men half of those with CVD report some form of disability (Ebrahim et al., 2000). Physical disability among older men is not necessarily progressive and irreversible. Modifiable cardiovascular lifestyle risk factors such as physical activity, cigarette smoking, obesity and heavy drinking have been associated with increased risk locomotor disability (Ebrahim et al., 2000; Wannamethee, Ebrahim, Papacosta, & Shaper, in press). Light forms of activity readily achievable in older persons, e.g. walking, gardening or Do-it-yourself (i.e. domestic handiwork) has been associated with reduced onset and recovery of mobility limitation suggesting that promotion of a light or moderate physical activity program may be an effective strategy in not only reducing CVD but increasing disability-free life expectancy in older adults (Ebrahim et al., 2000; Wannamethee et al., 2005).

7. STRATEGIES FOR CHD PREVENTION AMONG OLDER ADULTS

In primary prevention two major theoretical approaches have been advocated—the "population strategy" which aims to reduce the risk in the whole population and the "high risk strategy" which focuses on subjects at high risk of CVD (Rose, 1992). Current strategies for the prevention of CHD emphasise the importance of identifying subjects at high risk of developing CHD and offering timely advice and treatment to reduce disease risk. Defining the optimal balance of preventive strategies among older subjects who are at exceptionally high risk of CVD and in whom high levels of established risk factors are widespread is particularly important if the population burden of CVD is to be reduced. Adverse lifestyle trends are a cause for concern and low levels of risk factors are also related to healthy lifestyles. Reduction of obesity through physical activity and dietary changes may have favourable effects on blood pressure, the lipoprotein profile, hyperglycaemia, and insulin resistance. Cigarette smoking is an addictive behaviour and stopping smoking often requires clinical intervention. Thus prevention programs aimed at reducing adverse risk behaviours on a population-wide basis as well as high risk strategies remain a high priority in the elderly.

8. SUMMARY

In summary, the goals of CVD prevention in older people are not only to prevent morbidity and mortality but to reduce and minimise disability in older people. Interventions aimed at lifestyle and dietary changes including smoking cessation, physical activity, maintaining healthy weight, prevention of diabetes in combination with effective clinical treatment will almost certainly increase the quantity and quality of life.

AFFILIATION

Royal Free and University College Medical School, London, UK

REFERENCES

American Heart Association. (2005). Heart Disease and Stroke Statistics 2005 update. www.americanheart.org.

Collins, R., Armitage, J., Parish, S., Sleigh, P., & Peto, R. (2003). MRC/BHF Heart Protection Study of cholesterol lowering with simvastatin in 5963 people with diabetes: a randomised placebo controlled trial. *Lancet, 361*, 2005–2016.

Corrao, G., Rubbiati, L., Bagnardi, V., Zambon, A., & Poikolainen, K. (2000). Alcohol and coronary heart disease: a meta-analysis. *Addiction, 95*, 1505–1523.

Critchley, J., & Capewell, S. (2003). Smoking cessation for the secondary prevention of coronary heart disease. Cochrane Database Systematic Review, CD003041.

Dornbrook-Lavender, K. A., Pieper, J. A., & Toth, M. T. (2003). Primary prevention of coronary heart disease in the elderly. *Ann Pharmacother, 37*, 1654–1663.

Ebrahim, S., Wannamethee, S. G., Whincup, P., Walker, M., & Shaper, A. G. (2000). Locomotor disability in a cohort of British men: the impact of lifestyle and disease. *International Journal of Epidemiology, 29*, 478–486.

Grundy, S. M., Pasternak, R., Greenland, P., Smith, S., & Fuster, V. (1999). Assessment of cardiovascular risk by multiple-risk-factor assessment equations. *Circulation, 100*, 1481–1492.

Haffner, S. M., Lehto, S., Ronnemaa, T., Pyorala, K., & Laakso, M. (1998). Mortality from coronary heart disease in subjects with type 2 diabetes and in nondiabetic subjects with and without prior myocardial infarction. *New England Journal of Medicine, 339*, 229–234.

Heart Protection Study Collaborative Group. (2002). MRC/BHF Heart Protection Study of cholesterol lowering with simvastatin in 20,536 high-risk individuals: a randomised placebo-controlled trial. *Lancet, 360*, 7–22.

Hiranic, V., & Malbut, K. (2002). Disability among older people. In G. Prior & P. Primatesta (Eds.), *Health Survey for England 2000* (Chapter 3). London: The Stationary Office.

Hirvensalo, M., Rantanen, T., & Heikkinen, E. (2000). Mobility difficulties and physical activity as predictors of mortality and loss of independence in the community living older population. *Journal of the American Geriatrics Society, 48*, 493–498.

Houterman, S., Boshuizen, H. C., Verschuren, W. M. M., Giampoli, S., Nissinin, A., Menotti, A., et al. (2002). Predicting cardiovascular risk in the elderly in different European countries. *European Heart Journal, 23*, 294–300.

Law, M. R., Wald, N. J., & Thompson, S. G. (1994). By how much and how quickly does reduction in serum cholesterol concentration lower risk of ischaemic heart disease? *BMJ, 308*, 367–372.

Lewington, S., Clarke, R., Qizilbash, N., Peto, R., & Collins, R. (2002). Age-specific relevance of usual blood pressure to vascular mortality: a meta-analysis of individual data for one million adults in 61 prospective studies. *Lancet, 360*, 1903–1913.

Manolio, T. A., Pearson, T. A., Wenger, N. K., Barrett-Connor, E., Payne, G. H, & Harlan, W. R. (1992). Cholesterol and heart disease in older persons and women. Review of an NHLBI workshop. *Annals of Epidemiology, 2*, 161–176.

Muntwyler, J., Hennekens, C. H., Buring, J. E., & Gaziano, J. M. (1998). Mortality and light to moderate alcohol consumption after myocardial infarction. *Lancet, 352*, 1882–1885.

Pearson, T. A., Blair, S. N., Daniels, S. R., Eckel, R. H., Fair, J. M., Fortmann, S. P., et al. (2002). AHA guidelines for primary prevention of cardiovascular disease and stroke: 2002 update. *Circulation, 106*, 388–391.

Petersen, S., Peto, V., & Rayner, M. (2004). Coronary heart disease statistics 2004. London: British Heart Foundation.

Progress Collaborative Group. (2001). Randomised trial of a perindopril-based blood-pressure-lowering regimen among 6,105 individuals with previous stroke or transient ischaemic attack. *Lancet, 358*, 1033–1041.

Rayner, M., & Petersen, S. (2005). European cardiovascular disease statistics 2005 edition. London: British Heart Foundation.

Rose, G. (1992). Strategies of prevention. Oxford: Oxford Medical Publications.

Rossner, S. (2001). Obesity in the elderly—a future matter of concern. *Obesity Reviews, 2*, 183–188.

Selmer, R. (1992). Blood pressure and twenty year mortality in the city of Bergen, Norway. *American Journal of Epidemiology, 136*, 428–440.

Shaper, A. G., & Wannamethee, S. G. (2000). Alcohol intake and mortality in middle aged men with diagnosed coronary heart disease. *Heart, 83*, 94–399.

Shepherd, J., Blauw, G. J., Murphy, M. B., Bollen, E. L., Buckley, B. M., Cobbe, S. M., et al. (2002). Pravastatin in elderly individuals at risk of vascular disease (PROSPER): a randomised controlled trial. *Lancet, 360*, 1623–1630.

Turner, R., Holman, R., Stratton, I., Cull, C., Frighi, V., Manley, S., et al. (1998). Tight blood pressure control and risk of macrovascular and microvascular complications in type 2 diabetes. UKPDS 38. UK Prospective Diabetes Study Group. *BMJ, 317*, 703–713.

Wald, N. J., & Law, M. R. (2003). A strategy to reduce cardiovascular disease by more than 80%. *BMJ, 326*, 1419.

Wannamethee, S. G., Ebrahim, S., Papacosta, O., & Shaper, A. G. (2005). From a postal questionnaire of older men, healthy lifestyle factors reduced the onset of and may have increased recovery from mobility limitation. *Journal of Clinical Epidemiology, 58*, 831–40.

Wannamethee, S. G., & Shaper, A. G. (2001). Physical activity in the prevention of cardiovascular disease: an epidemiological perspective. *Sports Medicine, 31*, 101–114.

Wannamethee, S. G., & Shaper, A. G. (2002). Taking up regular drinking in middle age: effect on major coronary heart disease events and mortality. *Heart, 87*, 32–36.

Wannamethee, S. G., Shaper, A. G., & Lennon, L. (2004). Cardiovascular disease incidence and mortality in older men with diabetes and in men with coronary heart disease. *Heart, 12*, 1398–1403.

Wannamethee, S. G., Shaper, A. G., & Lennon, L. (2005). Intentional and unintentional weight loss and mortality in older men. *Archives of Internal Medicine, 165*, 1035–1040.

Wannamethee, S. G., Shaper, A. G., & Walker, M. (2005). Overweight and obesity and weight change in middle-aged men: impact on cardiovascular disease and diabetes. *Journal of Epidemiology and Community Health, 59*, 134–139.

Wannamethee, S. G., Shaper, A. G., & Whincup, P. H. (2004). Overweight and obesity and the burden of disease and disability in elderly men. *International Journal of Obesity, 28*, 1374–1382.

WHO. (1998). Obesity: preventing and managing the global epidemic. Report of a WHO consultation on obesity. Geneva: World Health Organisation, 3–5 June, 1997.

Williams M. A., Fleg, J. L., Ades, P. A., Chaitman, B. R., Miller, N. H., Mohiuddin, S. M., et al. (2002). Secondary prevention of coronary heart disease in the elderly with emphasis on patients >75 years of age. AHA Scientific Statement. *Circulation, 105*, 1735–1743.

Wilson, J. F. Should doctors prescribe alcohol to adults? (2003). *Annals of Internal Medcine, 139*, 711–714.

Zimmet, P., Alberti, K. G., & Shaw, J. (2001). Global and societal implications of the diabetes epidemic. *Nature, 414*, 782–787.

HERIBERT RAMROTH,[1] NORBERT SPECHT-LEIBLE,[2]
HANS-HELMUT KÖNIG[3] and HERMANN BRENNER[4]

MEDICAL CARE FOR NURSING HOME RESIDENTS: NATIONAL PERSPECTIVES IN INTERNATIONAL CONTEXT

The present foreseeable demographic development in Germany shows a strong increase in the proportion of older people in the total population, which is even stronger than in most other developed countries (Statistisches Bundesamt, 2001a, 2003). There is a widespread belief that health care systems spend more and more to provide intensive and aggressive care to older patients (Canadian Health Service Research Foundation, 2003). On the other hand, recent studies indicate that approaching death, rather than age, may be the main demographic driver of health care costs (Seshamani & Gray, 2004; Yang, Norton, & Stearns, 2003).

In this debate, medical care for nursing home residents is of particular interest. In 2001, two million Germans have been in need of care and 604,000 persons have been institutionalised in 9,165 nursing homes (NHs), with a decreasing trend for family care and an increasing trend for institutional care at the end of life (Statistisches Bundesamt, 2001b). Thus, provision of adequate medical care for frail disabled older persons is of particular relevance for the health care system. In Germany, a relatively comprehensive system of social insurance has been built in the past, with nursing care insurance being responsible for nursing care, and health insurance for acute hospital care. NHs serve personal care needs (support in the activities of daily living) and specialised nursing needs (e.g. wound care). They do not provide primary health care (which is the domain of general practitioners), and nearly all cases of acute illness are referred to acute hospital, which is different in the United States and in Great Britain.

In the United States the relationship between NHs for older persons and acute care hospitals, particularly the transfer of patients between these institutions, has been studied over years (Bergman & Clarfield, 1991; Covinsky et al., 2003; Joseph & Boult, 1998; Murtaugh & Freiman, 1995; Saliba et al., 2000). By contrast, little is known about hospitalisations and their determinants among NH residents in Europe and especially Germany.

The aim of this study was to assess rates of hospitalisations and their determinants among NH residents in Germany before and after nursing home admission and during the last year of life of those who died.

H.-W. Wahl et al. (eds.), The Many Faces of Health, Competence and Well-Being in Old Age, 175–188.

1. METHODS

1.1. Study Design and Study Population

A retrospective cohort study was set up among 1,926 NH residents newly institutionalised between 1st of January and 31st of December 2000 in one of the 97 NHs in the cities of Heidelberg, Mannheim and the Rhine-Neckar area, a study region with 829.930 inhabitants who applied for benefits from the German statutory nursing insurance system (Figure 1). For logistic reasons, the sample was restricted to members in one of the eight largest health insurance plans, which cover about 80% of the population. A comparison of hospitalisation rates before and after nursing home admission (NHA) was possible for a subset of 1,361 participants from two of the largest health insurance plans, covering 70% of all study participants. In this analysis, we will refer to this sub-cohort of all study participants.

According to statutory regulations, the benefits from the statutory nursing insurance system are provided to those people who need support in the activities of daily living (ADLs). Frequency and duration of support determine the level of care benefits. About 98% of all NH residents in Germany receive such benefits (Statistisches Bundesamt, 2001b). The benefits are granted contingent upon the results of a standardised medical examination carried out by the medical service of the health insurance plans. In this retrospective cohort study, we linked socio-demographic data as well as data of these medical examinations with follow-up data regarding hospitalisations from the health insurance plans.

The study was approved by the Ethics committee of the University of Heidelberg and by the Baden-Württemberg state commissioner of data protection.

1.2. Baseline Examination

The standardised medical examinations by the medical service of the health care insurance plans consist of a physical examination as well as a detailed interview, carried out

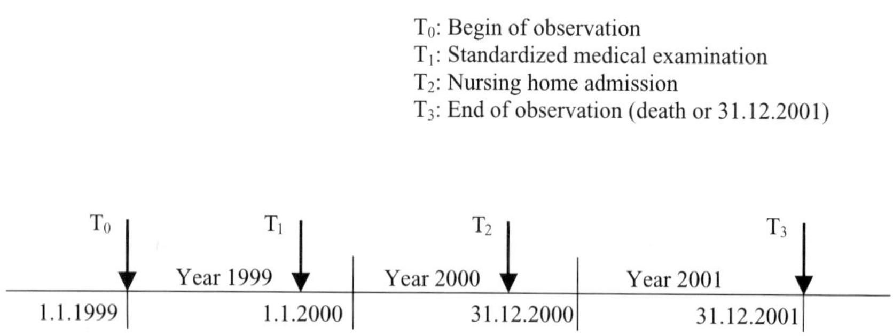

Figure 1. Time schedule for study design.

by trained physicians according to written guidelines that describe medical, functional and social aspects.

Medical diagnoses describing the underlying medical causes of dependency on permanent care are documented in rank order according to their relevance for impairment in the standardised medical examinations. For this analysis, the main medical cause (i.e. the diagnosis ranked first by the physician) was coded according to the International Classifications of Diseases 9 and 10.

The medical examination provided detailed information on the dependency and time of care required regarding basic ADLs, such as bathing, dressing, toileting, transferring and eating without assistance. In 10% of these medical examinations only a total time for need of help was given. Therefore, caused by a lower percentage of missing values, for this analysis the level of care dependency was determined by dividing the total time of care required regarding basic ADLs in quartiles.

Age was determined at the time when entering the NH.

1.3. Follow-Up Variables

Information on hospitalisations from 1st of January 1999 and deaths until 31st of December 2001 was extracted from records of the pertinent health insurance plan. Admissions to acute care hospitals with length of stay during the follow-up period were registered.

In addition to the dates of hospital entry and discharge, the leading diagnosis for hospitalisation as given by the acute care hospital at discharge was extracted from the records. The discharge diagnoses were classified according to the International Classifications of Diseases 9 and 10.

1.4. Statistical Methods

Relative time spent in hospital (RT), absolute rates of hospitalisations (HR) defined as the number of hospitalisations per person-year at risk, mean duration of hospital stay and total person-years (PY) under observation were calculated according to age, gender, level of care dependency, duration of NH residency, hospitalisation status immediately prior to NH admission and vital status at the end of the observation time.

The concept of rate comparison depends on the underlying definition of time windows and is therefore, potentially, somewhat arbitrary. The longer or shorter the distance from an important medical event, the higher or lower the calculated rates could be. Common models are the rate comparison of yearly or monthly periods. Here, rates are presented for 1-year periods before and after NH admission and during the last year of life. To show the trends of rates in context of nursing home admission and death, the relative time spent in hospital will be presented also in monthly or sometimes weekly time periods. For purposes of this analysis, the year was considered to consist of 360 days, divided into intervals of 30 days each.

For all analyses the statistical software SAS (Version 8.2) was used.

2. RESULTS

2.1. Sample Characteristics

The study population included 1,361 NH residents, newly institutionalised between 1st of January and 31st of December 2000. There were three times more women 1,026 (75.6%, mean age 83.5 years) than men $N = 335$, (24.4%, mean age 77.0 years), which reflects the considerably higher proportion of women among the older population caused by differences in life expectancy. More than 68% of the study participants (men 47.8%, women 75.1%) were older than 80 years. The leading medical diagnoses for dependency on permanent care were dementia ($N = 275$, 22.6%), cerebrovascular diseases (13.4%) and diseases of the nervous and sensory system (10.3%). Almost 80% of the participants were in need of nursing care for more than 1 h per day at the time of the standardised medical examination (Table 1).

Six hundred and eight persons (44.7%) had been transferred directly from acute care hospital into NH. In the observation period, 559 (41.1%) persons died (men 49.3%, women 38.4%). Insured and still living on 31st December 2001 were 763 (56.1%) of the participants. Thirty-nine (2.8%) persons left the study for other reasons.

2.2. The Year Before Nursing Home Admission

The whole study cohort ($N = 1{,}361$) was observed during the year before NHA. In this time, the overall percentage of time spent in hospital was 10.7% with a hospitalisation rate of 2.1 admissions into acute care hospital and a mean duration of hospital stay of 20.8 days (data not shown). These results do not show any changes in rates towards NHA. Therefore, it is much more informative to look at shorter time periods and additionally at monthly rates of RT. This way it can be seen that the relative time spent in hospital increased from 3.0% (12 months before NHA, HR = 0.8) to 42.4% (last month before NHA, HR = 12.2) (Figure 2). Therefore, when comparing hospitalisations before NHA, we separately analysed a time window of 3 months before NHA (Table 2). The increase was modest in the first 9 months and strongly accelerated afterwards. Thus, it seems obvious that the diseases during the last 3 months before NHA are the deciding ones which trigger NHA. During the last 3 months before NHA, people spent most time in hospital caused by psychiatric diseases (16.6%), injuries (16.2%) and cardiovascular diseases (14.6%) (Table 3).

2.3. The Year After Nursing Home Admission

In the first year after NHA, the mean duration under observation was 285 days per study participant (1062.4 PY), which reflects that 459 participants (33.7%) died during the first year after NHA (16.5% in the first 3 months).

Considering the overall rates for the first year after NHA, the hospitalisation rate was not lower (HR = 1.2) and the relative time spent in hospital only slightly lower (RT = 4.4%) than up to 3 months before NHA (HR = 1.1, RT = 5.1%). On the other hand, there is a steady decrease in RT after NH admission from 6.0% (first month after NHA)

Table 1. Distribution of age, main medical cause for dependency on permanent care, level of care dependency, observation time, transfer status and vital status

Factor	*Men*	*Women*	*Total*
Age (in years)			
<70	76 (22.7)	60 (5.8)	136 (10.0)
70–79	99 (29.6)	195 (19.0)	294 (21.6)
80–89	123 (36.7)	533 (51.9)	656 (48.2)
≥90	37 (11.0)	238 (23.2)	275 (20.2)
Main medical cause for dependency on permanent care (ICD-10/ICD-9)*			
Cancer (C00-D48/140-199, 210-239)	32 (10.7)	41 (4.5)	73 (6.0)
Hormone, nutrition and metabolic diseases (E00-E90, N18-N19/240-279,585-586)	3 (1.0)	26 (2.8)	29 (2.4)
Psychiatric diseases (F00-F99/290-319)	88 (29.4)	303 (33.0)	391 (32.1)
Among these: dementia (F00-F03/290)	54 (18.1)	221 (24.0)	275 (22.6)
Diseases of the nervous and sensory system (G00-G44, G47-G99/320-359)	36 (12.0)	89 (9.7)	125 (10.3)
Cerebrovascular diseases (G45-G46, I60-I69/430-438)	53 (17.7)	110 (12.0)	163 (13.4)
Cardiovascular diseases (D50-D89, I00-I59, I70-I99/200-208, 280-289, 390-429, 439-459)	17 (5.7)	52 (5.7)	69 (5.7)
Diseases of the musculoskeletal system (M00-M99/710-739)	12 (4.0)	92 (10.0)	104 (8.5)
Injuries and poisoning (R55, S00-T98/780, 800-999)	7 (2.3)	52 (5.7)	59 (4.8)
Other diseases	51 (17.0)	155 (16.7)	205 (16.9)
Level of care dependency (in minutes per day)[†]			
≤60	74 (22.1)	225 (21.9)	299 (22.0)
>60 to ≤120	52 (15.5)	188 (18.3)	240 (17.6)
>120 to ≤160	68 (20.3)	212 (20.7)	280 (20.6)
>160	63 (18.8)	189 (18.4)	252 (18.5)
Observation time			
≥1 Year (long-term residents)	199 (59.4)	703 (68.5)	902 (66.3)
Others	136 (40.6)	323 (31.5)	459 (33.7)
Transfer status			
Transferred from home into NH	169 (50.4)	584 (56.9)	753 (55.3)
Transferred directly from acute care hospital into NH vital status	166 (49.6)	442 (43.1)	608 (44.7)
Died before 31st of December 2001	165 (49.3)	394 (38.4)	559 (41.1)
Alive and under observation until 31st of December 2001	152 (45.4)	611 (59.6)	763 (56.1)
Censored before 31st of December 2001	18 (5.4)	21 (2.1)	39 (2.8)
Total	335 (100)	1,026 (100)	1,361 (100)

*143 persons with missing data.
[†]290 persons with missing data.

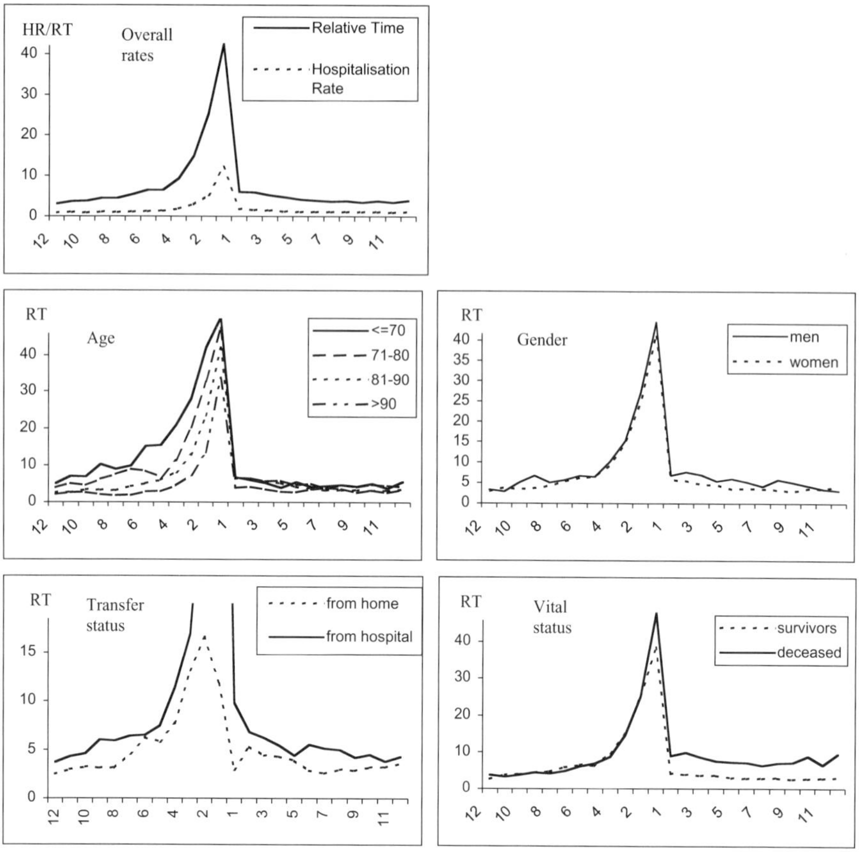

Figure 2. Relative time spent in hospital before and after nursing home admission (monthly rates)—(nursing home admission = month 0).

down to 3.9% (12 months after NHA) (Figure 2). Thus, analogously as before NHA, the time period of 1 year after NHA has been divided into two separate time windows, considering separately the first 3 months after NHA and the time more than 3 months after NHA. Relative time spent in hospital was 1.5-fold higher in the first (RT = 5.7%, HR = 1.5) than in the second time period (RT = 3.8%, HR = 1.1). There were no considerable differences in the mean duration of hospital stay (14.3 versus 13.9 days) (Table 2).

During the first year after NHA, people spent most time in hospital caused by cardiovascular diseases (15.6%), psychiatric diseases (14.2%) and injuries (13.1%) (Table 3).

2.4. The Last Year of Life

Following the concept presented in the former sections, we analysed rates in two different time windows during the last year of life, additionally illustrated through

Table 2. *Hospitalisations before and after nursing home admission and during the last year of life*

		12–3 Months before NH admission			≤3 Months before NH admission			≤3 Months after NH admission			3–12 Months after NH admission			12–3 Months before death			≤3 Months before death		
Person-years under observation		1021.7			339.3			305.0			757.4			155.3			105.1		
	N	*HR*	*MD*	*RT*	*HR*	*MD*	*RT*	*HR*	*MD*	*RT*	*HR*	*MD*	*RT*	*HR*	*MD*	*RT*	*HR*	*MD*	*RT*
Age (in years)																			
<70	136	2.0	22.8	10.9	9.0	27.1	40.0	1.8	13.0	6.0	1.1	16.6	4.6	2.1	13.7	7.3	5.3	12.3	15.0
70–79	294	1.4	19.4	6.9	7.5	24.0	33.2	1.5	15.8	6.3	1.1	15.4	4.6	1.8	13.3	6.2	5.4	11.4	14.5
80–89	656	1.0	17.0	4.3	6.0	21.3	25.9	1.6	14.7	6.1	1.0	13.2	3.6	1.4	14.5	5.4	4.6	11.9	13.0
≥90	275	0.6	16.2	2.5	4.3	18.9	18.1	1.2	11.9	3.9	1.0	12.0	3.1	1.2	13.5	4.2	3.8	9.4	8.9
Gender																			
Men	335	1.2	18.1	5.7	6.5	22.8	28.7	1.9	15.0	7.1	1.3	13.6	4.7	1.6	12.6	5.2	5.2	11.1	13.5
Women	1,026	1.0	18.7	5.0	6.1	22.1	26 8	1.4	14.0	5.2	1.0	14.0	3.6	1.4	14.6	5.3	4.3	11.3	11.8
Care level (in minutes)																			
0–≤60	299	1.3	18.9	6.2	5.7	22.2	25.8	1.2	14.0	4.4	1.2	14.1	4.4	1.6	12.3	5.2	5.2	10.9	13.5
>60–≤120	292	1.1	18.2	5.2	5 6	21.6	24.9	1.5	16.8	6.5	1.1	14.7	4.4	1.7	15.8	6.7	5.5	13.4	16.9
>120–≤160	286	1.1	18.0	5.1	5 8	20.5	24.6	1.4	14.2	5.3	0.9	13.2	3.3	1.1	16.0	4.8	3.8	10.0	9.4
160<	194	1.1	17.0	4 8	5 7	22.9	26.4	1.7	12.8	5.6	1.0	13.7	3.6	1.5	12.2	4.8	3.4	10.2	8.6
Long term																			
No	459	1.2	16.1	5.2	7.4	21.0	30.0	3.2	13.0	10.3	3.3	12.0	9.7	1.6	14.8	6.2	4.7	11.4	12.8
Yes	902	1.0	20.1	5.1	5.5	23.1	26.0	1.0	15.6	4.0	0.8	14.7	3.2	1.3	12.9	4.3	4.0	10.7	10.6
Transfer status																			
From home	753	0.9	18.4	4.3	2.9	20.0	13.8	1.2	13.8	4.2	1.0	12.8	3.3	1.4	13.9	5.2	4.5	11.2	12.2
From hospital	608	1.3	18.6	6.2	12.3	23.4	44.1	2.1	14.7	7.7	1.2	15.2	4.7	2.1	24.0	12.0	11.4	16.7	34.2
Vital status*																			
Dead	559	1.2	16.2	5.0	7.0	21.4	29.0	2.7	13.4	9.1	2.3	12.7	7.3						
Alive	802	1.0	20.5	5.2	5.6	23.0	26.1	0.9	15.6	3.9	0.8	14.7	3.0						
Total	1,361	1.1	18.5	5.1	6.2	22.3	27.3	1.5	14.3	5.7	1.1	13.9	3.8	1.4	14.0	5.3	4.5	11.2	12.3

N, number of study participants; HR, hospitalization rate per person-year at risk; MD, mean duration of stay (in days); RT, relative time spent in hospital (%).
* Vital status at study end.

Au: Please check the formatting of Table 2.

Table 3. Percentage of time spent in hospital according to the main diagnosis of hospital stay (%)

Main diagnosis of hospital stay	*1 Year before NH admission*	*3 Months before NH admission*	*1 Year after NH admission*	*1 Year before death*	*3 Months before death*
Infections (A00-B99, J10-J18, L00-L08, N30, N39/ 001-139, 480-487, 595, 599, 680-686)	4.5	4.2	10.9	12.9	14.2
Cancer (C00-D48/140-199, 210-239)	7.2	7.8	4.3	5.8	5.8
Hormone, nutrition and metabolic diseases (E00-E90, N18-N19/ 240-279, 585-586)	5.5	5.9	7.8	7.9	7.1
Psychiatric diseases (F00-F99/290-319)	16.6	16.6	14.2	11.4	8.2
Diseases of the nervous and sensory system (G00-G44, G47-G99/320-359)	3.6	4.4	3.1	2.5	2.4
Cerebrovascular diseases (G45-G46, I60-I69/430-438)	12.8	13.9	7.6	7.8	8.3
Cardiovascular diseases (D50-D89, I00-I59, I70-I99/200-208, 280-289, 390-429, 439-459)	15.9	14.6	15.6	17.2	18.4
Diseases of the musculoskeletal system (M00-M99/710-739)	3.3	2.4	1.0	0.2	0.4
Injuries and poisoning (R55, S00-T98/780, 800-999)	14.7	16.2	13.1	8.6	6.5
Diseases of the respiratory system (J00-J09, J19-J99/460-479, 488-519)	3.5	2.9	3.1	4.3	6.5
Diseases of the digestive system (K00-K93/520-579)	4.4	4.3	8.7	8.8	7.9
Other diseases	7.6	6.7	10.6	12.7	14.3

monthly and weekly calculated rates, to show the changes in rates towards the end of life (Figure 3). The overall rates during the last year of life of the 559 nursing home residents who died after NHA until 31st of December 2001 were RT = 8.1% and HR = 2.6. The mean duration under observation was 170 days per study participant (260.4 PY). Considering the different time windows from 12 to 9 months before death and the last 3 months before death, these rates were much lower in the former than in the latter (RT = 5.3% versus RT = 12.3%) HR = 1.4 versus HR = 4.5, (Table 2). The increasing trend of rates versus the end of life can be best illustrated by monthly and

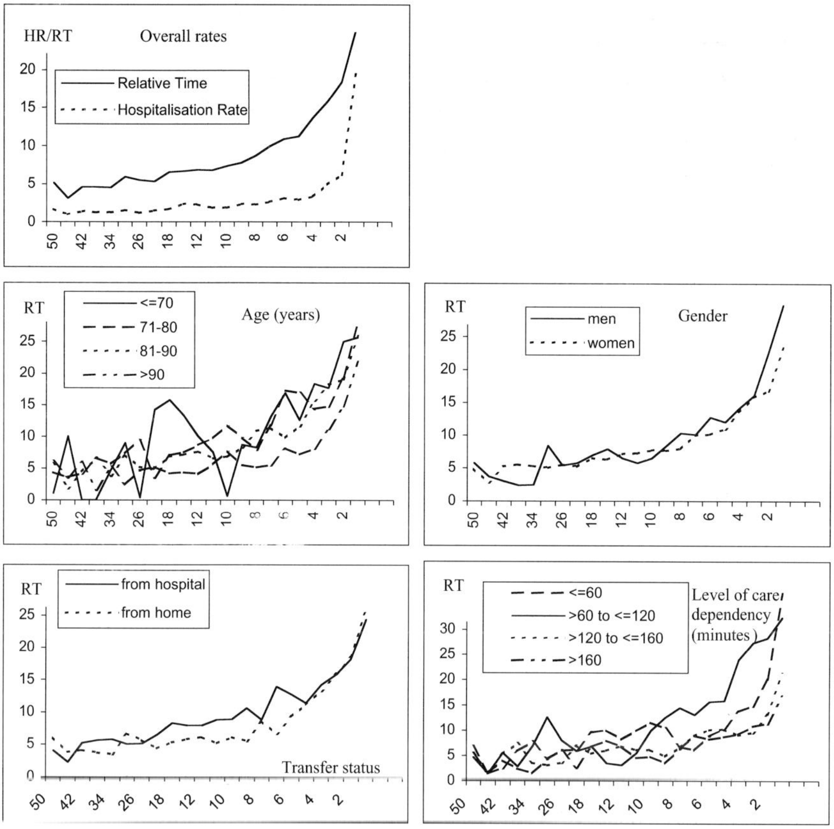

Figure 3. Relative time spent in hospital during the last year of life (weekly rates).

weekly rates which rose from 5.1% 12 months before death up to 25.3% during the last week of life (Figure 3). Nevertheless, percentages of time spent in hospital are not as high, as during the last 3 months before NHA. Additionally, the last year of life can be described by much more frequent, but shorter hospital admissions.

During the last 3 months of life, the largest share of time spent in hospitals was caused by cardiovascular diseases (18.4%), infections (14.2%) and cerebrovascular diseases (8.3%) (Table 3).

2.5. Subgroup Analyses

The following section presents results of analyses of different subgroups.

2.5.1. Age

In all observed time windows, relative time spent in hospital markedly decreased with age. However, the age gradient was much stronger up to 3 months before (≤70 years,

RT = 10.9%; >90 years, RT = 2.6%) than more than 3 months after NHA (≤70 years, RT = 4.6%; >90 years, RT = 3.1%) (Table 2, Figure 2).

During the last year of life, the relative time spent in hospital decreased with increasing age of the participants, from the twelfth to the fourth month before death. However, in the last 3 months before death, markedly different rates were found only for those aged over 90 (RT = 8.9%).

2.5.2. Gender

There were no considerable gender differences in hospitalisations before NHA, however, slight gender differences could be seen in both time windows after NHA, with higher rates for men than for women (≥3 months after NHA: RT = 4.7% for men, RT = 3.6% for women). These gender differences did not persist after additional control for age.

2.6. Time Level of Care Dependency

There was no clear relationship between level of care dependency and the rates of hospitalisation. If anything, a weak inverse trend was seen (namely the higher the dependence on permanent care, the lower the relative time spent in hospital), which persisted after control for age in multivariable analyses.

2.7. Transfer Status

As expected, RT for people with direct transfer from hospital into NH was more than three times higher than among other participants during the last 3 months before NHA, but not considerably higher in the time period before.

Differences between these groups diminished, but nevertheless persisted to some degree throughout the 12 months after NHA. The differences were particularly pronounced shortly before death.

2.8. Vital Status

People who died during the study period had been transferred more often into hospital but with shorter durations than others. The difference between deceased people and survivors was greatest up to 3 months after NHA (RT = 9.1% for people who died, RT = 3.9% for others).

3. DISCUSSION

A cohort of 1,361 persons who applied for benefits from the German statutory nursing insurance system and who were newly admitted to a NH in the year 2000, was retrospectively observed over a study period of 3 years. We presented results for the periods

1 year before and of 1 year after nursing home admission, and for the last year of life of those who died.

Excluding the last 3 months before NHA, the relative time (RT) spent in hospital was lower (4.4%) after than before NHA (5.1%), caused by shorter mean length of hospital stay, possibly because patients find a competent care network in NHs which was lacking at home. The last 3 months before NHA might be characterised by progression of chronic diseases or onset of new disability. Thus, it is not surprising that we found the by far most frequent and longest hospitalisations for this study period. RT increased up to 42.4% during the last months before NHA, i.e. rates were much higher than during the months before or after NHA. These data suggest that it is the medico-social problems occurring during the last 3 months before NHA that trigger NH placement. Lack of coordination between acute care and long-term care sectors may also be a reason for long hospitalisation directly before NHA.

Those NH residents who died spent one quarter of time in hospital during the last week of life. Hospitalisations were more common among men, the younger age groups and participants who died during follow-up. The relative time spent in hospital (RT) was somewhat lower for residents who stayed in NH for minimum 1 year (RT − 3.2%). However, for all observed subgroups rates increased strongly during the last weeks of life.

The inverse relationship between age and the rate of hospitalisation after NHA underlines findings in the general German population that with advancing age the utilisation of NHs and ambulatory services rose steeply, whereas the probability of hospital treatment decreased (Bickel, 1998; Brockmann, 2002). This might reflect a trend to deal more cautiously with hospital transfers of frail old people to avoid high-technology interventions (Covinsky et al., 2003; Kliebsch, Siebert, & Brenner, 2000) or "risky" treatments with uncertain benefit in the oldest old (Hamel et al., 2000; Perls & Wood, 1996). Interestingly, the inverse relationship with age was much weaker after than before NHA in our study. This might be due to the fact that the observed time window after NHA is much closer to death, and health care costs are more directly related to proximity to death than age (O'Neill, Groom, Avery, Boot, & Thornhill, 2000; Seshamani & Gray, 2004; Zweifel, Felder, & Meier, 1999).

The findings of higher hospitalisation rates among male than among female NH residents are consistent with results of analyses of aggregated data considering the general German population (Brockmann, 2002), and with studies from the US (Liao, McGee, Cao, & Cooper, 2000). The gender differences did not persist after control for age in additional, multivariable analyses; however, they might be ascribed to the observed age differences.

Like in a previous study among handicapped community-dwelling older people from Germany (Kliebsch et al., 2000), there was no clear relationship between level of care dependency and the rates of hospitalisation. If anything, a weak inverse trend was seen (namely the higher the dependence on permanent care, the lower the mean duration of stay per hospital transfer, and the relative time spent in hospital), which persisted after control for age in multivariable analyses.

People who died during the study period had been transferred more often to hospital but with shorter length of stay than survivors. The difference was particularly large after

NHA. RT strongly increased until the last week of life (RT = 25.3%). These findings are consistent with results of longitudinal studies from the US (Braithwaite, Col, & Wong 2003; Chelluri et al., 2003; Emanuel, 1996). During the last year of life, no considerable differences for the rates in long-term residents, i.e. those with NH stay for minimum 1 year, could be observed, which underlines the importance of proximity to death as the key trigger of increased hospitalisation rates.

The hospitalisation rates of NH residents found in our study are much higher than those reported from studies in the US, where hospitalisation rates ranged from 0.21–0.55 per NH bed and relative time spent in hospital ranged from 0.14% to 1.7% (Joseph & Boult, 1998). Besides the differences in health care delivery and payment systems, lower rates in the US may partly be explained by widespread use of do-not-resuscitate (DNR) orders (Zweig, et al., 2004), although DNR orders do not directly deal with hospitalisation. However, DNR orders are still quite uncommon in Germany even though their impact is discussed controversially. According to Teno (2004), subconscious benign neglect is a more likely explanation for these findings. Another reason for lower rates in the United States may be that skilled nursing homes in the US partially take over acute hospital care functions by having appropriately trained staff and well-equipped facilities.

The hospitalisation rates of NH residents found in our study are higher than those for severely handicapped but not institutionalised people in an earlier study from Germany and for the general German population according to national statistics (Kliebsch et al., 2000). On the one hand, higher rates for NH residents in comparison to handicapped community-dwelling older people might be expected, because the former are the most severely handicapped ones. Higher rates for NH residents than for the general German population are furthermore potentially caused by proximity to death (Busse, Krauth, & Schwartz, 1997; Seshamani & Gray, 2004). Thus, the time spent in hospital by NH residents may well be similar to the general population when proximity to death is taken into account.

On the other hand, NH care by well-trained staff could potentially result in fewer transfers to hospital. In our study, injuries, infections, cardiovascular diseases and psychiatric diseases were the leading causes of hospitalisation. Some intervention trials have suggested that measures to control or manage infections, closer monitoring of cardiovascular disease, prevention of falls and fractures and methods of geronto-psychology have the potential to reduce hospitalisations in NH residents (Bourbonniere & Evans, 2002; Chang et al., 2004; Joseph & Boult 1998; Kane et al., 2003; Murtaugh & Freiman, 1995; Ouslander, Weinbert, & Phillips, 2000; Saliba et al., 2000; Zimmer & Hall, 1997). Thus, there seems to be a potential for further reductions of hospitalisations by pertinent interventions.

People who have been transferred directly from acute care hospital into NH had higher rates during all observed time periods. Issues for further research could be to characterise newly admitted NH residents according to risk factors associated with hospitalisation or mortality (Flacker & Kiely, 2003). Further research should also address the following topics: Are hospitalisation rates of NH residents different form others, when proximity of death is taken into account? Can hospitalisation be reduced by NH providing (sub-)acute hospital care, and would this be cost-effective? Can extensive hospitalisation before NHA be reduced by improving coordination between acute care and long-term care sectors? Are there effective strategies for preventing illness that causes hospitalisation of NH residents?

Notwithstanding the need to address these further questions, our study extends the scarce database on hospitalisations among elderly disabled persons in Europe. It will be an important basis for assessing the impact of major changes in the social security system which are currently implemented in Germany, including implementation of a DRG-based prospective payment system.

ACKNOWLEDGEMENTS

The authors thank the health insurance companies involved with this study and the medical service of these companies for their cooperation.

AFFILIATIONS

[1]*German Centre for Research on Ageing at the University of Heidelberg*

[2]*Bethanien-Hospital, Geriatric Centre at the University Hospital*

[3]*Health Economics Research Unit, Department of Psychiatry, University of Leipzig*

[4]*1 (DZFA—University of Heidelberg)*

REFERENCES

Bergman H., Clarfield A. M. (1991). Appropriateness of patient transfer from a nursing home to an acute-care hospital: A study of emergency room visits and hospital admissions. *Journal of the American Geriatrics Society, 39*, 1164–1168.

Bickel H. (1998). Das letzte Lebensjahr. Eine Repräsentativstudie an Verstorbenen. Wohnsitutation, Sterbeort und Nutzung von Versorgungsangeboten. *Zeitschrift fur Gerontologie und Geriatrie, 31*, 193–204.

Bourbonniere M., Evans L. K. (2002). Advanced practice nursing in the care of frail older adults. *Journal of the American Geriatrics Society, 50*, 2062–2076.

Braithwaite R. S., Col N. F., Wong J. B. (2003). Estimating hip fracture morbidity, mortality and costs. *Journal of the American Geriatrics Society, 51*, 364–370.

Brockmann H. (2002). Why is health treatment for the elderly less expensive than for the rest of the population? Health care rationing in Germany. *Social Science and Medicine, 55*, 593–608.

Busse R., Krauth C., Schwartz F. W. (2002). Use of acute hospital beds does not increase as the population ages: Results from a seven year cohort study in Germany. *Journal of Epidemiology and Community Health, 56*, 289–293.

Canadian Health Service Research Foundation. (2003). http://www.chsrf.ca/mythbusters/pdf/myth10_e.pdf, assessed January 2005.

Chang J. T., Morton S. C., Rubenstein L. Z., Mojica W. A., Maglione M., Suttorp M. J., et al. (2004). Interventions for the prevention of falls in older adults: Systematic review and meta-analysis of randomised clinical trials. *BMJ, 20*, 328:680.

Chelluri L., Mendelsohn A. B., Belle S. H., Rotondi A. J., Angus D. C., Donahoe M. P., Sirio C. A., Schulz R., Pinsky, M. R. (2003). Hospital costs in patients receiving prolonged mechanical ventilation: Does age have an impact? *Critical Care Medicine, 31*, 1746–1751.

Covinsky K. E., Palmer R. M., Fortinsky R. H., Counsell S. R., Stewart A. L., Kresevic D., Burant C. J., Landefeld C. S. (2003). Loss of independence in activities of daily living in older adults hospitalized with medical illness: Increased vulnerability with age. *Journal of the American Geriatrics Society, 51*, 451–458.

Emanuel, E. J. (1996). Cost savings at the end of life: What do the data show? *JAMA, 275*, 1907–1914.

Flacker J. M., Kiely D. K. (2003). Mortality-related factors and 1-year survival in nursing home residents. *Journal of the American Geriatrics Society, 51*, 213–221.

Hamel M. B., Lynn J., Teno J. M., Covinsky K. E., Wu A. W., Galanos A., Desbiens N. A., Phillips R. S. (2000). Age-related differences in care preferences, treatment decisions, and clinical outcomes of seriously ill hospitalized adults: Lessons from SUPPORT. *Journal of the American Geriatrics Society, 48*, 176–182.

Joseph A., Boult C. (1998). Managed primary care of nursing home residents. *Journal of the American Geriatrics Society, 46*, 1152–1156.

Kane R. L., Keckhafer G., Flood S., Bershadsky B., Siadaty M. S. (2003). The effect of evercare and hospitalization use. *Journal of the American Geriatrics Society, 51*, 1427–1434.

Kliebsch U., Siebert H., Brenner H. (2000). Extent and determinants of hospitalization in a cohort of elderly disabled persons. *Journal of the American Geriatrics Society, 48*, 289–294.

Liao Y., McGee D. L., Cao G., Cooper R. S. (2000). Quality of the last year of life of older adults: 1986 vs 1993. *JAMA, 283*, 512–518.

Murtaugh C. M., Freiman M. P. (1995). Nursing home patients at risk of hospitalization and the characteristics of their hospital stay. *Gerontologist, 35*, 35–43.

O'Neill C., Groom L., Avery A. J., Boot D., Thornhill K. (2000). Age and proximity to death as predictors of GP care costs: Results from a study of nursing home patients. *Health Economics, 9*, 733–8.

Ouslander J. G., Weinbert A. D., Phillips V. (2000). Inappropriate hospitalization of nursing facility residents: A symptom of a sick system of care for frail older people. *Journal of the American Geriatrics Society, 48*, 230–321.

Perls T. T., Wood E. R. (1996). Acute care costs of the oldest old: They cost less, their care intensity is less, and they go to nonteaching hospitals. *Archives of Internal Medicine, 156*, 754–760.

Saliba D., Kington R., Buchanan J., Bell R., Wang M., Lee M., Herbst M., Lee D., Sur D., Rubenstein L. (2000). Appropriateness of the decision to transfer nursing facility residents to the hospital. *Journal of the American Geriatrics Society, 48*, 154–163.

Seshamani M., Gray A. M. (2004). A longitudinal study of the effects of age and time to death on hospital costs. *Journal of Health Economics, 23*, 217–235.

Statistisches Bundesamt. (2001a). *Statements zu Pressekonferenz Mikrozensus 2000*. http://www.destatis.de/presse/deutsch/pm2001/p1441031.htm, Bonn, assessed January 2005.

Statistisches Bundesamt. (2001b). *Online-Publikationen—Fachveröffentlichungen, Pflegestatistik 2001*. http://www.destatis.de/allg/d/veroe/d_pflege99.htm, Bonn, assessed January 2005.

Statistisches Bundesamt. (2003). *Bericht: "Bevölkerung Deutschlands bis 2050"*. www.destatis.de, Pfad: Presse/Presseveranstaltungen, Bonn, assessed January 2005.

Teno J. M. (2004). Do-not-resuscitate orders and hospitalization of nursing home residents: Trumping, neglect, or shared decision-making at the eleventh hour. *Journal of the American Geriatrics Society, 52*, 159–160.

Yang Z., Norton E. C., Stearns S. C. (2003). Longevity and health care expenditures—The real reasons older people spend more. *Journal of Gerontology Series B, 58*, 2–10.

Zimmer J. G., Hall W. J. (1997). Nursing home-acquired pneumonia: Avoiding the hospital. *Journal of the American Geriatrics Society, 45*, 380–381.

Zweifel P., Felder S., Meier M. (1999). Ageing of population and health care expenditure: A red herring? *Health Economics, 8*, 485–496.

Zweig S. C., Kruse R. L., Binder E. F., Szafara K. L., Mehr D. R. (2004). Effect of do-not-resuscitate orders on hospitalization of nursing home residents evaluated for lower respiratory infections. *Journal of the American Geriatrics Society, 52*, 51–58.

SIEGFRIED WEYERER and MARTINA SCHÄUFELE

COMMENTARY: MEDICAL CARE FOR NURSING HOME RESIDENTS: NATIONAL PERSPECTIVES IN INTERNATIONAL CONTEXT

Care provided by old-age homes has changed greatly in Germany over the last 20 years: The original focus on residential care has since given way to a focus on nursing care. Most recent statistics (Statistisches Bundesamt, 2005) indicate that this trend persists; the number of nursing homes increased from 9,165 (2001) to 9,700 (2003). Parallel to this development, the number of nursing home residents rose from 604,000 (2001) to 640,000 (2003).

1. MEDICAL INPATIENT CARE OF NURSING HOME RESIDENTS

In Germany, the hospitalisation of nursing home residents is a growing problem that is poorly defined and reported. Therefore, the present study by Ramroth, Specht-Leible, König, and Brenner (2006) focusing on hospitalisation and its determinants among nursing home residents before and after home admission is especially important. Also, it is of particular interest that the authors concentrate on the last year of life, since it is well known that costs of health care are generally highest in the year preceding death (Daviglus et al., 2005). Hospital discharge data from Germany's largest health insurer also show that costs for patients during their last year of life make up a large part of total health care expenditures (Brockmann, 2002).

2. ADVANTAGES OF A COHORT STUDY OF NEW HOSPITAL ADMISSIONS

The study by Ramroth et al. (2006) has several advantages. First of all, it is based on a cohort of new admissions. Most of the studies on medical care for home residents are cross-sectional studies. However, cross-sectional data obtained for residents in nursing homes are of limited use in planning geriatric services. They over-represent the long-stay residents because short-stay residents from earlier admission cohorts selectively either have died or have been transferred to other facilities. Such data do not elucidate, for example, whether the high prevalence of psychiatric disorders in nursing homes is due to selection (i.e. residents who already have mental health problems at the time of admission or who have been transferred from mental hospitals) or to the home environment, which may be an important factor in the development and course of health problems (Weyerer, Häfner, Mann, Ames, & Graham, 1995). Given

H.-W. Wahl et al. (eds.), The Many Faces of Health, Competence and Well-Being in Old Age, 189–196.

the rapidly expanding options for outpatient and semi-outpatient care, and in the wake of the new statutory long-term care insurance in Germany, a high prevalence of severe chronic illness and need for care can be expected even among newly admitted home residents.

Another strong point of the study is that the population is a cohort of new admissions to all 97 nursing homes that can be generalised to a region in the Rhine-Neckar area with over 800,000 inhabitants. This presents a more balanced picture of the mix of residents being cared for in nursing homes and their use of acute-care hospitals.

A further advantage is that the findings on the utilisation of medical care are based on longitudinal data, which strengthens the possibility that a temporal relationship might exist between the characteristics of nursing home residents at admission and their subsequent use of health services. The authors were able to obtain data for members of the eight largest health insurance plans, which together cover about 80% of the population. The advantage of using routine statistics such as health and social insurance data sets for epidemiological research stems from their volume and the minimal time lag between collection of the data and their availability. It is probably the only efficient and reliable way to obtain a complete picture of new admissions with regard to the number of and duration of hospitalisations, the duration of nursing home residency, hospital status prior to nursing home admission and vital status at the end of the observation period.

3. SHORTCOMINGS OF ROUTINE MEDICAL DATA

With regard to medical diagnoses and the amount of time spent on care required by basic activities of daily living (ADL), the value of routine data may be compromised by incomplete or inaccurate recording. For these variables, the number of missing data is relatively high (Table 1 in Ramroth et al., 2006). In addition, considering the multi-morbidity among elderly persons it seems to be difficult, and in many cases arbitrary, to determine the main medical cause for dependency on permanent care. As for primary data sets, data quality can be controlled by the investigator; the quality of secondary data is usually not documented because epidemiological quality requirements cannot be anticipated at the time of data gathering (Schach, 1992).

Due to the limitations of the database available to Ramroth et al. (2006), their study covers only hospitalisations but not other health care sectors, e.g. medical outpatient care, medical care capacities in the nursing homes and use of medication. Another shortcoming is that due to the limitations of registered diagnoses the impact of dementia, the most frequent diagnosis among nursing home residents, on medical care could not be assessed adequately. Also, the high costs of dementia disorders suggest particular observation of this disease. A recent publication (Statistisches Bundesamt Gesundheit, 2004) states that in terms of individual diagnostic groups, in the year 2002 mental and behavioural disorders accounted for 10% of the total costs of illness (22.4 billion Euro). The lion's share was spent on dementia (5.6 billion Euro), followed by depression (4.0 billion Euro) and neurotic, stress and somatic disorders (2.8 billion Euro).

Table 1. Cross-sectional study in 11 nursing homes in the city of Mannheim over time

Year of assessment *Number of residents in 11 nursing homes*		*1995/1996* *N = 1,283*	*1997/1998* *N = 1,286*	*2002/2003* *N = 1,276*	*p*
Gender	% female	74.9	74.8	74.6	ns (*X2-Test*)
Age (years)	M (SD)	79.8 (11.1)	80.3 (11.7)	80.3 (11.5)	ns (ANOVA)
Length of stay (years)	M (SD)	4.1 (4.7)	4.1 (4.8)	3.9 (4.8)	ns (ANOVA)
Limitation in ADL activities	% moderate/ severe	78.1	82.4	86.0	*<.001 (X2-Test)*
Transfer from hospital (before home admission)	%	48.8	54.0	58.4	*<.001 (X2-Test)*
Use of primary care physician (last 4 weeks)	%	95.7	97.0	96.3	ns (*X2-Test*)
Use of psychiatrist (last 4 weeks)	%	12.3	15.6	22.2	*<.001 (X2-Test)*
Transfer to hospital (last 4 weeks)	%	8.4	7.7	4.5	*<.001 (X2-Test)*
Diagnosis of dementia (ICD 10: F00-F03)	%	12.0	13.3	27.2	*<.001 (X2-Test)*
Diagnosis of dementia/other organic psychiatric disorders (ICD 10: F00-F09)	%	34.0	36.7	39.8	*<.05(X2-Test)*
Screening for moderate/ severe dementia	%	54.7	60.1	65.3	*<.001 (X2-Test)*

4. NURSING HOME RESIDENTS SUFFERING FROM DEMENTIA: RESULTS FROM PRIMARY DATA SETS

In order to gain a broader view of the medical care available to nursing home residents, we would like to present additional data from international and national studies. Although dementia (at a rate of 22.6%) was the leading medical diagnosis with regard to dependency on permanent care in the study by Ramroth et al. (2006), the prevalence of the recorded medical diagnosis of dementia certainly does not mirror the true prevalence of dementia. Recent results for the city of Mannheim, based on systematic assessments of cognitive impairment, indicate that over 60% of the residents in nursing homes suffer from dementia (Weyerer, Schäufele, Hendlmeier, Kofahl, & Sattel, 2005). Studies carried out since the early 1980s in Scandinavia, Great Britain and North America corroborate that between 51% and 72% of all nursing home residents suffer from dementia (Bickel, 1997).

Bickel (1995) had earlier pursued the question of whether or not dementia disorders were the reason for admission to a nursing home, or if instead they were to be understood as concurrent disorders, respectively, perhaps even developed only after admission to a nursing home. Not only did home residents frequently suffer from dementia, but this was also by far the most common reason for admission to a nursing home. In over half of all cases, dementia was the primary cause of the admission. This result was corroborated by a representative study carried out in the nineties in old-age and nursing homes in the city of Mannheim that compared newly admitted residents at the time of home admission to those studied cross-sectionally who had resided in the home for about 4 years. In both populations over half of the residents suffered from moderate to severe dementia (Weyerer & Schäufele, 1999). Studies carried out in Mannheim using identical instruments showed that meanwhile, approximately two-thirds of all nursing home residents suffer from some type of dementia. This is true of both residents studied cross-sectionally and the new admissions (Weyerer et al., 2005). Given the growing number of options for outpatient care and in the wake of the new statutory long-term care insurance, a high prevalence of chronic psychiatric and somatic disorders is to be expected even among newly admitted nursing home residents.

In general, dementia very often goes undetected among elderly medical inpatients. A comprehensive geriatric assessment by Joray, Wietlisbach, and Bula (2004) revealed for instance that almost two-thirds of cognitively impaired inpatients aged 75 years and older (Mini-Mental-State Examination <24) were not detected. In order to avoid underreporting, in a study by Burton et al. (2001) focusing on medical care for nursing home residents, the dementia diagnosis was not based only on medical records. Rather, baseline data were collected from multiple sources: structured interviews with a significant other and a nursing staff informant, and a Mini-Mental-State Examination (Folstein, Folstein, & McHugh, 1975). Psychiatrists and neurologists made a dementia diagnosis based on these sources and according to the criteria of the Diagnostic and Statistical Manual III (American Psychiatric Association, 1987). Almost 50% of the study population was designated as having dementia. Nursing home residents with dementia had significantly lower annual rates of physician visits and hospitalisations than those without dementia, virtually the same rate of visits to the emergency department, and similar lengths of stay in the hospital.

5. MEDICAL CARE OF NURSING HOME RESIDENTS IN THE CITY OF MANNHEIM

With 325,929 residents (status: 2003), Mannheim is by far the largest city in the catchment area studied by Ramroth et al. (2006). Compared to the entire Federal Republic (5.0%), the percentage of Mannheim residents aged 65 years and older who are cared for in nursing homes is only slightly higher (5.7%). Based on a random sample of 20 of the 26 old-age and nursing homes in Mannheim in the nineties, Weyerer and Schäufele (1999) studied cross-sectionally all home residents ($N = 1{,}927$) and—over a period of 6 months—all new home admissions ($N = 187$). There were no significant differences between the two populations as far as the medical diagnosis of organic disorders/dementia disorders (ICD 10: F 00–F 09); in each group over one-third of the home residents (cross-sectional study: 36.5%; new admissions: 36.4%) were affected. In reality, the true prevalence of dementia disorders among home residents was underestimated. Numerous epidemiological studies indicate that primary physicians frequently fail to diagnose dementia and other mental disorders. In order to gain a realistic picture of the prevalence of dementia, we systematically assessed all residents with the aid of qualified nursing staff. The assessment yielded a much higher rate of dementia disorders (cross-sectional study: 50.6%; new admissions: 53.1%). Major factors that significantly increase the risk of institutionalisation for demented patients include, in addition to the severity of the dementia, incontinence as well as the presence of non-cognitive symptoms such as disorders of the sleep-wake rhythm, agitation and aggressiveness. In addition to the cognitive disorders, dementia patients in nursing homes in Mannheim exhibited a substantial number of behaviour problems.

If a greater number of mental disorders than usual occur among residents of old-age and nursing homes compared to elderly people living in private households, then a very high rate of use of psychotropic drugs among home residents is to be expected. Studies carried out in old-age and nursing homes in different countries since 1987 (NSW Ministerial Taskforce, 1997) reveal that on average 56% of home residents are treated with psychotropic drugs. In Mannheim as well, over half of the home residents (cross-sectional study) used psychotropic drugs (58.0%, with regard to a period of 4 weeks). These were followed by diuretics (45.4%), cardiac drugs (32.6%), analgesic drugs (32.2%), beta-receptor blockers (24.4%) and gastrointestinal preparations (21.6%). This list of the most frequently administered medication (prevalence >20%) clearly illustrates that multi-medication plays a large role in nursing homes: 43.2% of all home residents take more than five or more medications daily, thus manifold interactions among the various medications are likely to occur. Categorisation of psychotropic drugs according to indication groups shows that antipsychotic drugs (37.4%) are the most common, followed at a distance by antidepressants (12.7%), tranquillisers (10.9%) and hypnotics/sedatives (8.0%). Although the use of psychotropic drugs in nursing homes was high, by no means had all patients with mental disorders received medical treatment. For example, over one-third of home residents with depression were not treated with any psychotropic drug. Among dementia patients as well—similar to patients over 70 years and older studied in the Berlin Study on Ageing (Helmchen et al., 1996)—insufficient medical treatment was obvious.

The literature often tends to regard the high use of psychotropic drugs in nursing homes as a consequence of institutionalisation. In Mannheim, however, we found no evidence of this. There was no correlation between the use of psychotropic drugs and the length of stay in the homes, on average 3.5 years. The rate of use of psychotropic drugs among newly admitted nursing home residents was similar to that of home residents who had already lived in the home for several years.

The higher-than-average occurrence of falls among the elderly frequently requires medical intervention. In the study by Ramroth et al. (2006), injuries and poisoning, at almost 5%, were the main medical cause for dependency on permanent care. A particularly serious side effect of psychotropic drug use among the elderly is the increased risk of falling. The percentage of home residents (cross-sectional study) who had experienced at least one fall during the 6-month observation period was 34.1%. Particularly severe falls with fractures occurred among 4.0%. In order to identify the influence of psychotropic drug use on the frequency of falls, we controlled for a number of confounding variables: age, gender, limitations to mobility, impairment of vision, dementia, depression, alcohol abuse, as well as the need for help or nursing care.

With regard to psychotropic drugs as a whole, the risk of falling increased by 46%—independent of all other risk factors. In terms of individual indication groups, the values lay between 33% (antidepressants) and 62% (tranquillisers/hypnotics/sedatives). The Mannheim results concur with those of studies carried out in nursing homes abroad (Mustard & Mayer, 1997). There, too, the risk of falls among nursing home residents who had been prescribed psychotropic drugs increased by 50%, with relatively minor differences between antidepressants, tranquillisers/hypnotics and antipsychotic drugs.

We were able to study the cross-section population of residents of 11 nursing homes with, for the most part, identical survey instruments at three time-points: in 1995/1996 and—following introduction of statutory long-term care insurance on July 1, 1996—in 1997/1998, and again in 2002/2003 (Table 1).

The number of nursing home residents changed only slightly over time. There were no substantial changes with regard to gender, age or length of stay of home residents. Approximately three-fourths were women; at the time of assessment the average age was about 80 years, and the length of stay was 4 years. However, we did find a marked increase in the number of home residents who were moderately or severely limited in their ADL. We also found an increasing percentage of residents who had been directly transferred from a hospital to a nursing home. In the study by Ramroth et al. (2006), there is also a relatively high proportion of newly admitted residents (44.7%) who had been transferred directly from acute care in hospital to a nursing home. The corresponding percentage in Mannheim was even higher; besides other factors this difference may be due to the fact that the data in Mannheim are based on a cross-sectional population and not on new admissions.

At all three waves the use of primary care physicians during the 4 weeks prior to assessment was, at over 95%, very high. With regard to psychiatrists, there was a significant increase in the consultation rate over time. In 2002/2003, and within 4 weeks, about every fifth resident was treated by a psychiatrist. The number of transfers to hospital based on a 4-week period also decreased over time.

Among dementia and other organic mental disorders diagnosed by the primary physicians, a significant increase from 34.0% to 39.8% is noted. Particularly, conspicuous is the increase in the percentage of dementia diagnoses (e.g. Alzheimer's Disease) over the course of 7 years from 12.0% to 27.2%. As in our earlier studies, the percentage of residents with a dementia disorder, as assessed by nursing staff, was also much higher this time than the percentage identified by primary care physicians and documented in nursing home records. Over the course of the entire 7-year observation period, the percentage of residents with signs of a moderate to severe dementia disorder increased significantly. In 1995/1996, according to dementia screening administered by nursing staff, 54.7% of residents suffered from a moderate to severe dementia disorder; in 2002/2003 their number had increased to 65.3%. As for all home residents, the percentage of those residents with a dementia disorder who had been transferred from a hospital within 4 weeks decreased significantly over time from 9.1% in 1995/1996, to 8.2% in 1997/1998, to 4.7% in 2002/2003.

6. HOSPITALISATION OF NURSING HOME RESIDENTS AND FUTURE RESEARCH

Because the transfer from a nursing home to the hospital for acute care can be a traumatic experience, particularly for patients with dementia, it is important to provide targeted prevention measures and case management in the nursing homes (Specht-Leible, Bender, & Oster, 2003). Medical care capacity and clinical resources in nursing homes may be important factors to limit hospital admissions. Intrator, Castle, and Mor (1999) tested the effect of facility characteristics on the probability of hospitalisation of nursing home residents. They found that homes with special care units, a greater number of physicians, nurse practitioners or physician assistants were less likely to hospitalise their residents. Health care reforms that integrate acute and long-term care may reduce, if not fully prevent, the need to hospitalise nursing home residents (Barker et al., 1994).

Since the health profile of nursing home residents, as well as medical service models, may change in Germany in the coming years, we would like to encourage Ramroth, Specht-Leible, König and Brenner to continue their methodologically sound approach in future studies.

AFFILIATION

Central Institute of Mental Health in Mannheim

REFERENCES

American Psychiatric Association. (Ed.). (1987). *Diagnostic and statistical manual of mental disorders, III-R.* Washington, DC: American Psychiatric Association.

Barker, W. H., Zimmer, J. G., Hall, W. J., Ruff, B. C., Freundlich, C. B., & Eggert, G. M. (1994). Rates, patterns, causes, and costs of nursing home residents: A population-based study. *American Journal of Public Health, 84*(10), 1615–1620.

Bickel, H. (1995). Demenzkranke in Alten- und Pflegeheimen: Gegenwärtige Situation und Entwicklungstendenzen. In Forschungsinstitut der Friedrich-Ebert-Stiftung (Ed.), *Medizinische und gesellschaftspolitische Herausforderung: Alzheimer Krankheit. Der langsame Zerfall der Persönlichkeit* (pp. 49–68). Bonn: Friedrich-Ebert-Stiftung.

Bickel, H. (1997). Epidemiologie psychischer Erkrankungen im Alter. In H. Förstl (Ed.), *Lehrbuch der Gerontopsychiatrie* (pp. 1–15). Stuttgart: Enke.

Brockmann, H. (2002). Why is health treatment for the elderly less expensive than for the rest of the population? *Social Science and Medicine, 55*, 593–608.

Burton, L. C., German, P. S., Gruber-Baldini, A. L., Hebel, R., Zimmerman, S., & Magaziner, J. (2001). Medical care for nursing home residents: Differences by dementia status. *Journal of the American Geriatrics Society, 49*, 142–147.

Daviglus, M. L., Liu, K., Pirzada, A., Yan, L. L., Garside, D. B., Greenland, P., et al. (2005). Cardiovascular risk profile earlier in life and Medicare costs in the last year of life. *Archives of Internal Medicine, 165*(9), 1028–1034.

Folstein, M. F., Folstein, S. E., & McHugh, P. R. (1975). "Mini mental state". A practical method for grading the cognitive state of patients for the clinician. *Journal of Psychiatric Research, 12*, 189–198.

Helmchen, H., Baltes, M. M., Geiselmann, B., Kanowski, S., Linden, M., Reischies, F. M., et al. (1996). Psychische Erkrankungen im Alter. In K. U. Mayer & P. B. Baltes (Eds.), *Die Berliner Altersstudie* (pp. 186–219). Berlin: Akademie Verlag.

Intrator, O., Castle, N. G., & Mor, V. (1999). Facility characteristics associated with hospitalization of nursing home residents: Results of a national study. *Medical Care, 37*(3), 228–237.

Joray, S., Wietlisbach, V., & Bula, C. J. (2004). Cognitive impairment in elderly medical inpatients: Detection and associated six-month outcomes. *American Journal of Geriatric Psychiatry, 12*(6), 639–647.

Mustard, C. A., & Mayer, T. (1997). Case-control study of exposure to medication and the risk of injurious falls requiring hospitalization among nursing home residents. *American Journal of Epidemiology, 145*, 738–745.

NSW Ministerial Taskforce. (1997). *Psychotropic medication use in nursing homes.* Report of the NSW Ministerial Taskforce. Sydney, Australia.

Ramroth, H., Specht-Leible, N., König, H.-H., & Brenner, H. (2006). Medical care for nursing home residents. National and international perspectives. In H. W. Wahl, H. Brenner, H. Mollenkopf, D. Rothenbacher, & C. Rott (Eds.), *The many faces of health, competence and well-being in old age: Integrating epidemiological, psychological and social perspectives.*

Schach, E. (1992). Data collection and processing. In J. Olsen & D. Trichopoulos (Eds.), *Teaching epidemiology* (pp. 56–74). Oxford: Oxford University Press.

Specht-Leible, M., Bender, M., & Oster, P. (2003). Die Ursachen der stationären Aufnahme von Alten- und Pflegeheimbewohnern in einer Geriatrischen Klinik. *Zeitschrift für Gerontologie und Geriatrie, 36*, 274–279.

Statistisches Bundesamt Gesundheit. (2004). *Krankheitskosten 2002.* Wiesbaden: Statistisches Bundesamt.

Statistisches Bundesamt. (2005). *Bericht Pflegestatistik 2003—Pflege im Rahmen der Pflegeversicherung—Deutschlandergebnisse.* Zweigstelle Bonn: Statistisches Bundesamt.

Weyerer, S., Häfner, H., Mann, A. H., Ames, D., & Graham, N. (1995). Prevalence and course of depression among elderly residential home admissions in Mannheim and Camden, London. *International Psychogeriatrics, 7*(4), 479–493.

Weyerer, S., & Schäufele, M. (1999). Epidemiologie körperlicher und psychischer Beeinträchtigungen im Alter. In A. Zimber & S. Weyerer (Eds.), *Arbeitsbelastung in der Altenpflege* (pp. 3–23). Göttingen: Verlag für Angewandte Psychologie.

Weyerer, S., Schäufele, M., Hendlmeier, I., Kofahl, C., & Sattel, H. (2005). *Demenzkranke Menschen in Pflegeeinrichtungen: Besondere und traditionelle Versorgung im Vergleich.* Stuttgart: Kohlhammer.

PART IV

SYNERGIES BETWEEN SOCIAL-ECOLOGICAL, PSYCHOLOGICAL AND EPIDEMIOLOGICAL RESEARCH

MARINA SCHMITT,[1] FRANK OSWALD,[2] DANIELA JOPP,[1]
HANS-WERNER WAHL[2] and HERMANN BRENNER[3]

THE IMPACT OF INTERNAL AND EXTERNAL RESOURCES ON HEALTH, COMPETENCE AND WELL-BEING: LONGITUDINAL FINDINGS FROM THE ILSE

Resources represent personal characteristics or goods that an individual uses or has access to in everyday life or in specific life situations. According to Diener and Fujita (1995, p. 926), resources include "material, social or personal characteristics that a person possesses that he or she can use to make progress towards his or her goals. Resources can be external possessions (e.g. money), social roles (e.g. being a chair person) and personal characteristics (e.g. intelligence)". The concept of resources thus represents an umbrella term, including variables that are assumed to have positive effects on the individuals' goal pursuit and development.

Because heterogeneous variables are summarised under the resource term, further classification is called upon. One common classification of resources includes the distinction between internal and external resources. Internal resources represent variables such as personality, health or intelligence, whereas external resources represent factors that are linked to the external world of the individual such as social network, finances or environmental conditions.

Given that resources facilitate goal pursuit, resources are considered to be positively related to developmental outcomes. A number of studies showed that internal resources such as cognitive status, personality or economics are positively linked to developmental criteria such as subjective well-being over the life span. Among external resources effective for health, competence and well-being in later life are socio-physical characteristics of the living environment, like social network, living space or housing standard (e.g. Schaie, Wahl, Mollenkopf, & Oswald, 2003; Wahl, Scheidt, & Windley, 2004). In contrast to internal resources, the resource quality of external socio-physical characteristics appears to be more blurred. A similar condition (e.g. having much living space) can, in one case, be a resource, and in another case, a risk factor that may eventually influence health and well-being in later life in manifold ways.

However, resource status might not be the only crucial factor to development, but also resource change. According to Hobfoll's Conservation of Resources theory (COR-theory; 1989, 2001), loss of resources is assumed to be the most influential driving force. In several studies, perceived resources loss was found to be highly related

H.-W. Wahl et al. (eds.), The Many Faces of Health, Competence and Well-Being in Old Age, 199–209.

to negative developmental outcomes such as high depression. Resource loss was also found to be predictive for low subjective well-being (Jopp & Leipold, 2004). However, when it comes to predicting well-being, it seems to be the case that resource status has a higher predictive power than resource loss. When comparing the resource status and loss with respect to some basic resource domains, status explained a larger proportion of the variance than loss in a sample of young and old individuals (Jopp & Leipold, 2004).

Changes in resources are also considered as important determinants of positive developmental outcomes. Hobfoll's COR-theory (1989, 2001), for example, assumes that individuals are characterised by an inherent need to enhance and maintain their resources. If this need is violated, either by losing resources or by anticipating resource loss, negative reactions can be observed such as high levels of depression (e.g. Wells, Hobfoll, & Larvin, 1999) or low subjective well-being (e.g. Jopp & Leipold, 2003). In comparison to negative resource change, resource gain is expected to have less powerful effects than resource loss. Hobfoll (2001) argues that resource gains play a protective role in the context of resource loss. However, Holahan, Moos, Holahan, and Cronkite (1999) found that resource loss as well as resource gains were significantly related to depressive symptoms over a time period of 10 years. Regarding the relation between resource status and resource loss, those individuals who lost a considerable amount of resources over the 10 years were found to have had more resources at the first measurement occasion than the resource gain group.

Concerning developmental outcomes, the constructs of health, competence and well-being are particularly good candidates to consider. For example, Rowe and Kahn (1998) argue that successful ageing is characterised by high physiological (and cognitive) functioning, a low risk for age-related diseases and disabilities and active involvement in life. Moreover, a considerable number of theories and studies have proposed the use of subjective well-being as the central indicator of positive development and ageing (e.g. Butt & Reiser, 1987; Lawton, 1975; Neugarten, Havighurst, & Tobin, 1961). However, many authors argue that successful development and ageing should be assessed with multiple dimensions, including subjective and objective measures, and focusing on stable as well as dynamic indicators (e.g. Baltes & Carstensen, 1996; Schulz & Heckhausen, 1996; Steverink, Lindenberg, & Ormel, 1998).

Therefore, this investigation addresses the following core question: What impact do internal and external resources and their longitudinal changes have on multiple dimensions of ageing such as health, competence and well-being in middle-aged and older adults?

The potential of the Interdisciplinary Longitudinal Study on Adult Development (with the German acronym ILSE; Martin, Grünendahl, & Martin, 2001) is used to address this question: With its interdisciplinary and longitudinal approach, changes throughout the process of adult development can be examined using a wide range of data on internal and external resources as well as on health, competence and well-being measures.

1. METHOD

1.1. *Participants*

The data collection for this study was part of the ILSE study. Data were gathered between September 1993 and April 1996 (T1) and between September 1997 and April 2000 (T2) in two data-collection centres in East and West Germany (T1–T2: 4.1 years). The sample was stratified by age and gender. At T1, addresses of 4,800 participants were obtained from the respective local registries. On the basis of this listing, addresses were randomly drawn from this pool and the persons were contacted. This procedure was followed until samples of 500 participants from East and West Germany of each age group (born 1930–1932 and 1950–1952, respectively) were obtained. Half of the data from each age group were collected in the former East Germany, and half in West Germany. In both age groups, 52% were men. With the reliance on a random drawing from central registries addresses, and based on comparisons with the family status, income and housing status of the same age groups of the overall population in Germany, our sample is largely representative of the German-speaking population of Germany and comparable with other samples used in longitudinal studies (Martin, Grünendahl, & Martin, 2001).

The sample used in this analysis includes 449 middle-aged (mean age at T1 = 44.2 years) and 449 older persons (mean age at T1 = 63.0 years) who participated at both measurement occasions of the ILSE. Dropout analysis revealed no significant differences between participants and non-participants at T2 concerning educational attainment, income, health, depression and crystallised intelligence.

1.2. *Materials*

Several instruments were applied to collect data on internal and external resources, health, competence and well-being.

1.2.1. *Internal Resources*

Personality and cognition were considered internal resources. Concerning personality, neuroticism, extraversion and openness measured by the German version of Costa and McCrae's NEO-Five-Factor Inventory (NEO-FFI; Borkenau & Ostendorf, 1993) were included. To narrow down the scope of cognitive functioning for the purpose of this study, a factor analysis was conducted including participants' scores on knowledge drawn from the German version of Wechsler Adult Intelligence Scale (Tewes, 1991) as well as the Picture Memory Test, the Digit Memory Test and the Digit Symbol Test drawn from the Nuremberg Ageing Inventory—a test battery including questionnaires on cognition, autonomy, age-related changes and ageing satisfaction (Oswald & Fleischmann, 1993). The factor analysis revealed one general cognitive performance factor with an eigenvalue above 1. Explained variance was 45.4%.

1.2.2. *External Resources*

As external resources, socio-physical environmental factors, finances and education were examined. Concerning socio-physical environmental factors, participants indicated the amount of persons they have close contact to (network size), the number of persons per household (household size), their housing standard (1 = without toilet to 4 = with toilet, bath and central heating), their living space (1 = less than 40 m^2 to 6 = 120 m^2 and more, adjusted for the number of persons living in the household) and the possibility to retreat within their own apartment (ranging from 1 = no possibility to retreat to 5 = high possibility to retreat). Housing tenure was assessed by the dichotomous variable ownership versus non-ownership (mostly tenants). Concerning financial resources, the respondents were asked to give the categorical income of their household (1 = lower than 255 € to 11 above 3,070 €). By dividing the centre of this non-metric information by the size of each household, a pseudo-metric income per person was generated. Education was measured by the number of years of educational attainment.

1.2.3. Health

Health status was measured using subjective health and number of diseases as indicators. Subjective health was scored by asking participants for an overall subjective evaluation of their current health on a 6-point scale (1 = very good to 6 = very bad). Concerning number of diseases, the German version of the Cumulative Illness Rating Scale (CIRS; Parmelee, Thuras, Katz, & Lawton, 1995) was used. The physicians presented participants a checklist of 13 items and asked them to report the actual occurrence of each of the listed diseases. The participants could answer "Yes" or "No" to each item. A sum score ranging from 0 to 13 was built.

1.2.4. Competence

Competence was measured based on the participants' leisure activities. The participants were asked to report how often they perform each of 26 leisure activities (e.g. visiting family and friends, museums, or sporting events, needleworks, photographing, reading, dancing, painting) on a 10-point rating scale ranging from 0 = never to 10 = every day. As an indicator of competence, a mean frequency score of activities was calculated. Data on competence were only available at the second measurement point.

1.2.5. Well-being

Additionally, different dimensions of subjective well-being (life satisfaction, morale) were included as outcomes. Participants completed the German Version of the revised standardised Philadelphia Geriatric Center Morale Scale (PGCMS; Lawton, 1975). The participants could answer "Yes" or "No" to each item. Data were recoded so that each high morale response received a score of "1" and each low-morale response received a "0". Summed scores could range from 0 to 17. The items are scored so that a higher value indicates a higher level of morale. Concerning life satisfaction, the participants were asked to rate their current satisfaction in different domains (family, friends, housing and finances) on 5-point rating scales ranging from 1 = very unsatisfied to 5 = very satisfied. In the next step, a factor analysis including the participants' satisfaction scores with family, friends, housing and finances was conducted. Factor analysis revealed one factor with an eigenvalue above 1 and an explained variance of 42.3%.

To facilitate the comparison between T1 and T2, resource and outcome variables were standardised. First, for every resource variable and outcome variable, the total sample mean score at T1 was set at 50 and the standard deviation was set at 10. Second, T2-scores of internal and external resources as well as the outcome variables were standardised at T1-scores. Third, differences scores (T2–T1) were calculated for resources. Except for competence, changes in successful ageing were considered in autoregressive models including T1 outcomes as covariates. Autoregressive models allow for a partition of the T2 outcome variance into a part attributable to the stability of the variable over time (i.e. variance due to the T1 outcome) and into another part reflecting changes between T1 and T2 attributable to "exogeneous" sources, which might be included into the model as predictor variables to estimate these variables unique influence on the outcome's change.

2. RESULTS

To examine the role of internal and external resource status and resource changes in predicting changes in health and well-being after controlling for outcome status at T1, gender, age and region, we conducted a series of regression analyses. With respect to competence, outcome status at T1 could not be included as a covariate because data on leisure activities were only collected at T2. As independent variables, internal and external resources at T1 as well as change scores of internal and external resources (T2–T1) were considered. As dependent variables, standardised T2 indicators of health, competence and subjective well-being were included. On account of missing data for some of the variables used in the present analyses and due to listwise deletion, the sample size ranges from $N = 641$ to $N = 649$.

Table 1 summarises the results of the regression models for the prediction of health indicators. Two health indicators were addressed, i.e. subjective health and number of diseases at T2 (Table 1). After controlling for subjective health and number of diseases at T1 (due to high inter-correlations between both variables), only neuroticism at T1 and change in neuroticism significantly predicted change in subjective health. The total amount of explained variance was 33%. Concerning the changes in the number of diseases at T2, the predictors were number of diseases at T1 and subjective health at T1. Besides, age has a significant effect, with older persons having more diseases. Among the external resources, the possibility to retreat contributed slightly but significantly to the number of diseases: A lower possibility to retreat was significantly associated with a higher number of diseases.

With respect to competence (Table 2), age, region, external and internal resource status variables at T1 and resource changes played a significant role. The complete model explained 17% of the variance. Being a member of the older age group or living in West Germany was significantly associated with higher competence in the sense of more optional activities. Results indicate that among the internal resources at T1, higher extraversion, higher openness and higher cognitive functioning predicted competence at T2. Additionally, resource change in extraversion (in the sense of an increase in extraversion over time) contributed significantly to competence in terms of leisure activities. Among external resources, network size at T1 and—with respect to resource changes—an increase in network size over time contributed significantly to competence.

Table 1. Regression analyses summary for internal and external resources and their longitudinal changes predicting health indicators

	Subjective health		Number of diseases	
Variable	*STB*	*Semi-partial R^2*	*STB*	*Semi-partial R^2*
Subjective health T1	0.41***	0.13	0.13***	0.01
Number of diseases T1	0.14***	0.14	0.46***	0.17
Sex	−0.02	0.00	0.02	0.00
Age group	0.00	0.00	−0.23***	0.04
Region	−0.06	0.00	−0.03	0.00
Internal resources T1				
Neuroticism	0.12**	0.01	−0.01	0.00
Extraversion	−0.03	0.00	−0.05	0.00
Openness	0.03	0.00	0.03	0.00
Cognition	−0.03	0.00	0.01	0.00
External resources T1				
Network size	−0.05	0.00	0.03	0.00
Household size	−0.02	0.00	−0.10	0.00
Number of children	0.03	0.00	0.00	0.00
Housing tenure	0.01	0.00	−0.02	0.00
Living space	−0.09	0.00	0.06	0.00
Housing standard	−0.08	0.00	−0.01	0.00
Possibility to retreat	0.05	0.00	−0.09*	0.00
Income	−0.04	0.00	−0.02	0.00
Education	−0.05	0.00	−0.01	0.00
Change in internal resources T1–T2				
Neuroticism	0.14***	0.14	0.03	0.00
Extraversion	−0.04	0.00	−0.01	0.00
Openness	0.04	0.00	0.04	0.00
Cognition	−0.06	0.00	0.01	0.00
Change in external resources T1–T2				
Network size	−0.06	0.00	0.06	0.00
Household size	0.01	0.00	0.00	0.00
Number of children	0.01	0.00	−0.04	0.00
Housing tenure	0.03	0.00	0.03	0.00
Living space	−0.03	0.00	0.00	0.00
Housing standard	0.00	0.00	0.00	0.00
Possibility to retreat	−0.02	0.00	−0.06	0.00
Income	−0.05	0.00	0.02	0.00
Adjusted R^2	0.33***	($N = 644$, p < 0.01)	0.42***	($N = 648$, p < 0.01)

$^{*}p < 0.05$.
$^{**}p < 0.01$.
$^{***}p < 0.001$.

Table 2. *Regression analysis summary for internal and external resources and their longitudinal changes predicting competence*

Variable	Competence	
	STB	*Semi-partial* R^2
Sex	0.03	0.00
Age group	−0.26***	0.03
Region	−0.18***	0.02
Internal resources T1		
Neuroticism	−0.06	0.00
Extraversion	0.11*	0.01
Openness	0.12*	0.01
Cognition	0.15*	0.01
External resources T1		
Network size	0.17***	0.02
Household size	−0.02	0.00
Number of children	−0.02	0.00
Housing tenure	0.05	0.00
Living space	−0.01	0.00
Housing standard	−0.02	0.00
Possibility to retreat	0.08	0.00
Income	0.02	0.00
Education	0.06	0.00
Change in internal resources T1–T2		
Neuroticism	−0.06	0.00
Extraversion	0.09*	0.01
Openness	0.05	0.00
Cognition	0.05	0.00
Change in external resources T1–T2		
Network size	0.10*	0.01
Household size	0.04	0.00
Number of children	−0.06	0.00
Housing tenure	0.03	0.00
Living space	−0.06	0.00
Housing standard	0.01	0.00
Possibility to retreat	0.06	0.00
Income	0.06	0.00
Adjusted R^2	0.17***	($N = 647$, $p < 0.01$)

$^{*}p < 0.05$.
$^{**}p < 0.01$.
$^{***}p < 0.001$.

In the next step, predictors of morale and life satisfaction as indicators of subjective well-being were examined (Table 3). Morale at T1, neuroticism scores at T1 and a change (in the sense of decrease) in neuroticism were the most important predictors of morale. Additionally, status of extraversion and change of extraversion played a

Table 3. *Regression analyses summary for internal and external resources and their longitudinal changes predicting indicators of subjective well-being*

	Morale		*Life satisfaction*	
Variable	*STB*	*Semi-partial R^2*	*STB*	*Semi-partial R^2*
Morale T1	0.35***	0.07		
Life satisfaction T1			0.43***	0.14
Sex	−0.01	0.00	0.10**	0.01
Age group	0.04	0.00	−0.21***	0.02
Region	0.02	0.00	−0.01	0.00
Internal resources T1				
Neuroticism	−0.31***	0.04	−0.14***	0.01
Extraversion	0.12**	0.01	0.11**	0.01
Openness	0.04	0.01	−0.04	0.00
Cognition	−0.03	0.00	−0.04	0.00
External resources T1				
Network size	0.01	0.00	0.05	0.00
Household size	0.15*	0.01	0.15*	0.01
Number of children	−0.05	0.00	−0.08*	0.01
Housing tenure	−0.02	0.00	0.09*	0.01
Living space	−0.08	0.00	−0.05	0.00
Housing standard	−0.01	0.00	0.04	0.00
Possibility to retreat	0.12**	0.01	0.05	0.00
Income	0.11**	0.01	0.14**	0.01
Education	−0.02	0.00	−0.01	0.00
Change in internal resources T1–T2				
Neuroticism	−0.30***	0.06	−0.14***	0.01
Extraversion	0.11**	0.01	0.14***	0.02
Openness	−0.02	0.00	0.01	0.00
Cognition	−0.01	0.00	−0.05	0.00
Change in external resources T1–T2				
Network size	0.10*	0.01	−0.02	0.00
Household size	0.14***	0.01	0.13**	0.01
Number of children	0.00	0.00	−0.04	0.00
Housing tenure	−0.05	0.00	0.06	0.00
Living space	−0.06	0.00	−0.05	0.00
Housing standard	0.01	0.00	0.06	0.00
Possibility to retreat	0.15***	0.01	0.03	0.00
Income	0.10**	0.01	0.09*	0.01
Adjusted R^2	0.44***	($N = 649$, $p < 0.01$)	0.41***	($N = 641$, $p < 0.01$)

*$p < 0.05$.
**$p < 0.01$.
***$p < 0.001$.

significant role: Higher extraversion at T1 and an increase in extraversion were associated with higher morale. Concerning external resources, household size at T1 (as a status variable) and an increase in household size (as a change variable) contributed significantly to morale. Additionally, a higher possibility to retreat and a higher income at T1 were significant predictors of morale. Here again, positive changes in both variables significantly predicted well-being. Furthermore, an increase in network size had a positive effect on morale. The model explained 44% of the total variance of morale. Interestingly, region, age group and gender had no predictive effect on morale.

The predictor pattern of life satisfaction was somewhat different (Table 3). In contrast to morale, beside life satisfaction at T1, gender and age group were significant predictors for life satisfaction with women and older persons being more satisfied with their actual living situation compared to men and younger participants. Again, neuroticism and extraversion as internal resources at T1 as well as positive changes in both variables over time were important predictors of life satisfaction. Concerning T1 status variables of external resources, living together with more persons in the same household, having, however, fewer children, being a homeowner and having a higher income were positively associated with life satisfaction. Additionally, changes in external resources played an important role, too: An increase of persons per household and an increase in income contributed significantly to higher life satisfaction. The complete model explained 41% of the variance.

3. DISCUSSION

Since successful development and ageing is considered a multidimensional and multidirectional construct, influenced by stable as well as dynamic indicators, the aim of this study was to examine the influence of internal and external resources and resource changes on changes in health, competence and well-being.

In the overall picture, our results show that internal and external resources are positively linked to changes in developmental outcomes of health, competence and well-being, while simultaneously controlling for other predictors and status of health, competence and well being at T1. However, the amount of variance explained by resources differed in health, competence and well-being, as well as different predictor patterns, was revealed. Whereas both internal and external resources played a minor role in predicting subjective health and number of diseases after controlling for outcome status at T1, they played an important role in competence, life satisfaction and morale. As to subjective well-being, personality traits (neuroticism, extraversion) were important predictors as internal resources are concerned. Concerning external resources, both constructs were predicted differently. While household size, the possibility to retreat and income were positively linked to morale, life satisfaction was predicted by household size, number of children, housing tenure and income. Thus, well-being to a greater extent than health depends on socio-physical external as well as internal resources from a longitudinal perspective. Concerning competence, internal resources like extraversion, openness and cognition were significant predictors, while—as an external resource—only network size played an important role.

Going further, our results indicate that longitudinal changes in external and internal resources may have an additional effect on different aspects of successful ageing—with the exception of health indicators in which resource changes do not play any role in predicting health status. A possible explanation for the fact that neither resource status nor resource changes predicted the overall health status might be that the ILSE participants are basically relatively healthy, assuming that resources might not yet have an impact. Concerning competence and subjective well-being, the results indicate that both resources and resource gains in the internal and in the external domain were important predictors, not to be underestimated in the ageing process. An increase in extraversion (as an internal resource) and in network size (as an external resource) significantly predicted competence. Additionally, internal resource gains (in the sense of a decrease in neuroticism and an increase in extraversion) were positively linked to morale and life satisfaction. With respect to external resources, an increase in household size and in income were significant predictors of subjective well-being indicators, with possibility to retreat as an additional external change predictor of morale. These results are in contrast to Hobfoll's COR-theory (1989, 2001) which points to less powerful effects of resource gain compared to resource losses.

In conclusion, the results demonstrate that considering both internal and external resources and their changes adds important information on an explanative level and should be included in further research on health, competence and subjective well-being. Given the fact that, for the time being, participants in ILSE are basically relatively healthy, one might assume that the impact of internal and external resources should increase even more when they need to cope with more developmental risks and losses in the future.

More research needs to address differentiated effects for subgroups of participants, e.g. in terms of differences (a) between persons with high and low resource status and (b) with resource losses and gains to analyse their differential effect on indicators of successful ageing. Additionally, dependent upon resource status, resource gains or resource losses might affect indicators of successful ageing differentially. Furthermore, age differential effects of resources and resource changes would shed light on the developmental changes in health, competence and well-being.

ACKNOWLEDGEMENTS

The preparation of the manuscript was supported in part by the German Federal Ministry of Family, Senior Citizens, Women and Youth (BMFSFJ) and the Baden-Württemberg Ministry of Science, Research and Art (MWK) Grant Ref. 314-1722-102/16.

AFFILIATIONS

[1]*Department of Adult Development, German Centre for Research on Ageing at the University of Heidelberg*

[2]*Department of Social and Environmental Gerontology, German Centre for Research on Ageing at the University of Heidelberg*

[3] *Department of Epidemiology, German Centre for Research on Ageing at the University of Heidelberg*

REFERENCES

Baltes, M. M., & Carstensen, L. L. (1996). The process of successful aging. *Aging and Society, 16*, 397–422.

Borkenau, P., & Ostendorf, F. (1993). *NEO-Fünf-Faktoren-Inventar nach Costa und McCrae.* Göttingen: Hogrefe.

Butt, D. D., & Reiser, M. (1987). Successful aging: A theme for international psychology. *Psychology and Aging, 2*, 87–94.

Diener, E., & Fujita, F. (1995). Resources, personal strivings, and subjective well-being: A nomothetic and idiographic approach. *Journal of Personality and Social Psychology, 68*, 926–935.

Hobfoll, S. E. (1989). Conservation of resources: A new attempt at conceptualizing stress. *American Psychologist, 44*, 513–524.

Hobfoll, S. E. (2001). The influence of culture, community, and the nested-self in the stress process: Advancing conversation of resources theory. *Applied Psychology: An International Review, 50*, 337–370.

Holahan, C. J., Moos, R. H., Holahan, C. K., & Cronkite, R. C. (1999). Resource loss, resource gain, and depressive symptoms: A 10-year model. *Journal of Personality and Social Psychology, 77*, 620–629.

Jopp, D., & Leipold, B. (2003, November). *Perception of resources and their relationship to subjective well-being: Exploring age differences.* Poster presented at the 56th Annual Meeting of the Gerontological Society of America, San Diego, CA.

Jopp, D., & Leipold, B. (2004). *Perceptions of resources and their age-differential relationship to subjective well-being.* Poster represented at the 1st Conference "The many faces of health, competence, and well-being in old age: integrating epidemiological, psychological, and social perspectives", Heidelberg.

Lawton, M. P. (1975). The Philadelphia geriatric center morale scale: A revision. *Journal of Gerontology, 30*, 85–89.

Martin, M., Grünendahl, M., & Martin, P. (2001). Age differences in stress, social resources, and well-being in middle and older age. *Journals of Gerontology, 56B*, P214–P222.

Neugarten, B. L., Havighurst, R. S., & Tobin, S. S. (1961). The measurement of life-satisfaction. *Journal of Gerontology, 16*, 134–143.

Oswald, W. D., & Fleischmann, U. (1993). *Das Nürnberger Altersinventar (NAI).* Göttingen: Hogrefe.

Parmelee, P.A., Thuras, P.D., Katz, I., & Lawton, M. P. (1995). Validation of the Cumulative Illness Rating Scale in a Geriatric Residential Population. *Journal of the American Geriatrics Society, 43*, 130–137.

Rowe, J. W., & Kahn, R. L. (1998). *Successful aging.* New York: Pantheon Books.

Schaie, K. W., Wahl, H.-W., Mollenkopf, H., & Oswald, F. (Eds.). (2003). *Aging independently: Living arrangements and mobility.* New York: Springer.

Schulz, R., & Heckhausen, J. (1996). A life span model of successful aging. *American Psychologist, 51*, 702–714.

Steverink, N., Lindenberg, S., & Ormel, J. (1998). Towards understanding successful aging: Patterned chance in resources and goals. *Aging and Society, 18*, 441–467.

Tewes, U. (1991). Hamburg-Wechsler Intelligenztests für Erwachsene Revision—Handbuch und Testanweisung. Bern: Huber.

Wahl, H.-W., Scheidt, R., & Windley, P. (Ed.). (2004). *Annual Review of Gerontology and Geriatrics, 23* ("Aging in Context: Socio-Physical Environments"). New York: Springer Publication.

Wells, J. D., Hobfoll, S. E., & Larvin, J. (1999). When it rains, it pours: The greater impact of resource loss compared to gain on psychological distress. *Personality and Social Psychology Bulletin, 25*, 1172–1182.

DIETRICH ROTHENBACHER,[1] CHRISTOPH ROTT,[2]
DANIELA JOPP,[2] and HERMANN BRENNER[1]

DETERMINANTS, PROGNOSTIC RELEVANCE AND DEVELOPMENT OF ANXIETY AND DEPRESSION IN PATIENTS WITH CORONARY HEART DISEASE: AN INTERDISCIPLINARY APPROACH WITHIN THE KAROLA STUDY

Cardiovascular diseases are the leading cause of disability and death in developed countries and about half of all cases are directly attributable to coronary heart diseases (National Heart Lung and Blood Institute, 1998), which are a direct consequence of coronary atherosclerosis. The Framingham Study and other large-scale cohort studies have initiated the identification of a number of determinants and risk factors for atherosclerosis, such as male sex, obesity, smoking, physical inactivity, blood lipids, family history and others (Dawber, 1980).

In addition to somatic risk factors, psychological factors such as depression and anger are also thought to play a role in the etiology of coronary heart disease (CHD). That depression is an adverse prognostic factor for patients with acute myocardial infarction (MI) has been demonstrated in several studies (Rozanski, Blumenthal, & Kaplan, 1999). About 15–20% of patients with myocardial infarction experience major depression shortly after the manifestation of coronary artery disease in the case of MI. An independent inverse association of depressive symptoms after acute MI and five-year survival has been demonstrated (Lésperance, Frasure-Smith, Talajic, & Bourassa, 2002).

Because symptoms of anxiety and depression frequently coincide, as recently shown in patients with stroke (Aben, Verhey, Lousberg, Lodder, & Honig, 2002), and because the most common form of affective disorder is mixed anxiety-depression (Jenkins et al., 1997), a division and separate consideration of symptoms of anxiety and depression may not always be adequate (Shorter & Tyrer, 2003).

However, less clear is to what degree symptoms of anxiety and depression are present weeks after the acute phase of the first cardiovascular manifestation and whether these symptoms also affect prognosis. Several studies investigated the long-term development of symptoms of anxiety and depression in patients with coronary heart disease (Herrmann-Lingen & Buss, 2002; Lésperance et al., 2002). The study by Lespérance and colleagues on average revealed a slight decrease within a time period of 1 year in a group of patients with coronary heart disease, but also indicated interindividual differences in intraindividual change. Even if a change in depressive symptoms within

H.-W. Wahl et al. (eds.), The Many Faces of Health, Competence and Well-Being in Old Age, 211–221.

a 1-year period may not show a prognostic value (Lésperance et al., 2002), it would be very important to know the overall development of these symptoms and to identify differential patterns of change and their determinants in order to better understand the psychological process of dealing with a severe chronic disease over time. Several studies have demonstrated the impact of psychosocial resources on the course of coronary heart disease (e.g. Frasure-Smith et al., 2000; Lésperance et al., 2002, Slesina & Werdon, 2003). But patients with a limited amount of such resources (e.g. with a higher age, lower education, no job training and limited social support) may also be vulnerable for increased scores of symptoms of anxiety and depression. Thus, the investigation of the impact of resources on the course of symptoms of anxiety and depression after a severe cardiovascular event may also shed some light on the course of the coronary heart disease itself.

Furthermore, the prognostic relevance of symptoms of anxiety and depression in patients with coronary heart disease (CHD) would have important implications as it is currently largely unappreciated in clinical practice, although both effective pharmacological and psychotherapeutic interventions exist.

We conducted a prospective study in a large group of patients with coronary heart disease who were participating in an in-patient rehabilitation program to investigate the prevalence of symptoms of anxiety and depression within 3 months after first diagnosis of CHD and to determine the association of these symptoms with fatal and non-fatal cardiovascular disease events during a 1-year follow-up period. Furthermore, we wanted to investigate the course of symptoms of anxiety and depression and explore determinants of the symptom course.

1. DESCRIPTION OF THE KAROLA STUDY POPULATION

All patients with coronary heart disease (CHD) (International Classification of Diseases, 9th Rev. pos. 410–414) aged 30–70 years and participating in an in-patient rehabilitation program between January 1999 and May 2000 in one of two rehabilitation clinics in Germany (Schwabenland-Klinik, Isny and Klinik im Südpark, Bad Nauheim) were enrolled in the study (initial response 58%). In Germany, all patients with acute manifestation or surgical treatment of CHD are offered a comprehensive in-hospital rehabilitation program after discharge from the acute care hospital. The aim of this 3-week program is the reduction of cardiovascular disease risk factors, improvement of health related quality of life, and the preservation of the ability to work (latter only if a subject was at work at onset of the disease). This in-patient rehabilitation program begins approximately 3 weeks after the acute events or cardiac surgery but this time interval may be longer in some cases. In the current study only patients who were admitted within 3 months after the acute event or cardiac surgery were included. A follow-up was conducted 1 year later. All subjects gave written informed consent. The study was approved by the Ethics Boards of the Universities of Ulm and Heidelberg and of the Physicians' chamber of the States of Baden-Wuerttemberg and Hessen.

1.1. Data Collection

At the beginning of the in-patient rehabilitation program all subjects filled out a standardised questionnaire containing sociodemographic information and medical history. In addition, information was taken from the patients' hospital charts. In all patients a 12-lead ECG was recorded and they were submitted to a bicycle stress test at the beginning of the rehabilitation programme.

1.2. Follow-Up and Evaluation of Adverse Cardiovascular Events

In all patients follow-up was conducted 1 year after discharge from the rehabilitation clinic. Information was obtained from the patient himself by a mailed standardised questionnaire. A standardised questionnaire regarding cardiovascular disease events and treatment since discharge from the in-patient rehabilitation clinic was also obtained from the primary care physician. If a subject died during follow-up, the death certificate was obtained from local Public Health departments and the main cause of death was coded according to the International Classification of Diseases, 9th Revision.

Cardiovascular disease (CVD)-events during the first year of follow-up were defined as CVD as main cause of death, physician diagnosed non-fatal myocardial infarction, ischemic cerebrovascular event, or a coronary-revascularisation procedure, all as reported by the primary care physicians.

1.3. Assessment of Anxiety and Depressive Symptoms

Anxiety and depressive symptoms were evaluated at the end of rehabilitation (baseline) and after 1 year of follow-up by the German version of the Hospital Anxiety and Depression Scale (HADS-D). The HADS-D is a well-standardised self-assessment questionnaire containing 14 questions to identify and quantify generalised anxiety and depression (seven items each) in medical patients (Herrmann, 1997). All items are scored on a four point Likert scale from 0 to 3 points. A summary score is calculated both related to anxiety and depressive disorders. A test value $\geq$11 points is associated with a manifest anxiety or depressive disorder, values from 8 to 10 are of borderline significance, and values below 8 are regarded as normal (Herrmann, 1997). Reliability (Cronbach's alpha) of the anxiety subscale was $\alpha = 0.85$, the respective score for the depression subscale was $\alpha = 0.84$.

2. STATISTICAL METHODS

After describing the study population with respect to various sociodemographic and medical characteristics, the prevalence of anxiety and depressive symptoms and the distribution of the pertinent scores were determined. The relation of baseline anxiety and depression with CVD-events during follow-up was assessed by means of a chi-square test.

A multivariable analysis approach (unconditional logistic regression) was then employed to assess the independent association of symptoms of anxiety and depression on the risk of CVD-events. The following potential confounders were considered: body mass index, smoking status, duration of school education, family status, history of diabetes mellitus, HDL-cholesterol and additionally for severity of cardiovascular disease (number of affected vessels), history of myocardial infarction, treatment with beta-blockers, ACE-blockers, (as latter two might cause symptoms of depression as side effects), and antidepressants.

The changes of symptoms of anxiety and depression within a 1-year period were evaluated with an individual growth modelling technique (Raudenbush & Bryk, 2002; Singer & Willet, 2003). These models yield estimates of fixed effects, which describe the intercept and slope of the overall sample trajectory, and random effects, which describe the person-level trajectory in terms of their deviations (in intercept and slope estimates) from the overall trajectory. Because individual growth models do not allow the determination of a specific direction of a person's development, significant change on the individual level was determined using the one standard error of measurement approach (Schaie, 1996). This confidence band estimate provides a critical difference and is established by the reliability of the test and the variation of the respective variable at the first measurement point. If an individual score at follow-up had varied more than the critical difference this change is regarded as "significant." The predictors of patterns of change were evaluated by means of chi-square tests. All statistical procedures were carried out with the SAS statistical software package (version 8.2).

3. RESULTS

Overall, 1206 patients with a diagnosis of a CHD were included in the study at baseline during the in-patient-rehabilitation program. All patients had a newly diagnosed CHD within past 3 months. One-year follow-up information was complete for 981 patients (81.3%). Table 1 shows the main sociodemographic and medical characteristics of the study population.

Of the 981 patients with a diagnosis of CHD 58.5% had suffered from a myocardial infarction and 42.7% of the patients had a three-vessel disease including main stem stenosis. The mean age of CHD-patients was 58.9 years and most of them (56.6%) were between 60–70 years old, 85.2% were male and 84.3% were married. Most patients had a body mass index between 25 and 30 kg/m^2.

During the follow-up time of the first year, 133 (13.6%) fatal and non-fatal CVD-events occurred (combining fatal CVD, myocardial infarction, stroke or TIA without revascularisation procedures resulted in 42 events, or 4.3%). Of the 18 patients (1.8%) who died during follow-up, 13 died due to cardiovascular diseases. A revascularisation procedure was done in 103 (10.5%) of the patients, 29 (3.0%) and 8 (0.8%) patients suffered a non-fatal myocardial infarction, stroke or TIA, respectively

Table 2 shows the prevalences of symptoms of anxiety and depression at baseline and their relationship to fatal and non-fatal CVD-events. Of all patients with CHD, 16.0%

Table 1. Sociodemographic and medical characteristics of the patients with coronary heart disease

Characteristics at baseline	*CHD patients total = 981*
History of myocardial infarction, *n* (%)	574 (58.5)
Clinical score (angiographic evaluation)	
1 Vessel disease	264 (26.9)
2 Vessel disease	254 (25.9)
3 Vessel disease	419 (42.7)
Unknown	44 (4.5)
Age (yr)*, *n* (%)	58.9 ± 7.88
30–39	22 (2.2)
40–49	117 (11.9)
50–59	287 (29.3)
60–70	555 (56.6)
Male, *n* (%)	835 (85.2)
School education <10 yr, *n* (%)	589 (60.0)
Family status married, *n* (%)	827 (84.3)
Body mass index (kg/m^2)	27.2 ± 4.0
<25	289 (29.5)
25–30	518 (52.8)
>30	172 (17.5)
Cigarettes smoked (yes)	666 (67.9)
History of high blood pressure, *n* (%)	546 (55.7)
History of diabetes, *n* (%)	169 (17.3)

showed a borderline and 8.2% a manifest anxiety symptoms score, whereas 11.4% and 6.0% showed a borderline and manifest depressive symptoms score, respectively.

Of the patients who showed manifest anxiety symptoms, 22.5% experienced a CVD-event during follow-up compared to 13.5% and 12.2% of patients with a borderline or

Table 2. Prevalence of anxiety and depressive symptom score at baseline and relation to fatal and non-fatal CVD-events during 1-year follow-up

	N (Column %) Total = 973	*Fatal and non-fatal CVD-events during 1-year follow-up, n(Row%)*
Anxiety symptom score		
<8 (normal)	737 (75.8)	90 (12.2)
8–10	156 (16.0)	21 (13.5)
≥11	80 (8.2)	18 (22.5) P = 0.02
Depressive symptom score		
<8 (normal)	804 (82.6)	105 (13.1)
8–10	111 (11.4)	13 (11.7)
≥11	58 (6.0)	11 (19.0) P = 0.40

Table 3. Association of anxiety and depressive symptom score with fatal and non-fatal CVD-events during 1-year follow-up

	Results of multivariate analysis, OR (95% CI)		
	Adjusted for age and gender	Adjusted for multiple covariates*	Adjusted for multiple covariates†
Anxiety symptom score			
<8	1 Reference	1 Reference	1 Reference
8–10	1.09 (0.67–1.82)	1.12 (0.66–1.87)	1.05 (0.62–1.77)
≥11	1.95 (1.10–3.46)	1.91 (1.04–3.50)	2.11 (1.12–3.98)
Depressive symptom score			
<8	1 Reference	1 Reference	1 Reference
8–10	0.89 (0.48–1.65)	0.85 (0.46–1.59)	0.84 (0.44–1.59)
≥11	1.45 (0.73–2.91)	1.43 (0.70–2.91)	1.50 (0.71–3.14)

*Adjusted for body mass index, smoking status, duration of school education, family status, history of diabetes mellitus and HDL-cholesterol.

† Adjusted for above listed variables and additionally for severity of cardiovascular disease (number of affected vessels), history of myocardial infarction, treatment with beta-blockers, ACE-blockers and antidepressants at hospital discharge (baseline).

normal anxiety symptom score, respectively ($p = 0.02$). Of the patients who showed manifest depressive symptoms, 19.0% experienced a CVD-event during follow-up compared to 11.7% and 13.1% of patients with a borderline or normal symptom score, respectively ($p = 0.40$).

We then employed a multivariate analysis strategy to estimate the independent relationship of symptoms of anxiety and depression at baseline with the risk of a CVD-event during follow-up after adjustment for potentially confounding variables (Table 3). Compared to patients with a normal anxiety symptom score at baseline, patients having a borderline anxiety symptom score had an odds ratio (OR) of 1.09 (95% confidence interval (CI) 0.67–1.82) and patients with an increased symptom score had an OR of 1.95 (95 % CI 1.10–3.46) for a CVD-event during follow-up after adjustment for age and gender. The OR associated with an increased anxiety symptom score was similar after adjustment for multiple covariates and it was 2.11 (95% CI 1.12–3.98) after further adjustment for severity of CVD, history of myocardial infarction, treatment with beta-blockers, ACE-blockers and antidepressive medication (latter was taken by only $n = 18$ (1.8%) of the patients).

Compared to patients with a normal depressive symptom score at baseline, patients having a borderline depressive symptom score had an OR of 0.89 (95% CI 0.48–1.65) and patients with an increased symptom score had an OR of 1.45 (95 % CI 0.73–2.91) for a CVD-event during follow-up after adjustment for age and gender. After full adjustment the OR for a CVD-event associated with an increased depressive symptom score was 1.50 (95% CI 0.71–3.14).

The investigation of the course of symptoms of anxiety and depression over the 1-year follow-up period by means of individual growth curve modelling revealed an estimated mean level of 4.82 points for anxiety and of 4.34 points for depressive

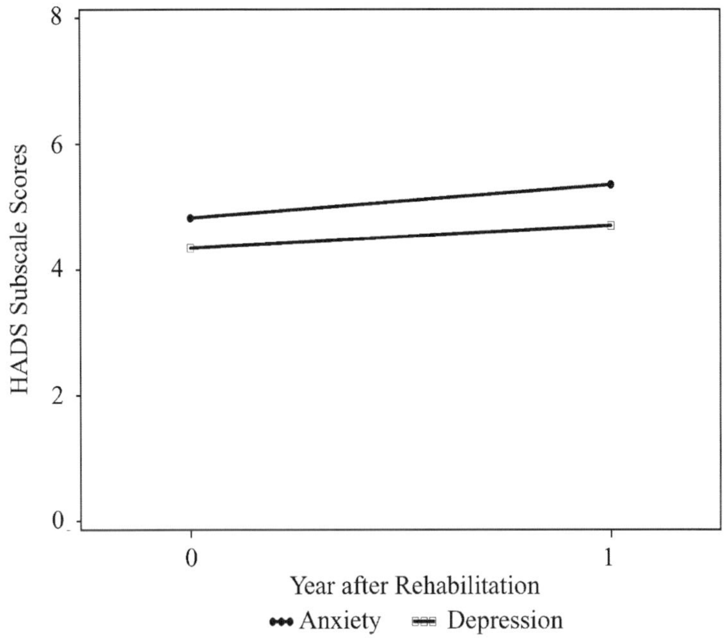

Figure 1. One year change in symptoms of anxiety and depression.

symptoms at baseline (end of rehab). The correlation between both affective disorders was substantial ($r = 0.74$, $p < 0.001$). Within both affective disorders, scores did not decline but increased significantly (see Figure 1), 0.53 for anxiety and 0.36 for depressive symptoms (both $p < 0.001$). In both domains the rate of change was uncorrelated with the initial level.

We then investigated whether the severity of the disease and basic sociodemographic factors made a difference in level and rate of change in symptoms of anxiety and depression. Patients suffering from a myocardial infarction had significantly higher anxiety scores compared to those with other coronary heart diseases (5.02 vs. 4.52, $p < 0.05$). The small difference in symptoms of depression failed to reach the 5% significance level. In both areas no differential change with respect to the kind of illness was evident. When assessing the impact of age and gender, only differences in level of anxiety and depressive symptoms occurred with no differences in change. Patients in their sixties had the lowest anxiety scores. All other age groups showed significantly elevated values compared to this reference group ($p < 0.001$ for age 40–49 and age 50–59). The difference for those under the age of 40 did not reach statistical significance. Regarding symptoms of depression, patients under the age of 40 and above age of 60 scored lowest. Compared to the reference group age 60 and above, subjects in their forties and fifties revealed significantly higher values (both $p < 0.05$). Men had lower anxiety scores compared to women ($p < 0.05$) but no gender differences in symptoms of depression emerged.

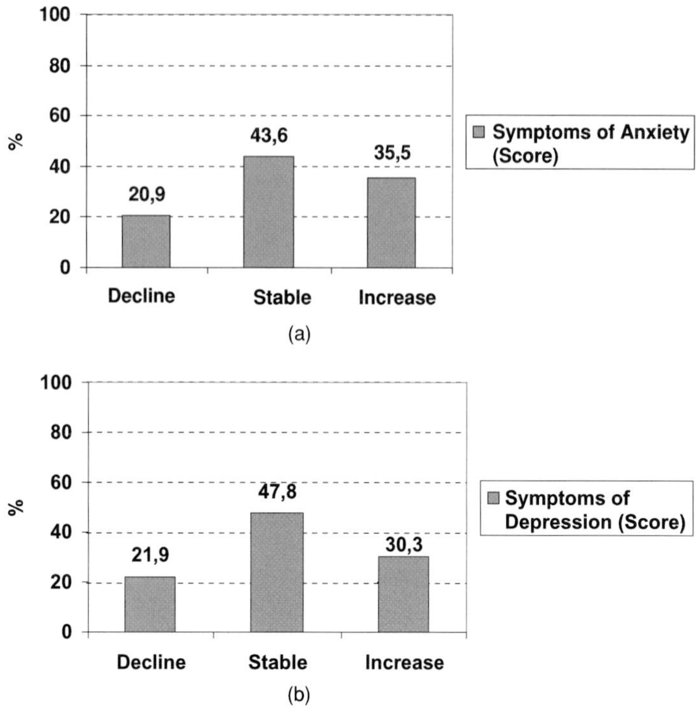

Figure 2. (a) Distribution of patients with declining, stable and increasing anxiety scores. (b) Distribution of patients with declining, stable and increasing depression scores.

Patients who have completed their job training had significantly lower scores in anxiety than those who did not receive any training ($p < 0.05$). No effect of job training was seen with respect to the level of symptoms of depression. However, in this area we found a trend that patients without job training had a steeper increase of depressive symptoms than those with job training ($p = 0.06$).

To evaluate significant changes in symptoms of anxiety and depression on the individual level, we first calculated the critical differences applying the one standard error of measurement approach. For anxiety it is 1.98, for depressive symptoms 1.91. This means that an individual change of two points or more on either scale is regarded as a "significant" change. With respect to anxiety, 20.9 % had declining scores, 43.6 % remained stable and 35.5 % revealed increasing scores (see Figure 2a). Regarding change in symptoms of depression, a similar pattern emerged: The scores of 21.9% declined, 47.8 % remained stable and 30.3 % showed higher scores at follow-up compared to baseline (see Figure 2b).

Because the symptoms of anxiety and depression showed a strong correlation we also defined correlated patterns of change, which represent increasingly negative change profiles. The first group consisted of patients with improvement in at least one symptom area and no increasing scores in the other (28.0 %). The second group (25.7%) consisted of patients with stable scores in anxiety and depression. The third group comprised patients who increased in one symptom score while showing stable or declining scores in the other. The proportion of this group amounts to 26.8 %. Pattern four characterises patients with deterioration in scores of anxiety as well as in scores of symptoms of depression, which was seen in 19.5 %. In a final step we evaluated whether the severity of the coronary heart disease (MI or other CHD) and the basic sociodemographic characteristics were differently distributed across the four patterns of change. However, none of these predictors was related to the patterns of change (all $p > 0.05$).

4. DISCUSSION

This prospective cohort study including 981 patients with recently diagnosed CHD aged 30–70 years demonstrated that symptoms of anxiety and depression were present in a considerable proportion of patients weeks after first diagnosis of CHD, and that these symptoms might be independent determinants of an increased risk for subsequent adverse cardiovascular events. The risk was twice as high in patients with generalised anxiety symptoms and it increased up to 50% in patients with a manifest depression, however, the latter association was only tentative.

The results of this study are in agreement with findings of others and add to the evidence (Barefoot et al., 1996; Connerney, Shapiro, McLaughlin, Bagiella, & Sloan, 2001; Kawachi et al., 1994; Lésperance et al., 2002; Rozanski et al., 1999; Stansfeld & Fuhrer, 2002) that affective disorders such as anxiety and depression are indeed independent determinants for prognosis in patients with CHD. A dose response relationship was found between phobic anxiety (which might represent, however, a very special form of anxiety) and fatal CHD in the US Health Professional's follow-up study (Kawachi et al., 1994). A small study including 207 men and 102 women who underwent coronary artery bypass graft surgery also demonstrated that depression is common among these patients and is an independent determinant for cardiac events recorded within 12 months (Connerney et al., 2001). Evidence has also been delivered that these effects not only mirror an early selective mortality, they rather seem to persist until later stages of the follow-up (Barefoot et al., 1996). This is in line with our findings as the overall course of both anxiety and depressive symptoms did not decline but slightly increased within 1 year after. The observation that only the level of the symptoms, especially that of anxiety but not the rate of change, was influenced by the severity of the illness and selected sociodemographic factors points also in the same direction. The identification of different patterns of change within one domain and across the two domains suggests that the slight overall increase in both symptoms over 1 year of follow-up may have various origins. Patients may have a quite different course. Only about one-third of the patients showed more symptoms in each domain compared to baseline results and one-fifth deteriorated in both. These groups may be especially physically and psychologically vulnerable for reasons that we do not yet understand.

The following limitations of our study should be considered. Although we had a large sample of patients with CHD (over 50% with a MI), fatal-CVD events were rare in this study population. This might be explained by the fact that mortality of MI is highest within the pre- and early in-hospital phase. As the acute events leading to diagnosis of CHD or MI had occurred at least 3 weeks before inclusion in this study, we were dealing with a selection of patients with a better prognosis compared to a patient population within the early phase of a newly diagnosed CHD. Furthermore, not all patients of course are willing or able to participate in a rehabilitation program. This is another reason why severely ill-patients are probably underrepresented in our study sample.

Furthermore, the present study did not have the power to find a weak association between e.g. depressive symptoms and CVD-events; it had a power of 80% to detect an OR of 2.7 ($\alpha = 0.05$) or larger and this may explain why the 95% CI of the point estimate of the depressive symptom score for risk of future CVD-events, although increased to 50%, included the null-value. From a developmental perspective, another limitation is that only two measurement points were available, which is a limited basis for individual growth modelling. In addition, we have not yet investigated whether individual psychological resources that have been found to serve as protective buffers in stress and coping studies also operate with respect to anxiety and depressive symptoms in cardiovascular patients, such as positive subjective health, the absence of worrying or social support.

In conclusion, the results of this study and the so far available evidence from the literature have clinical and therapeutic implications and suggest that depression and anxiety are also present weeks, months and perhaps years after a newly diagnosed CHD. Therefore, we suggest that anxiety and depression should be regularly evaluated on a routine basis and be part of secondary prevention like other established risk factors, such as lipids and blood pressure. And finally, more research should be focussed on psychological resources and processes that may play a role in coping with such a severe illness like coronary heart disease in order to improve both the quality of life and the prognosis of affected respective patients.

AFFILIATIONS

[1]*Department of Epidemiology*

[2]*Department of Adult Development, German Centre for Research on Ageing at the University of Heidelberg*

REFERENCES

Aben, I., Verhey, F., Lousberg, R., Lodder, J., & Honig, A. (2002). Validity of the Beck Depression Inventory, Hospital Anxiety and Depression Scale, SLC-90, and Hamilton Depression Rating Scale as screening instruments for depression in stroke patients. *Psychosomatics, 43*, 386–393.

Barefoot, J. C., Helms, M. J., Mark, D. B., Blumenthal, J. A., Califf, R. M., Haney, T. L., O'Connor, C. M., Siegler, I. C., & Williams, R. B. (1996). Depression and long-term mortality risk in patients with coronary artery disease. *The American Journal of Cardiology, 78*, 613–617.

Connerney, I., Shapiro, P. A., McLaughlin, J. S., Bagiella, E., & Sloan, R. P. (2001). Relation between depression after coronary artery bypass surgery and 12-month outcome: A prospective study. *Lancet, 358*, 1766–1771.

Dawber, T. R. (1980). *The Framingham study: The epidemiology of atherosclerotic disease*. Cambridge, MA: Harvard University Press.

Frasure-Smith, N., Lespérance, F., Gravel, G., Masson, A., Juneau, M., & Talajic, M. (2000). Social support, depression and mortality during the first year after myocardial infarction. *Circulation, 101*, 1919–1924.

Herrmann, C. (1997). International experiences with the hospital anxiety and depression scale-a review of validation data and clinical results. *Journal of Psychosomatic Research, 42*, 17–41.

Herrmann-Lingen, C., & Buss, U. (2002). *Angst und Depressivität im Verlauf der koronaren Herzkrankheit*. Frankfurt: Verlag für Akademische Schriften.

Jenkins, R., Lewis, G., Bebbington, P., Brugha, T., Farrell, M., & Gill, B. (1997). The national psychiatric morbidity surveys of Great-Britain—initial findings from the household survey. *Psychological Medicine, 27*, 775–789.

Kawachi, I., Colditz, G. A., Ascherio, A., Rimm, E. B., Giovannucci, E., Stampfer, M. J., & Willett, W. C. (1994). Prospective study of phobic anxiety and risk of coronary heart disease in men. *Circulation, 89*, 1992–1997.

Lésperance, F., Frasure-Smith, N., Talajic, M., & Bourassa, M. G. (2002). Five-year risk of cardiac mortality in relation to initial severity and one-year changes in depression symptoms after myocardial infarction. *Circulation, 105*, 1049–1053.

National Heart, Lung and Blood Institute. (1998). *Morbidity & mortality: 1998 chartbook on cardiovascular, lung, and blood diseases*. Rockville, MD: National Institute of Health.

Raudenbush, S. W., & Bryk, A. S. (2002). *Hierarchical linear models: Applications and data analysis methods (2nd ed.)*. Thousand Oaks, CA: Sage.

Rozanski, A., Blumenthal, J. A., & Kaplan, J. (1999). Impact of psychological factors on the pathogenesis of cardiovascular disease and implications for therapy. *Circulation, 99*, 2192–2217.

Schaie, K. W. (1996). Intellectual development in adulthood. The Seattle Longitudinal Study. Cambridge: Cambridge University Press.

Shorter, E., & Tyrer, P. (2003). Separation of anxiety and depressive disorders: Blind alley in psychopharmacology and classification of disease. *British Medical Journal, 327*, 158–160.

Singer, J. D., & Willet, J. B. (2003). *Applied longitudinal data analysis*. New York: Oxford University Press.

Slesina, W., & Werdon, K. (2003). *Psychosoziale Faktoren der koronaren Herzkrankheit*. Stuttgart: Schatthauer.

Stansfeld, S., & Fuhrer, R. (2002). *Depression and coronary heart disease*. London, UK: BMJ Books.

K. WARNER SCHAIE

COMMENTARY: INTERDISCIPLINARY LONGITUDINAL STUDIES OF AGEING

If one is interested in exploring the antecedent variables that differentiate groups of individuals with different demographic characteristics such as age, gender, or region of residence, one needs to look for data sets that have followed such groups over time. Hence, multi-disciplinary studies are increasingly common and two prime examples the ILSE and KAROLA studies are described in this volume (Rothenbacher, Rott, Jopp, & Brenner; Schmitt, Oswald, Jopp, Wahl, & Brenner). Before commenting on these studies, I will raise some issues common to interdisciplinary studies in general, and show a conceptual framework from my own Seattle Longitudinal study to illustrate how any major longitudinal study investigating aging processes is likely to become interdisciplinary whether it started in that manner or not. I then comment on some design issues relevant to both ILSE and KAROLA. Finally, I comment briefly on the power of interdisciplinary longitudinal studies of aging.

1. ISSUES IN INTERDISCIPLINARY STUDIES

1.1. Different Levels of Reductionism

One of the major issues in the design of interdisciplinary studies is to deal with the levels of reductionism involved. The principal initiator of the study will generally perceive the data of his discipline to provide the basic dependent variables. Nevertheless, as soon as other disciplines are added, one or more of the original dependent variables may well be perceived by another discipline instead as the their independent variables. While there may be many levels of potential influences (e.g. environmental, societal, individual, physiological system or cellular levels), the use of more than two or three levels of reductionism may be problematic, especially when each level may exert direct and/or indirect influences or may serve as a moderator of influences at other levels.

1.2. Communication Problems

Most interdisciplinary studies include scientists whose technical vocabulary may differ widely. Hence, one of the first issues for effective collaborative relationships across disciplines consists of gaining a full understanding of the technical terms of neighbouring disciplines. The same terms may denote rather different constructs.

H.-W. Wahl et al. (eds.), The Many Faces of Health, Competence and Well-Being in Old Age, 223–230.

1.3. Asymmetrical Advances in State-of-the-Art

Different disciplines advance in an asymmetric fashion. Constructs that remain at a taxonomic level in one field may have attained precise and reliable measurement in another. Sampling strategies at a macro-societal level may aspire to obtain representative populations while studies of individual differences may instead call for sampling the entire range of the phenomenon studied. Likewise, state-of-the-art statistical analyses will differ markedly across different disciplines. Hence, compatibility of data across different disciplines may be compromised with respect to reliability of measurement, comparability of sampling approaches as well as precision of data analyses. Most of these issues, of course, require some compromises in order to enable interdisciplinary research approaches.

2. EXAMPLE FROM THE SEATTLE LONGITUDINAL STUDY

Figure 1 shows a conceptual framework for the Seattle Longitudinal Study (Schaie, 2005) that illustrates both the advantages and disadvantages of operating within an interdisciplinary framework of longitudinal research. The Seattle study began as a narrow inquiry on the relationship of age differences in cognitive abilities to age differences in personality and cognitive styles (Schaie, 1958). Given the scientific climate of the times it was seen as a strictly intra-disciplinary inquiry. It soon became clear that the questions raised required a longitudinal approach that allowed definition of alternative patterns of antecedents of change in cognitive function across adulthood. These concerns soon led to the recognition that data collection and analysis strategies had to move beyond those available to a single discipline.

To understand intellectual development from early adulthood to old age we tried to embed what we know about such development within the context of changing environmental influences and changes in individuals' physiological infrastructure. Figure 1 contains two endpoints: The first is concerned with those influences that affect the level of late-life cognitive functioning. A second endpoint of interest, however, is the

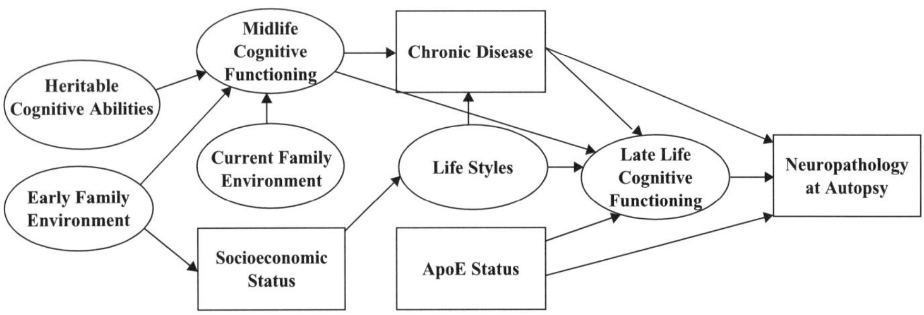

Figure 1. Conceptual framework for the Seattle Longitudinal Study (adapted from Schaie, 2005, p. 8)

status of the cortex at life's end that would describe the neural infrastructure required for the maintenance of cognitive functioning; often determinable only at post mortem. Figure 1 should be interpreted as a conceptual path model; rectangles are used to identify indicators that are observed directly while ovals indicate the latent constructs that would be inferred from measurement models for sets of observed variables.

Let me now try to explicate some of the attributes of the heuristic model in Figure 1 in terms of their implications for the need of interdisciplinary inquiry. First, the initial bases for the development of adult intelligence must be attributed to both heritable (genetic) influences as well as to early environmental influences typically experienced within the home of the biological parents. Although some of the behaviour genetic literature suggests that much of the early environmental variance is non-shared (e.g. Plomin & Daniels, 1987), there is recent retrospective evidence of some early shared environmental influences upon later cognitive performance (Schaie & Zuo, 2001). Both generic and early environmental factors influence midlife cognitive functioning. Early environmental influences also exert influences on midlife social status (Nguyen, 2000). By contrast, virtually no correlations have been found between retrospective accounts of family environments in the family of origin and the current family, although the current family environment does influence midlife cognitive performance (Schaie & Willis, 1995). Genetic factors are also likely to be implicated in the rate of cognitive decline in adulthood. The best-studied gene in this context is the *Apo-E* gene, one of whose alleles is thought to be a risk factor for Alzheimer's disease. *Apo-E* status is therefore also added as a factor in midlife; the expression of this gene is probably not important prior to midlife.

A number of causal influences can be specified that determine level of intellectual functioning in late life as well as cortical status at autopsy. The direct influences to be implicated in addition to genes that are turned on in late life, most likely originate in midlife. They include level of cognitive functioning in midlife, midlife life styles and the incidence and severity of chronic disease. There are also indirect influences attributable to the effects of midlife cognitive function and life styles upon chronic disease, as well as shared family influences on midlife cognition and of social status upon midlife life styles.

Recognition of these relationships in the Seattle study was largely influenced by the investigators being imbedded in interdisciplinary settings and being influenced by colleagues in other disciplines. Our work on to the impact of social structures and individual micro-environments on cognitive change (cf. Schaie & O'Hanlon, 1990) was influenced early on by the writing of Matilda Riley (Riley, 1985; Riley, Johnson, & Foner, 1972) and later on by the work of Schooler (1972, 1987, 1990), as well as many other sociologists, anthropologists and epidemiologists. Colleagues conducting research on chronic disease furthermore convinced us that we needed to consider the relation between chronic disease and cognitive change (Bosworth & Schaie, 1997, 1999; Gruber-Baldini, 1991; Hertzog, Schaie, & Gribbin, 1978, Schaie, 2005).

Collaboration with Robert Plomin, a noted developmental behaviour geneticist, allowed us to take advantage of our longitudinal database to collect data to implement a study of cognitive family resemblance in adulthood. We did this by adding a large number of adult offspring and siblings of our longitudinal panel members (Schaie, Plomin, Willis, Gruber-Baldini, & Dutta, 1992; Schaie et al. 1993; Schaie & Willis, 1995; Schaie & Zuo, 2001).

Collaboration with Sherry Willis, an educational psychologist, resulted in mounting a major intervention study to implement educational training as a procedure designed to slow or reverse loss in cognitive function with age (Schaie & Willis, 1986; Willis & Schaie, 1986, 1988).

Finally, we expanded into the fields of neuropsychology and neuropathology to consider end-of-life outcomes by expanding our efforts into the clinical assessment of cognitive impairment and collaborative work on neural correlates of behaviour change involving collaboration with colleagues in neuropsychology, neurology, neuro-imaging and neuropathology (cf. Schaie et al. 2005, for an early example of this work).

Each of the expansions into adding the expertise of additional disciplines has raised new problems in trying to bridge assumptions and methods of different disciplines. Nevertheless, we could not have fully exploited the potential of our work without taking the interdisciplinary approach.

3. THE ILSE STUDY

I will first comment briefly on the particular advantages and limitations of the ILSE study design and then address some of the substantive issues.

3.1. Design Issues

The ILSE Study represents an application of the minimal requirements of the *cross-sequential* design (Schaie, 1977). It includes two birth cohorts differing on average by 16 year who were followed over the same time period (i.e. 4 years on average, from 1993/1996 to 2000/2003). It should be noted that this design confounds age with both cohort and time. Although it is not possible in this design to resolve this confounds, conclusions will be valid when comparing intra-cohort changes over time, while disregarding age. In other words, differences in change over 4 years observed in the study cannot be directly attributed to the age difference between the two cohorts, but are more likely attributable to the differential prior experience of these cohorts ILSE.

The *cross-regional sampling* is one of the major strengths of the ILSE Study. Because of the natural experiment of differential prior experiences across the two regions for one of the two cohorts, it would be possible to conduct an independent test of the age vs. cohort differences hypothesis. To do so one would merely need to enter the age group by region interaction into the regression analyses.

The methods section of this paper indicates that only study participants who were available at both T1 and T2 entered the analyses. Unfortunately, no data were provided on participant attrition. Unless attrition is trivial (say <5% of original participants) it would be important to consider attrition differences in initial performance with respect both age group and region.

3.2. *Substantive Issues*

Internal resources appear to be rather narrowly restricted to four of Costa and McCrae's (1992) personality factors and a single omnibus measure of cognitive functioning. In particular, it should be noted that the first factor extracted from a WAIS type intelligence scale has generally been identified as being overdetermined by *Gf* (fluid intelligence) in prior research. However, previous studies of the relationship between cognitive abilities and health and/or well-being outcomes (cf. Bosworth, Schaie, & Willis, 1999) have found that measures of *Gc* (crystallized intelligence) involving culturally acquired skills are the best outcome predictors. It is likely, therefore, that an index based on the WAIS sub-scales that reflect *Gc* would account for a greater proportion of outcome variance than the single-factor score entered into the analyses reported in this paper. Other intrinsic psychological factors that warrant further investigation might involve variables such as ego-strength and group dependency, or Costa and McCrae's fifth factor a*greeableness*.

The variables chosen to define external resources are not unreasonable. They vary, however, from items where respondents should be expected to have adequate information to provide semi-objective information (e.g. education, income, housing characteristics), to rather subjective scales where each respondent has to form their own scale reference (e.g. health, well-being). As a consequence scales must vary substantially in reliability (nor reported in this paper), which along could account for some of the low or non-significant predictive value of these resource characteristics.

It is not clear why well-being, measured in this study, was not used as an outcome criterion. All the more curious is the decision to characterize participation in leisure activities as a measure of "competence," and use this measure as an outcome variable. Recently there has been an interest in studying participation in leisure activities as a possible mechanism of maintaining "cognitive competence" in the elderly (cf. Wilson et al., 2002). However, leisure activities are typically used as an independent rather than as an outcome variable. In a normal well functioning population sample such as ILSE it seems more likely that high involvement in leisure activities could be an expression of "busyness" or of an extroversive temperament, as is suggest by the reported values in Table 2 (Schmitt et al., this volume).

The ILSE Study is a useful example of the added power obtained when different disciplines (in this case behavioural and social scientists as well as epidemiologists interact with each other). It could, however be strengthened markedly, if more objective health and behavioural outcomes were investigated directly.

4. THE KAROLA STUDY

As a cognitive psychologist I feel a lot less comfortable in providing substantive comments on the KAROLA study. However, there are a number of design and analysis issues that seem important of attention.

Design Issues. The KAROLA study is a large longitudinal follow-up of patients with coronary heart disease participating in two German rehabilitation clinics. The

Schooler, C. (1987). Psychological effects of complex environments during the life span: A review and theory. In C. Schooler & K. W. Schaie (Eds.), *Cognitive functioning and social structure over the life course* (pp. 24–49). Norwood, NJ: Ablex.

Schooler, C. (1990). Psychosocial factors and effective cognitive functioning in adulthood. In J. E. Birren & K. W. Schaie (Eds.), *Handbook of the psychology of aging* (3rd ed., pp. 347–358). San Diego, CA: Academic Press.

Willis, S. L., & Schaie, K. W. (1986). Training the elderly on the ability factors of spatial orientation and inductive reasoning. *Psychology and Aging, 1*, 239–247.

Willis, S. L., & Schaie, K. W. (1988). Gender differences in spatial ability in old age: Longitudinal and intervention findings. *Sex Roles, 18*, 189–203.

Wilson, R., Mendes de Leon, C. F., Barnes, L. L., Schneider, J., Buenias, J. L., Evans, D. A., et al. (2002). Participation in cognitively stimulating activities and risk of incident Alzheimer disease. *Journal of the American Medical Association, 287*, 720–748.

PART V

APPLICATIONS AND SOCIAL POLICY IMPLICATIONS

ALAN WALKER

AGEING EUROPE: CHALLENGES FOR POLICY AND RESEARCH

This chapter (based on a public lecture) provides an overview of the research and policy challenges facing European societies as they age—a tall order—and it was tempting to jettison one-half of the brief that I was given. However it is essential to connect science and policy. In fact it is remarkable how often scientific evidence is neglected in discussions on social policy and nowhere is this more true than with regard to population ageing. Here unsubstantiated rhetorical assertions have frequently dominated the policy process. The chapter critically assesses the most common assertions that are made about population ageing and argues that the label "crisis" is misplaced and that the idea that ageing is a threat to health care systems is a fallacy. Then it examines briefly the five major challenges that are created by the ageing populations of the European Union (EU) and argues that, in some respects they are also opportunities. There are five common policy challenges being faced by the EU: safeguarding economic security in old age; maintaining intergenerational solidarity; combating age discrimination; providing social care in the context of changes in the family and residence patterns and ensuring that older people experience full citizenship and are not socially excluded. Each of them pre-existed the enlargement on 1 May 2004 but this has extended the range of institutions and practices in the EU and made more urgent the need for action.

Following this brief review the chapter is equally brief about the relationship between science and policy. Then, finally, it looks at the challenges facing research in this field and how we might begin to create an integrated research agenda in Europe. This section draws on the work of the FORUM project which, for the past 2 years, has been working with scientists and end users of research to try to develop common European research priorities. To start with, it is important in a public lecture such as this to address the so-called ageing crisis.

1. CONSTRUCTING THE AGEING CRISIS: APOCALYPTIC DEMOGRAPHY

As a result of the unique combination of declining fertility and falling death rates leading to increasing longevity, the EU is ageing—though the rate differs between Member States and, especially, between regions. In a large number of the 'old' EU15 regions the population had stopped growing by the end of the last century. This will extend to the majority of these EU regions which will see their population levelling off or declining before 2015. The younger generation, the 0–24 age group, represented 31.1% of the population in 1995, and this will decline to 27% in 2015 (some 11 million

H.-W. Wahl et al. (eds.), The Many Faces of Health, Competence and Well-Being in Old Age, 233–244.

less). The older generation (65+) will increase, significantly and unevenly, throughout the EU. In some regions of France, Italy and Spain the 80 plus generation will represent between 7% and 9% of the population (compared with an average 3.9% in 1995). As a consequence the average age of the EU15's population will increase from 38.3 years in 1995 to 41.8 in 2015. The additional impact of migration means that, in some regions in eastern Germany, northern Italy, central France and northern Spain, the average age will be between 44 and 50 years in 2015.

The growth of the very old (80+) will be the strongest, in terms of intensity. A large share of the total increase in this cohort over the next 25 years (plus 62% between 1995 and 2025) is taking place within the 5-year period 2000–2005. Within these 5 years the increase will be above 25% in Belgium and France, and almost as much in Italy and Austria. The average increase in the EU will be 18.6%. Italy leads the way (yet again in demographic terms): in 2025, 7.1% or one in every 14 Italians, will be over 80. Germany comes next, due to the pre-war baby boom, and Denmark, Sweden and Ireland will follow after 2020. In Germany those over the age of 60 will comprise nearly two-fifths of the population by 2050 (compared with just under a quarter today) while those over 80 will be around one in every eight Germans. Life expectancy at birth is 81 years for women and 75 years for men. Centenarians are a key indicator of longevity and, in this country now there are some 7,200 people aged 100 or more. By 2050 this number will have grown 16 times to 115,000 or roughly one in every 600 Germans. The gender division in this story is the same here as in other EU countries: by 2050 nearly one in every six women will be aged 80 and over compared with one in 10 men.

The Eastern European countries are also experiencing demographic ageing. All of them, except Poland, will see a decline in the total population (and that of working age) before 2010. The EU shares demographic ageing with other world regions though, with Japan, it has the most pronounced trend over the next 20 years.

These are remarkable transformations in age structures but there are very few signs that policy makers and the public in general grasp their revolutionary nature. In practice sensible debate about what it means to be an ageing society is prevented by the crisis mentality that exists among some policy makers on this topic. Ageing populations are seen as a threat to health care systems (and pension systems too). Apocalyptic demography has prevented rational debate about the challenges of ageing and, in some countries, has led to short-term fixes rather than longer term planned solutions. However ageing populations are not a crisis. All of the challenges ageing societies face are subject to policy influence.

First of all it must be remembered that increasing longevity is an indicator of social and economic progress: the triumph of science and public policy over many of the causes of premature death which truncated lives in earlier times. The EU and the whole developed world should take pride in the fact that increasing numbers of citizens are able to reach advanced old age and to do so in relative economic security. Secondly nowhere is there is a simple connection between demographic change and the demand for spending on social policy and welfare, still less with the *levels* of such spending.

In fact with regard to health and social care systems demography, by itself, is a secondary element in the increase in health spending. The key factor is the use of technology and the cost of medical inputs, combined with the high level of care at older ages. Significant too is the extent to which social care is provided within institutions (Jacobzone, 1999). Thus, although there is a strong cross-sectional relationship between age and health based on individual data, at the aggregate level there is no connection between the proportion of the population aged 65 and over and the relative levels of health expenditure as a share of GDP. In other words, there is no demographic imperative (Scherer, 1996) and it is a fallacy that ageing is a threat to health and social care systems.

When we look at the need and demand for formal health and social care services it is not ageing that is the main issue but, rather, health status and a range of social factors as well, especially family relationships: marriage patterns, fertility, household composition and living arrangements. For example we know that those living alone tend to make greater use of formal services than those living with others (partly because of the correlation between advanced old age and living alone) and the proportion living alone is rising. The impact of divorce is less clear: who will care for tomorrow's step-grandmothers and step-grandfathers? In certain instances there is a more direct connection between health in old age and the demand for formal services, including acute episodes such as stroke and long-term impairment such as dementia. Cognitive impairment is one of the main reasons why older people enter long-term institutional care. The prevalence of moderate or severe cognitive impairment rises steeply with age—from 2.3% in those aged 65–74, to 7.2% in those aged 75–84, and to 21.9% in those aged 85 and older. Undoubtedly dementia causes acute problems for family carers and there is a need for special measures to support the care of this group. Moreover the under-diagnosis of depression in old age is well known (and linked to other morbidities and suicide among men).

Another danger of apocalyptic demography is that, when confronted with current evidence on the incidence of functional incapacity, including cognitive impairment, this is simply projected into the future: more very elderly people means much more disability. But the scientific evidence tells a rather different story. In fact what is happening in all developed countries is that, not only is life expectancy increasing but so to is disability-free life expectancy. Moreover there is a parallel increase in very severe disability-free life expectancy.

In other words there is a clear unambiguous trend to increasing disability-free life expectancy. Thus Manton, Stallard, and Riggan's (1982) theory of dynamic equilibrium which suggested that, with a decline in mortality, the prevalence of chronic diseases increases but the diseases are on average less severe and result in disability less often, has been demonstrated by the time series data on disability-free life expectancy. As Robine (2003) has shown the decline in mortality among the very elderly in the 1980s and 1990s was accompanied by an increase in the prevalence of chronic diseases, however these conditions were, on average, less severe and less often led to severe levels of disability. The implications of this development are massive, not only in terms of undermining the apocalyptic case. It suggests that each future generation may use less services than the previous one. If European countries had based current provision on the disability projections of 20 years ago they might have had 50–70% more long-term beds.

While the negative implications of population ageing have been over-stated there is no doubt that it presents some key challenges for policy and it is to those that the chapter now turns.

2. AGEING EUROPE: THE POLICY CHALLENGES

Turning to the five key policy challenges facing Europe, it is important to emphasise the advantageous position of the EU in responding to them. All of the world's major public welfare systems are found in the EU and it has some of the longest established institutions with regard to old age.

First, although they boast the most superior pension systems in the world the EU countries are still unable to ensure that all older people experience economic security. Poverty is a persistent problem among a minority (and this varies substantially by group) and there are large inequalities between the incomes of older and middle-aged people. In addition there are two major divisions in economic security, based on age and gender, that pension systems have reinforced rather than reduced. On the one hand older pensioners tend to have lower incomes than more recently retired and, in some countries, are excluded from pension provision. On the other hand, older women are likely to have lower incomes than older men and are much more likely to be poor. Putting together these age and gender influences means that very elderly women are usually the most deprived and excluded.

With regard to pension system sustainability the main issue is not population ageing *per se* but its combination with changes in the structure of employment and especially the practice of retirement. In a very short space of time there has been a major restructuring of the life course in most developed countries resulting from the ending of employment prior to pension ages (Kohli, Rein, Guillemard, & van Gunsteren, 1991; Walker, 1997, 1999). In some EU countries this was a trend openly encouraged by public policy. Thus, paradoxically, as longevity has increased, the age at which people exit from economic activity has fallen. This means that a gradual restoration of employment among older workers and a postponement of retirement, coupled with other modest reforms, can ensure the sustainability of pension systems in the EU, and these provide the highest public pensions in the world.

Secondly because intergenerational relations are not only a basic building block of social cohesion but also crucial for both pension and health care funding *and* for family care, the challenge for ageing societies is to ensure that, as the age structure changes, the preservation of intergenerational solidarity becomes a clear objective of policy. For example, Austria has an explicit generational impact assessment for new policy proposals. What is required is a new approach to intergenerational relations. Rather than seeing generations as competing for welfare it is more helpful to adopt a life course perspective, such as that proposed by Daniels (1998) in his concept of the "prudential life-span account". This approach allows for the development of guidelines for distribution and redistribution between the life stages under the assumption that everyone can expect the same treatment over their life course. This sort of approach would facilitate a more open and active management of resource distribution between the generations than is presently the case. It would also allow the long-term generational impact of policies to be better integrated in decision-making.

Thirdly, age discrimination represents a huge challenge. It is a source of stigma, social exclusion and the denial of full citizenship and, in the labour market, it denies older people the chance of making an economic contribution. The prevention of age discrimination in employment is, of course, a matter of social justice. But, in an ageing society, this imperative is reinforced by the need to respond to the ageing of the workforce.

Fourthly, with regard to social care, the main policy challenge is how to fill the care gap left by the unique combination of increased longevity and declining fertility? It is not realistic to expect the family to shoulder the sole responsibility for care. The fear that providing support to families will weaken their commitment to care and result in a massive burden on the public finances has led some policy makers to ignore the obvious fact that the family is changing rapidly and requires new forms of support if it is to continue to care. But currently in the EU there are major variations between countries in their provision for long-term care, for example in the field of home care.

What is needed now is an expansion of social care support, in the community, to enable care to be shared between the family and the formal sector. The boomer generation is likely to want both high quality and tailor made community support and certainly not large-scale residential care. When the boomers call for residential care they will be very severely disabled. The most effective form of support is likely to be multi-skilled community workers who are capable of both basic nursing and social care tasks, thereby overcoming the common barrier between health and social care. In addition care systems need to restore their preventative role and their rehabilitation role. Methods of paying for this expansion of long-term care are likely to be country-specific. Thus, there are different models in the EU based on taxation (Scandinavia) and social insurance (Germany), which are designed to share the costs and pool the risks between the individual and society.

Lastly there are the policy challenges presented by the new politics of old age—the main question here is what roles should older people occupy in the older, more age-balanced societies we are heading towards? The main challenge is to develop new roles and statuses and new attitudes commensurate with the transformation of age structures.

There is undoubtedly already a new mode of political activism on the part of older people which is almost guaranteed to be stepped up by the boomer generation. The advent of self-advocacy and a strong consumerist orientation among the new generation of older people poses a clear challenge to service providers. That is, how can they develop approaches that enable service users and carers to genuinely participate in decision-making? In some care systems this basic human right is lost in the process of becoming a client and even well intentioned professionals may, in effect, disenfranchise older people from making crucial decisions about their own lives. This challenge to policy makers and service providers is how to create a more equal and effective partnership with the citizens they serve?

Looking beyond the health and social services, ageing societies demand that policy makers explore new ways of involving older people in decision-making (there are plenty of examples in EU countries, see Naegele & Walker, 1999) and new roles to ensure that continuing opportunities are available for participation and self-fulfilment. This also requires a recognition by policy makers of the contribution already being made by older people to families, to communities and to wider society.

In essence, these five policy challenges are indicative of the Rileys' (Riley, Kahn, & Foner, 1994) famous structural lag thesis, because they demonstrate that Europe's policy and practice systems have not yet adjusted to the ageing of societies. They have not grasped the fundamental, far-reaching implications of this radical change in age structures. At the same time, therefore, they represent opportunities to change the nature of European societies to make them more age friendly, for example, in the labour market, in building design, in transport, in cultural pursuits and so on. Elsewhere I have argued that the strategy to achieve this is active ageing (Walker, 2002).

3. CONNECTING SCIENCE AND POLICY

How can science contribute to meeting these policy challenges? Let me acknowledge at once that some scientists do not want to engage with the policy and practice worlds but see their role as purely one of generating robust evidence which policy makers and practitioners may take up if they wish. This is a matter of individual choice but it is important to recognise that this position relies heavily on enlightenment in the policy and practice worlds if progress is to be made, for example, in improving the quality of life of older people. Other scientists regard it as a matter of duty to try to realise the benefits of research for older people by engaging with policy makers and practitioners, but this can be a frustrating and time-consuming business. Moreover there are few personal rewards in terms of scientific recognition and professional standing associated with what is regarded by many scientists as peripheral activity.

Nonetheless the goal surely should be for policy and practice in the ageing field to be as strongly evidence-based as possible. If scientists do not engage in this task, who will? Even for those scientists committed to this endeavour there is no guarantee whatsoever that even the most unequivocal research findings will be used by policy makers and practitioners. One reason for this is the complexity of the relationship between science and policy/practice. In fact it is often characterised by misunderstandings on both sides. On the one hand policy makers sometimes have completely unrealistic expectations about research (assuming they consider it all), especially with regard to time frames. On the other hand researchers often mistakenly expect scientific rationality from the policy making process: the engineering model where evidence leads automatically to changes in policy and practice. This is almost never the case and, therefore, many research findings miss their target.

In the absence of a simple rational model of policy making the best that scientists can do is to try to permeate the process to try to influence the *context* in which policies are made, as well as more direct methods such as taking part in policy initiatives such as official investigations. The UK Growing Older Programme used a range of strategies to try to ensure that research findings made their way into the policy system—targetted workshops, summary findings, briefings—but this demanded both central resources and commitment from the researchers involved (http://www.shef.ac.uk/uni/rojects/gop/) (Walker and Hagan Hennessy, 2005; Walker, 2005). We know that the findings reached their targets and that they have certainly had an impact on the context in which policy is being made, but any evidence of specific policy influence must await both time and an independent evaluation. On the policy making side there are many examples of politicians and administrators who are eager to use the latest research to inform their work. In other words, there is good practice to build on from both directions.

4. AGEING EUROPE: THE RESEARCH CHALLENGES

What are the major research challenges facing Europe? We might expect a very wide range of answers to this question depending on scientific disciplines and individual researcher's specialisms. But, what is remarkable, is the high level of consensus among scientists not only about the infrastructure required but also about the specific research priorities. This consensus has been revealed by a substantial programme of work over the past 2 years aimed at identifying the key priorities for ageing research in Europe. More than 150 scientists, including most of Europe's leading researchers in this field, have been engaged in this endeavour as well as end user groups, especially those representing older people. It has been conducted under the auspices of the European FORUM project and, therefore, a brief description of that project is necessary.

FORUM was an Accompanying Measure under Europe's Framework Programme 5 (FP5) which means it was a coordination initiative rather than conducting either basic or applied research. It was intended to address the four structural challenges facing research on ageing in Europe. First of all there are no systematic linkages between centres of excellence in most countries and none between countries. Thus, although Europe has some of the world's leading researchers in this field contacts between them are haphazard and mainly reliant on individual action. In other words the organisation of ageing research is atomised which, of course, means that there is both duplication of effort and a lost opportunity to realise the fruits of collaboration between countries. In some countries, such as Germany, research is regionalised, and this compounds the problem. Of course the European Congress of Gerontology is an important source of informal contacts but a sign of how far Europe lags behind the US in this respect is that the long-needed European Journal of Ageing (EJA) has only recently got off the ground (http://www.springeronline.com).

The converse of this diffusion, secondly, is the absence of a concerted European perspective. The European level framework programmes are bolted on to the national ones without considering how they might be integrated. Potential synergies between European and national programmes are not exploited and, therefore, added value is not gained. Even when there are European programmes, such as FP5, they are poorly coordinated and, again, potential added value is lost. This is perverse because the sharing of knowledge and experience in order to improve the quality of life of citizens is a basic building block of the EU and has played a role since the Treaty of Rome. This mutual exchange and comparison is an important aspect of being in the EU. As a result the cross-national element of research on ageing has become more formalised and attempts have been made to coordinate it over the last decade or so.

Thirdly, there is a growing recognition among scientists and policy makers and research funders that disciplinary research has artificially compartmentalised both the ageing process and older people's lives. There is a need for much more interdisciplinary research and especially so in the ageing field, where a holistic understanding of the ageing process requires inputs ranging from basic biology to clinical, social, psychological and cultural analyses. This is not to argue that all disciplinary boundaries should be broken down, which would be foolish, but those topics that lend themselves to interdisciplinary research should be approached in that way. The choice of methods should be led by the research problem and not imposed willy-nilly. In practice, however, research funding is strongly compartmentalised by disciplines and scientists gain esteem and advancement chiefly within narrow disciplines. In other words, just as in the policy world, the scientific one is not sufficiently "joined up".

Fourthly, there is a damaging detachment between science and society. This applies to policy makers and practitioners as noted previously but also to wider society. In the ageing field in Europe there is a growing interest in research among older people themselves. For some this is taking the form of a critique of the positivist model which excludes older people from participation in the research process beyond their role as subjects. There are parallel calls from other end users of research that their interests should be included as well. There is a challenge to scientific methods, in other words, to involve users.

While it cannot hope to provide the answers to these challenges they were the backdrop to the establishment of the FORUM project. It had five objectives:

- to promote European cooperation in ageing research;
- to develop synergies between European and national research;
- to improve channels of communication between European and national research;
- to encourage interdisciplinary research;
- to promote public awareness of the importance of scientific research on ageing.

The overall aim was to maximise the European value of ageing research.

With regard to the methods to achieve these objectives, at the heart of the whole process was the European Forum on Population Ageing Research. This body consisted of national research funders and policy makers, that is, those with the power to influence national research agendas. Feeding into the Forum were the results of six workshops on three key topics: quality of life; health and care management; genetics, longevity and demography. The workshops were multi-disciplinary scientific meetings designed to identify gaps in research and structural barriers to collaboration. In addition there was a user consultation conference involving policy makers, NGOs and public and private providers. The process was managed by an international steering committee. Finally there were a range of dissemination activities, including a website and newsletters.

The remainder of this chapter introduces some of the outputs from this work. The level of effort and commitment given by European scientists to this project has been remarkable. There is no doubt that there is widespread consensus among scientists on the need for a concerted European focus in ageing research. This summary cannot do justice to their high quality contributions (full reports available from the website: http://www.shef.ac.uk/ageingresearch) and it will simply emphasise some of the key issues.

First, with regard to research and methodology, the scientific workshops developed a set of recommendations on the need for new instruments and measures and research approaches. Emphasising the earlier point about the underdevelopment of comparative research in Europe, some of the basic tools necessary for such work are missing and, unless European-wide investment is made, added value will not be forthcoming. Key priorities for such investment are:

- a European longitudinal study;
- the development of comparative methods and common conceptual tools;
- European level coordination of data collection, for example, of biological samples;
- the development and validation of quality of life indicators appropriate to older people.

The diversity of European populations is a potential strength of comparative research but Europe lacks consensus on measuring concepts such as quality of life in a cross-cultural context. For example comparative studies should include both standardised instruments and culture-specific ones. Key priorities are:

- research on expectations and normative belief systems to shed light on how ageing individuals formulate their quality of life judgements and their expectations of services;
- predictors of active ageing;
- interdisciplinary approaches to the construction of genomic risks profiles;
- qualitative and quantitative measures of the effects of e-health and e-care;
- quality of care indicators; new evaluation approaches, for example to assess efficiency in social care and care outcomes;
- an international standard co-morbidity index;
- definitions of health and frailty in the oldest old.

Turning to the key priorities for methods and research approaches scientists across the disciplinary spectrum agreed on three general ones:

- the need to target sub-groups of the older population, such as ethnic and older migrant groups, the oldest old and youngest old;
- using European-wide population studies as a rich resource, for example, to increase the sample size of sub-groups;
- focussing on heterogeneity rather than averages.

Each of the pairs of workshops dedicated to quality of life, health and social care and genetics, longevity and demography made extensive recommendations that are too detailed to report here.

Second the scientific workshops and user consultation addressed the structural barriers to European research collaboration and how to overcome them. In particular they stressed the lack of infrastructure for support for cross-national and comparative research and the need for a systematic approach to European research collaboration. The priorities for action are:

- interdisciplinary collaboration across Europe to examine the portability of different approaches;
- training and support for young researchers;
- European funding capacity and journals;
- a database of European research;
- new dissemination strategies, including the translation of national research into other EU languages;
- the establishment of national institutes of ageing;
- a European institute on ageing to, among other things, coordinate national research, standardise data collection and storage, encourage interdisciplinary research between genetic, social, demographic and epidemiological fields, promote ageing research and fund research networks;
- an observatory on social care;
- the creation of a scientific community for the bio-demography of ageing to integrate understanding of demography, epidemiology, genetics and biology.

While there is a recognition of the need to maintain disciplinary identities, the scientists agree that a major challenge is to develop interdisciplinary research. They see the advantages of interdisciplinarity but they also are aware of the substantial barriers to achieving it. These barriers include the lack of common scientific languages, the lack of academic credit for such work and of funding dedicated to encouraging interdisciplinary research. A key to success on this front is the sharing of good practice. In terms of how interdisciplinary collaborations should be organised the key points are that the approach be determined by the research questions, that interdisciplinary skills are required as well as disciplinary ones, and the need for financial support for interdisciplinary centres that operate as transversal organisations.

There is also a strong commitment among scientists for the involvement of end users of research and good grasp of the dilemmas this entails. Although no consensus exists on precisely how to involve users there is agreement on the need for a partnership model for the formulation of research agendas, which involves as many stakeholders as possible. There is also agreement on the basic principles that should guide involvement: clarity about aims of users involvement and the definition of who the users are, and the aim to be inclusive of the wide diversity of older people. Scientists and user groups agree that a European review of good practice and models of users involvement in research is urgently needed.

The scientific workshops and users consultation formulated extensive recommendations for policy makers at both national and European levels. First there is a set of recommendations aimed at both national and European policy makers that are designed to overcome the structural deficiencies outlined earlier. To encourage and facilitate interdisciplinary research and European collaborations research funders must recognise the difficult and time-consuming nature of this work; create specific funding mechanisms that cross-national research council boundaries; improve funding for social sciences; create interdisciplinary networks and coordinate the collection of data at European level. To ensure that ageing research attracts young talented scientists there is a need for support structures, such as visiting studentships and post-doctoral fellowships, and for international training in ageing research. A strategically planned approach to dissemination at the European level is urgently needed, as are good practice examples of dissemination to wide audiences and new partnerships with NGOs. To involve users more extensively in research requires funding, for example, to support the making of links between research and policy. A number of specific initiatives are proposed, including a European Institute on Ageing to bring together all disciplines in the ageing field; European networks to connect scientists, user groups and older people; a European Observatory on Care for Older People to coordinate research and instruments and a European longitudinal study.

Specific recommendations for national research funders and policy makers include a commitment to fund a programme of research in this field; investment in networking infrastructures; balancing commercial and non-commercial interests to ensure that the former does not dominate priorities and support for interdisciplinary research centres.

Secondly, those aimed at European research funders and policy makers include using this body of work to develop Framework Programme 7 (FP7); supporting basic research on ageing; providing funding for European-wide NGOs to work with researchers; facilitating cooperation between policy makers, medics, social scientists and others involved in the ageing field; making application forms more user-friendly; providing budgets for interpretation and translation and supporting "high risk" research such as totally new projects and innovative methodologies. One such project would be a study of e-health/e-care focussing on the implementation of technological development into the health care system and how health professionals and older people manage their health through e-health/e-care.

All scientists and user groups agree that the EU has a fundamental role to play in supporting and encouraging national governments to develop their own research agenda on ageing. It is recognised that, without such measures, ageing research in Europe will never reach the organised levels achieved in the US and, therefore, will not realise its full potential. Having paid tribute to the massive investment of time and effort made by European scientists and said that it is impossible to do justice to the wealth of proposals and ideas they generate I am now going to pick just five recommendations, but do so in the knowledge that this is an artificial exercise.

- Use FORUM recommendations to construct FP7;
- establish a European Institute on Ageing;
- help to develop European multi- and interdisciplinary collaboration;

- a commitment to user involvement in research;
- attract and support new researchers to ageing.

Finally there are a few words about the next stage of this collaborative work in Europe. At the programme level a new venture is underway to coordinate these activities: The European Research Area in Ageing (http://www.shef.ac.uk/era-age). While at the level of science plans are being made to continue a network of scientists across different disciplines working in the field of quality of life in old age. If these two endeavours are successful, together they will pave the way for a genuinely European approach to ageing research.

5. CONCLUSION

This chapter has argued that while ageing is not a crisis for Europe, it demands a concerted policy strategy spanning a wide range of domains. It further argues that science should play a central role in providing the evidence-base for policy and practice but acknowledges that this is not straightforward. Finally, in summarising the results of a unique European collaboration between scientists, the chapter illustrates the remarkably high level of consensus that exists about how to create a concerted research agenda on ageing. We now have a major task to persuade the policy makers (not all of whom are reluctant)—an essential task if Europe is to adjust successfully to its ageing populations. Science matters, no doubt about that, but if it is to benefit older people it must be translated into policy and practice.

AFFILIATION

University of Sheffield

REFERENCES

Daniels, N. (1998). *Am I My Parent's Keeper?* New York: Oxford University Press.

Jacobzone, S. (1999) *Healthy ageing and the challenges of new technologies* (Mimeo).

Kohli, M., Rein, M., Guillemard, A. M., & van Gunsteren, H. (Eds). (1991). *Time for retirement.* Cambridge: CUP.

Manton, K. G., Stallard, E., & Riggan, W. (1982). Strategies for analysing ecological health date: Models of the biological risk of individuals. *Medical Statistics, 2*, 1863–1881.

Naegele G., & Walker A. (Eds.) (1999). *The politics of old age in Europe*. Buckingham: OU Press.

Riley, M., Kahn, R., & Foner, A. (1994). *Age and structural lag: Society's failure to provide meaningful opportunities in work, family and leisure*. New York: Wiley.

Robine, J. M. (2003). The relevance of population health indicators. *Journal of Epidemiology Community Health, 57*, 318.

Scherer, P. (1996). The myth of the demographic imperative. In C. Steurle & M. Kawai (Eds.), *The new world fiscal order* (pp. 61–83). Washington DC: Urban Institute.

Walker, A. (1997). *Combating age barriers in employment*. Luxembourg: Office for the Official Publications of the European Communities.

Walker, A. (1999). *Managing an ageing workforce—A guide to good practice*. Luxembourg: Office for the Official Publications of the European Communities.

Walker, A. (2002). A strategy for active ageing. *International Social Security Review, 55*(1), 121–140.

Walker, A. (Ed.) (2005). *Understanding Quality of Life in Old Age.* Maidenhead: McGraw Hill.

Walker, A. and Hagan Hennessy, C. (Eds) (2005). *Growing Older: Quality of Life in Old Age.* Maidenhead: McGraw Hill.

SVEIN OLAV DAATLAND

ON THE RELEVANCE OF AGEING RESEARCH FOR POLICY AND PRACTICE

Environmental gerontology and the man–environment interaction is a field where the trivialities of everyday life are indeed found significant. The smaller story may be about things and pieces, but they translate into large questions about autonomy, dignity and citizenship. Environmental barriers that are easily overcome by most people, to the extent that they are even overlooked, may have profound importance for persons with functional limitations. Steep stairs, narrow doors, even a tiny doorsill, may become barriers to moving outdoors at your own choice, or stop you from getting back home again by yourself. These and other types of barriers that are so trivial for the majority of the population, and may have been trivial for most of one's own life course, may grow significant and insurmountable in old age. They may become a constant reminder of one's shortcomings when they are blamed upon oneself, as they often are, because environments are often taken for granted, even when they in fact are man-made and blameable.

A substantial proportion of the population have some form of functional limitation, be it in mobility, in comprehension, or in sensory capacity. Some have multiple losses, others are more lightly affected. Some may have acquired these limitations early in life, others late, and the latter may be the most vulnerable as they have developed little competence in how to compensate for these limitations.

The risks of being affected increase with age, in particular in late life when hardly anyone is left untouched. Older people spend a larger part of the day in their dwelling than do any other adult age group, and increasingly so the older one gets. Some keep their health, energy and motivation much longer than others, but all are in time affected by ageing, and will eventually come to experience that our (physical) world will grow smaller, and we shall in late life have to validate our identities and self-esteem through the trivialities of daily life. Hence these are issues that at one time or another will affect us all, and are therefore of vital concern also for a responsive and inclusive society.

The issues are therefore important, but what about research? Can research help us solve the problems in this area, or at least help us compensate for them? The answer is yes, but a yes that needs to be qualified in a number of ways and directions, which is what this chapter is about.

Before I move into the meat of the matter, a brief looking back at the formative years of gerontology may be appropriate and set the stage for the arguments to follow. I shall therefore start there, and point to some dilemmas that emerged early in gerontology and are still confronting us. This excursion will lead me into a second section that explores the utility of research issue in more general terms, which in the third section will be explored more concretely with some illustrations from studies that have been

H.-W. Wahl et al. (eds.), The Many Faces of Health, Competence and Well-Being in Old Age, 245–254.

presented to us during these couple of days.[1] I shall conclude with some ideas about future constraints and opportunities in the field.

1. THE GERONTOLOGICAL IMAGINATION

1.1. Building a Discipline

In retrospect, gerontology needed to establish itself as a separate field of research because basic disciplines like medicine, psychology and sociology had little interest in ageing and older people. Pioneers had to invent a new research area, even to construct a distinct discipline. The pioneering efforts often transcended the basic disciplines. Elie Metchnikoff, who suggested the name "gerontology" for this field one hundred years ago, wrote about "The nature of man" (1903), and "The prolongation of life" (1908). Grand questions that needed equally grand theorising; in Metchnikoff's case with roots in both medicine, statistics and the emerging social sciences (Hendricks & Achenbaum, 1999).

I might in passing mention that Metchnikoff suggested that the pathologies of premature ageing were produced by microbes in the digestive tract, which may be among the reasons why cures of digestion became a fashion early in the former century. Those who have read the Swedish doctor Axel Munthe's international best-selling book about San Michele, will know that he made his career on the digestive problems among rich ladies in Paris, who may have hoped to find also the fountain of youth in this inner world.

Another pioneer was I. L. Nascher, who launched his book on "Geriatrics" in 1914, which eventually became the name also for the emerging clinical speciality on the diseases of later life.

Stanley Hall was a third pioneer with his book on "Senescence" in 1922, about the psychology of the second half of life. He argued for a developmental psychology that included the whole life course, but it should take many years to gain recognition for this, if it is indeed gained.

A fourth pioneering effort to be mentioned here is by the well-known physiologist Walter B. Cannon (1939), who in the late 1930s suggested that the explanations for ageing could be found in the failures of homeostasis. How *timing* may be important in research is illustrated here, as the biological balance theory of Cannon fitted well with the emerging balance paradigm in the social sciences, namely functionalism, which came to constitute the basic bones of one of the founding theories of social gerontology—disengagement theory (Cumming & Henry, 1961). The balance suggested in this theory was not between organs in the body as in Cannon's case, but between the individual and the society—a balance that was represented by a mutual withdrawal between the two in the approach of old age and death.

1.2. Dilemmas and Responses

These were years of general scientific optimism. So also in the new area of gerontology, that needed its own theories and institutions in order to claim territory and legitimity, which is part of the reason why the early years of gerontology were years of grand theorising and the construction of (gerontological) associations, journals and congresses. But being established, the ambitions later dropped from grand theories down to smaller scale modelling for applied purposes. This development raised two types of dilemmas.

Theoretically the dilemma concerned the distinctiveness of ageing as a process and old age as a phase of life, and then the very argument for a distinct discipline. On the one hand gerontology aimed to include ageing and old age into the normality of life in order to combat prejudice and ageism. On the other hand, gerontology needed a distinctiveness that justified its position as a separate discipline or at least as a distinct field of research.

Strategically the dilemma concerned the balance between theory and application. The best arguments for financial, moral and political support were found in the utility of research findings in policy and practice. This avenue made it possible to expand gerontology as an institution by including practitioners, and to integrate people and perspectives from several disciplines and professions. Gerontology therefore emerged as a multi-disciplinary, even an inter-disciplinary, field. But while problems and interventions are often multi-disciplinary, theorising is normally not, but is most often specific to each discipline. The attempt to make a synthesis of people and perspectives from a number of disciplines risks therefore to produce a tragic compromise, where all are playing away from home (Daatland, 2002).

To be sure, problems of ageing and older people are multilevel and complex, and therefore invite efforts from a number of disciplines and professions. But the rules of the game are specific to each discipline. Paradigmatic differences in designs and measurements, in levels of analysis and theoretical perspectives, are among the barriers to inter-disciplinarity—even to multi-disciplinarity. I will therefore argue for an organic rather than a mechanic integration, implying that joint research efforts are best served by *complementary* roles and positions that acknowledge the distinctive identity of each basic discipline.

Such a strategy may help gerontology avoid the relative isolation from the basic disciplines that has developed over the years. The reasons for this isolation are several, and may be blamed on both gerontology and the mother sciences (Bengtson & Dowd, 1980). One reason is the neglect of age and ageing by the basic disciplines. Another—and then blaming gerontology—is the preoccupation with applied knowledge and the correspondingly scant attention to theory. A third reason is a preoccupation with old age instead of ageing, which is another side of the priority of descriptions over explanations, and application over theory.

The solutions to these predicaments may be different in the longer and shorter term. While we in the longer term may be better served by having the phenomena of ageing and later life properly integrated into the basic disciplines, we are not there yet, and need to protect and promote ageing as a field of research through separate channels. The danger is then to downgrade our theoretical ambitions and our scientific status and standing. We must therefore play two horses, both the different worlds (disciplines) we come from, and the common ground (gerontology) we play on (Daatland, 2004).

1.3. Ideals and Realities

The proof of the pudding lies in the eating. So also as far as inter-disciplinarity is concerned. Some disciplines are close, and may share theories, concepts, and methodologies. Others represent different worlds. They may share their good intentions and focus on similar questions, but they differ in designs and theorising and hardly ever meet or read each other's publications.

There are considerable differences also *within* a discipline area. Take social gerontology as an example, where a focus on individual adaptation to ageing as in disengagement and continuity theory has competed with a macro level, structural approach, as in age-stratification and modernisation theory (cf. Bengtson & Schaie, 1999). We have also seen attempts to integrate macro and micro perspectives, but the different "schools" have tended to claim their territory by downgrading the other, be it for reductionism or for structuralism.

Borders are even clearer between the medical sciences on the one hand and the social sciences on the other, and power differentials are also more prominent here. Old age has in modern society come to be constructed first of all as a medical problem. This bio-medicalisation of ageing (Estes & Binney, 1989) may be part of a broader trend, and may interplay with popular perceptions about ageing as decline on the one hand, and the need for political and administrative control on the other. Gerontologists may have contributed to this in order to promote ageing research as a distinct field of research. Medical problems have high legitimity both among politicians and the general public, and is easier to convert from *private troubles* to *public issues* than are social problems and the societal conditions that may have produced them.

To be sure, later life may be tough, and poor health may for the majority of elders be the major threat to autonomy and well-being in late life. The bio-medicalisation of ageing has no doubt helped motivate funding and transfers to the benefit of older people, both in terms of treatment, care services, and for that matter in terms of research. But the dilemma lies in the very conception of older people as the problem, and in the implicit alienation of later life from the normal life course. We need to go beyond these conceptions and develop images that include ageing and later life into normality, as for example in the life-span developmental model of Baltes and Baltes (1990). In doing so, we also integrate older people into society as full citizens.

The ecology of ageing area is then an appropriate case in point, as it forces us to reflect on what normality indeed is, and where abnormality is located, in them or in us, in the person or in the environment, in the individual or in the society. Without this consciousness we would risk the classical danger of wasting our efforts in pulling an endless parade of people out of a rushing stream, without investigating who is upstream pushing them into it.

This excursion to the origins and dilemmas of gerontology may have been a slightly intricate way of pushing a very simple message, which is that our images of ageing and later life are truly real in their consequences. The implication is that conceptualisations and theory development may be equally consequential, and may in fact be the most powerful products of our research efforts, at least in the longer term. This leads me over to the second section of the chapter, about the utility of research.

2. THE UTILITY OF RESEARCH

The use and usability of research may be evaluated along several dimensions (Weiss, 1977). Research may for example be directly *instrumental* in the production of necessary tools and instruments. Model cases are the natural and medical sciences, for example, the development of new oil production technologies or new medical drugs and treatments. The quality and relevance of such research is more or less self-evident. It either works well or it does not. The true story is obviously far more complex, as a long list of initial failures may have been necessary on the road to success.

Conceptual utility is a more vague matter, as is also the utility of the social sciences that operate in these (conceptual) waters. To be sure, social research may be instrumental and (contribute to) produce new instruments, methods and techniques for industries and services. Social research is, however, more often conceptual, and may produce new knowledge about phenomena and processes that confirms or refutes earlier theories or ideas. Social research shall also inform and support public debate and political decision making, provide training and higher education for the labour market, and represent an intellectual capital for planning and evaluation. Modern bureaucracies and politics are hardly conceivable without the input from the social sciences.

Being more vague means, however, that the utility of social research is often questioned. Part of this is a scepticism towards theories in general, which are seen as "fiction" in contrast to "facts", and as abstractions from practical concerns and "real life". Theories and theorising are maybe also devalued by the impatience of modern times, where people want action first, thinking next. Today's politicians probably receive small credits for a suggestion for research, and more for crying out that "enough's enough, let's get things going". To be sure, research may be used as an excuse for non-action, when we in fact have already the knowledge needed to move forward, but research should normally be a sound investment, as we usually need a map to guide our steps. Theories are in fact very practical, mind you if they are good theories. After all, if you do not understand a problem, how can you solve it? And besides, it is not a question of theories or not, but about explicit or implicit theories. Any action is built on ideas of how things work, or they demand a justifying idea after the fact. Common sense theories are usually implicit and then beyond the critical reflections of public discourse. Formal and research based theories are not always better, but they are at least explicit and refutable. Research then represents an attitude to reality and a method for separating myths and realities. Of course we need dreams and visions, but we also need self-corrective reflections. Some researchers may be visionary, but most of us are in the self-correction business and should so be.

Why then is theory important? Theories are important because they integrate knowledge, they provide explanations, they make predictions possible or at least better than without theory and they function as guides and models for interventions in policy and practice (Bengtson, Rice, & Johnson, 1999). Theory then integrates the substance knowledge of a field, and what their implications for practice are.

One of these practices are *political*. It need be underlined that research is not politics, and researchers not politicians. They should at least not be politicians in their capacity as researchers. Research and politics play by different rules, but interplay and impact on each other as they indeed shall. But while politics is about negotiations and compromises to get decisions through, research is a more uncompromising business. Political decisions are produced via democratic negotiations. Scientific decisions are not, but should feed their findings and ideas into the political arena. Put grandly, the task of research is to draw a map of knowledge upon which political decisions may navigate. Research is in this sense a vital element in democracy, and should share findings and theories to all relevant parties, not reserve it for special interests, be they governmental or private.

Research and politics also differ in their orientation in time: Where politics looks forward and tries to form tomorrow's society by today's decisions, research tends to look back and to study the effects of yesterday's decisions. Planners and politicians may therefore come to look at research as outdated if not downright irrelevant: "I know what I know, don't bother me with facts!" Research may be associated to the already established practices and their limitations, and be criticised for breaking in already open doors, while the political system is looking towards the possible and probable futures: "Tell me what I don't know!" This brings me over to the third section of the chapter, with some illustrations of research utility as they have appeared at this conference.

3. ILLUSTRATIONS

The ecology of ageing—how ageing and later life is located in environments and places—is a vast subject area, and have stood particularly strong in the United States (Lawton, 1977; Parmelee & Lawton, 1990; Scheidt & Windley, 1985). Germany stands out in Europe, and the Heidelberg group stands out in Germany (Kendig, 2003; Schaie, Wahl, Mollenkopf, & Oswald, 2004; Wahl & Weisman, 2003), a position that is confirmed by this very conference.

The chapter on outdoor mobility by Mollenkopf and others illustrates how trivialities of daily life may indeed become existentially important when the often taken-for-granted ability to move around is not there. The chapter also illustrates the blindness of the majority society, and how citizenship rights presuppose a mobility that is not available to a substantial minority of the population.

Many of the empirical details of barriers to mobility are well known, but are often overlooked. The very documentation of these problems becomes an eye-opener, and illustrates the agenda-setting role of good research. Problems are presented to the public in a way that demand attention and action.

This study also illustrates the *limitations* of research; that knowledge is often not enough to produce changes. And finally, this study is an example of a classical three-step strategic research effort: First to uncover the problems, next to explain them and finally to suggest actions to have them solved. A natural extension of the study would have been to investigate why such knowledge is not always carried over into implementation and practice.

The chapter on the home environment by Oswald and others illustrates the potential impact of innovative conceptualisations. The power of new constructs is further illustrated by them being introduced here to a reality (the home) that is so well known to us all, to the extent that this familiarity may have made us blind. Hence new concepts may be an eye-opener, in this case for the home as an arena for identity management related to both *attachment* (belonging) and *agency* (coping). The two are seen as complementary processes.

Future extension of this model might benefit from the exploration of possible conflicts or ambivalences between the two. One solution to such ambivalence might be illustrated by Kruse's concept of "willingness to let go". *Detachment* is here seen as a functional strategy when environments and individual competencies are in conflict (see intro chapter by Kruse). Although ageing in place is an ambition for most in later life, Kruse finds that many older persons are strikingly unsentimental about their house and possessions when functional limitations make relocation a better option.

The final illustration is taken from the chapter on well-being in very old age by Rott and others, which also illustrates the importance of conceptualisations, but here in a more general fashion. The Valuation of Life approach to quality of life studies expands our traditional conceptions by integrating also the very frail into the debate about what a decent life is, and indeed by including the very weakest into humanity and as "one of us". By doing so, this approach offer them a dignity and a protection that they risk if they are not so included.

4. WHAT NEXT?

Let me conclude with some ideas about future directions. The studies presented have documented substantial barriers to participation and active citizenship, and these are barriers that are primarily located in (non-friendly) environments: In housing and physical surroundings that are not designed for people with functional limitations; in environments that represent barriers to equal opportunity and threats to a decent life in old age. This is not a new story; we have known about such barriers for some time, so what is in fact the problem? Is it a problem of knowledge, of resources, or more likely a lack of will?

A shortage of *resources* may be a primary limitation and poverty a major enemy within this. Substandard housing is part of the poverty problem, and when resources are scarce, priorities are correspondingly sharp and leave people excluded. Poverty may also be internalised as poor health, premature ageing, low aspirations and a lack of cultural capital. Poor people are more at risk in all walks of life, and they have less competence in the mastery of these risks. Initial disadvantages therefore accumulate over time. To provide equal opportunities therefore require a redistribution policy to the benefit of the less fortunate. This is motivated also as a compensatory measure for the low aspirations and control beliefs among the unprivileged. If not supported by others, they are often unable to achieve something better.

Not all countries and times do, however, support a redistribution policy; hence resources may be a necessary, but not a sufficient condition. We also need *knowledge*. If we do not understand the difficulty, how else can we untie it? To raise knowledge through research may therefore indeed make a difference—also more indirectly, for example, as a way to correct prejudices that tend to blame the disabilities on the individual. *Misplaced causality* is particularly frequent with reference to older persons. Any failure of mastery is then easily blamed on the victim, even among older people themselves (Levy, 2003). This is a case of "the enemy within"; a tendency to self-stereotyping and self-blame which affect people that are victims of devaluation. They tend to identify with these prejudices, and then reduce their control beliefs and capacity for mastery. Hence information should also be directed towards older people themselves in order to raise their self-efficacy and competence. A related mechanism is a tendency to project the problems onto others, maybe as a self-protective strategy, and to identify as younger than one's age. In so doing they tend to make themselves blind to the risks of old age for themselves.

So knowledge is indeed important, but again—knowledge is not enough, because the knowledge that is already there is often not taken seriously. There are different qualities of knowledge, and we need to move the present "surface knowledge" to "deeper knowledge" of a character that breaks through our defensive strategies and demands a corresponding action. Anyone who has tried to quit smoking will know the difference. How one could "know" that smoking is dangerous, and still not "know" it and therefore allow oneself to continue.

This brings me over to the third type of problems, those of *ideology*. By this I mean the ideas about what the problems are and how they should be solved. The will (or lack of will) to take on these challenges is rooted in a conception of what the problem is, how it has come about and whose responsibility it is. Both people and countries differ in how they conceive these problems, and therefore also in their "theories" about how they should be solved and by whom. Let me in this case only point to country differences, and then more precisely to differences between countries as welfare states. I would suggest that *social needs*, including services and housing for elders, is seen as more of a personal and family responsibility under a conservative welfare regime such as the German, and more of a public responsibility under a Scandinavian type of welfare state. Germany on the other hand gives relatively higher priority to *medical* needs and services. This difference is hardly explained by resources or knowledge, and more likely by tradition and ideology. Which is the better welfare state model shall not concern me here, simply that they have different priorities and different conceptions of how responsibilities should be distributed. In the final instance it boils down to a question about what should be respected as a citizen's rights, and how far the problems we are here talking about should be elevated from their status as private troubles to a status of public issues that deserve a collective and political response.

5. IN CONCLUSION

A responsive and inclusive society is one where all have access to the same basic *liberties* like freedom of speech, a free vote, and a right to be equally treated in law and by governments. Any *fair inequality* should come about through competition in open systems, not in closed rooms that are reserved for the privileged, be they privileged by class, gender, race or for that matter by age or functional ability.

As people are differentially advantaged in life, the responsive society needs mechanisms that are balancing out these inequalities. Countries differ in the extent to which such compensations are seen as a collective or a private responsibility, and in how ambitious these compensations and support systems should be. Welfare states vary in how broadly and far they reach out, and in what levels of inequality they accept. Risks that are universal and affect us all tend to be more generally recognised and hence as part of the welfare state. Other problems and groups are given a less protected status. Hence resources are not enough, not even knowledge. We need also a "story"—an ideology—that links problems, resources and responsibility.

Today's political climate does not favour an expanding welfare state, which is to the disadvantage of the problems we are here talking about, as they can hardly be solved by markets and the private sector alone. They need public monitoring and support through legislation and resource allocation if solutions shall be inclusive and not only cover the more advantaged. We need collective mechanisms, civic and public, to include the weaker and less fortunate as full citizens. An inclusive society needs to protect the weaker, and to the extent possible compensate for their weaknesses. Hence we need to know more about the barriers to participation and citizenship, and we need an ideology that makes this knowledge compellingly relevant for corrective action.

We need also recognise the limits of these ambitions and to respect differences that are reasonable. Needs and aspirations change over the life course, and so also do our orientations (Daatland & Biggs, 2004). We may for example willingly come to trade our autonomy for security in late life, and to trade the excitements of the external world for the comforts of the home, even the bed, when illness strikes. Things change, and they do so with great diversity both within and between countries, because people have different needs and tastes. We should respect these differences, but in doing so not accept any degrading barriers to the pursuit of reasonable needs and dreams.

AFFILIATION

Norwegian Social Research (NOVA)

NOTE

[1] Referring here to the Deutsches Zentrum für Alternsforschung (DFZA) conference, "The many faces of health, competence, and well-being in old age: Integrating epidemiological, psychological, and social perspectives", University of Heidelberg, June 18th–19th, 2004.

REFERENCES

Baltes, P. B., & Baltes, M. M. (1990). Psychological perspectives on successful aging: The model of selective optimization with compensation. In P. B. Baltes & M. M. Baltes (Eds.), *Successful aging: Perspectives from the behavioral sciences* (pp. 1–34). Cambridge: Cambridge University Press.

Bengtson, V. L., & Dowd, J. J. (1980). Sociological functionalism, exchange theory and life cycle analysis: A call for more explicit theoretical bridges. *International Journal of Aging and Human Development, 12*(1), 55–73.

Bengtson, V. L., & Schaie, K. W. (eds.). (1999). *Handbook of theories of ageing*. New York: Springer.

Bengtson, V. L., Rice, C. J., & Johnson, M. L. (1999). Are theories of aging important? Models and explanations in gerontology at the turn of the century. In V. L. Bengtson & K. W. Schaie (Eds.), *Handbook of theories of ageing* (pp. 3–20). New York: Springer.

Cannon, W. B. (1939). *The wisdom of the body*. New York: W. W. Norton & Co.

Cumming, E., & Henry, W. (1961). *Growing old*. New York: Basic Books.

Daatland, S. O. (2002). Time to pay back? Is there something for psychology and sociology in gerontology? In L. Andersson (Ed.), *Cultural gerontology* (pp. 1–11). London: Auburn House.

Daatland, S. O. (2004). Common arena, separate worlds? On the ideals and realities of multi-disciplinarity. Paper at the 17th Nordic Congress of Gerontology, Stockholm.

Daatland, S. O., & Biggs, S. (Eds.)(2004). *Ageing and diversity: Multiple pathways and cultural migrations*. Bristol: Policy Press.

Estes, C. L., & Binney, E. A. (1989). The biomedicalization of aging: dangers and dilemmas. *The Gerontologist, 29*(5), 587–596.

Hall, G. S. (1922). *Senescence: The last half of life*. New York: Appleton & Co.

Hendricks, J., & Achenbaum, A. (1999). Historical development of theories of aging. In V. L. Bengtson & K. W. Schaie (Eds.), *Handbook of theories of ageing* (pp. 21–39). New York: Springer.

Kendig, H. (2003). Development in environmental gerontology: A multidisciplinary field. *The Gerontologist, 43*(5), 611–615.

Lawton, M. P. (1977). The impact of the environment on aging and behaviour. In J. E. Birren & K. W. Schaie (Eds.), *Handbook of the psychology of aging* (pp. 276–301). New York: Van Nostrand Reinhold Co.

Levy, B. R. (2003). Mind matters: Cognitive and physical effects of aging self-stereotypes. *Journal of Gerontology, Psychological Sciences, 58B*(5) P203–P211.

Metchnikoff, E. (1903). *The nature of man [Etude sur la nature humaine]*. New York: Putnam.

Metchnikoff, E. (1908). *The prolongation of life: Optimistic studies*. New York: GP Putnam's Sons.

Nascher, I. L. (1914). Geriatrics: The diseases of old age and their treatment (Including *physiological old age, home and institutional care, and medico-legal relations)*. Philadelphia: Ayer Company Publishers.

Parmelee, P. A., & Lawton, M. P. (1990). The design of special environments for the aged. In J. E. Birren & K. W. Schaie (Eds.), *Handbook of the psychology of aging* (pp. 464–488). San Diego: Academic Press.

Schaie, K. W., Wahl, H-W., Mollenkopf, H., & Oswald, F. (Eds.) (2004). *Aging independently: Living arrangements and mobility*. New York: Springer.

Scheidt, R. J., & Windley, P. G. (1985). The ecology of aging. In J. E. Birren & K. W. Schaie (Eds.), *Handbook of the psychology of aging* (pp. 245–258). New York: Van Nostrand Reinhold Co.

Wahl, H-W., & Weisman, G. D. (2003). Environmental gerontology at the beginning of the new millennium: Reflections on its historical, empirical, and theoretical development. *The Gerontologist, 43*(5), 616–627.

Weiss, C. H. (ed.)(1977). *Using social research in public policy making*. Lexington: Lexington Books.

APPENDIX

ABSTRACTS OF POSTER SESSION

DUAL-EARNERS AND BREADWINNERS IN OLD AGE: DIFFERENCES IN MARITAL SATISFACTION?

BAAS, STEPHAN; LEINWEBER, JUDITH;
SCHMITT, MARINA
baas@dzfa.uni-heidelberg.de

Research on marital satisfaction in long-lasting partnerships is not well established. Recent research has been concentrating on younger couples; these results cannot be referred to long-lasting marriages. Additional research is necessary to examine the preconditions of marital satisfaction in long-lasting relationships. So far research figured out that dyadic coping is the most important prerequisite for marital satisfaction, but a comparison between different age groups shows that this strategy was least diffused in the older age group. Still unexplained is whether the lack of dyadic coping could be interpreted in terms of a cohort effect or what other reasons are responsible for these differences. One possible explanation can be found in the income distribution between both spouses and interrelated types of marriage—either dual career couples or traditional male breadwinners: According to recent research equal earnings of both wife and husband may have a disequilibrating effect on relationships. With this study we would like to respond to the following question: What are the effects of these types of marriages—dual earners or breadwinners—on marital satisfaction when both partners are retired? Based on this question 99 couples and accordingly 198 persons were interviewed by the German Centre for Research on Ageing. Results of structural equation models show that different aspects of relationships (type of marriage, dyadic coping and environmental mastery) have varying impacts on marital satisfaction: Male "dual earners" are more satisfied when compared with male "breadwinners", while female marital satisfaction depends more on dyadic coping and environmental mastery.

SILVER-SURFERS IN GERMANY: THE POTENTIAL OF A NEW MEDIUM

DOH, MICHAEL
doh@dzfa.uni-heidelberg.de

Since the end of the 1990s, the Internet has spread like wildfire through Germany. Since then, over half those 14 years and older belong to the Internet user community.

However, the use of the Internet is not distributed equally over societal groups. As data from of the nation-wide survey presented here show, Internet diffusion varies considerably along classical socio-structural lines; age, sex, education, income and occupation all predict Internet use. With respect to persons over 50 years—frequently called "silver-surfers"—about 25% are online, while this is true for only 5% of those of 70 years and older. The majority of silver-surfers is male, between the age of 50 and 59, well-educated and often still active in the labour force. As a consequence, the "older" adults already using the Internet at present still represent quite a selective group of persons with special interests, utilisation and behaviour (e.g. more selective, information-oriented Internet use compared to younger persons online). It seems that the vast majority of older persons offline does not realise the utility and surplus of this medium. High costs and lack of computer skills deter the older individual from using the Internet as well. In sum, the various possibilities and potentials that the Internet offers to ageing persons—such as communication, information, education, participation and maintenance of autonomy—remain greatly underutilised.

PHYSICAL ACTIVITY AND SELF-RATED HEALTH IN MIDDLE AND OLD AGE

EICHBERG, SABINE
eichberg@uni-bonn.de

It has been demonstrated that general physical activity and fitness positively influence current and later self-rated health. It is unclear whether this relation is valid for all age groups and for both sexes. Thus, the aims of this study were (a) to examine age and gender differences in physical activity, fitness and objective health and (b) to investigate the age and gender specific impact of these factors on self-rated health in current and later life. As part of the "Interdisciplinary Longitudinal Study of Adult Development" (ILSE) physical activity, fitness, objective health and self-rated health of 437 men and women at the ages of 44 and 64 years were assessed in 1994/95 (T1) and 4 years later (T2). There were no age and gender differences in self-rated health and physical activity at both measurement points. Younger persons were objectively healthier and revealed a better fitness. Men's fitness exceeded that of women. Only in younger men self-rated health was affected by physical activity and fitness at T1. At follow-up self-rated health at T1 and objective health at both measurement points were the most notable predictors. At T2 fitness of older men and physical activity of younger women were associated with self-rated health. The impact of physical activity on self-rated health is possibly mediated by objective health. Furthermore, the results suggest that physical activity and fitness have an impact on self-rated health in persons with a high level of or an increase in physical activity and fitness.

DETECTION OF COLORECTAL CANCER BY THE TUMOUR M2-PK STOOL TEST

HAUG, ULRIKE; ROTHENBACHER, DIETRICH; HARDT, PHILIP[1]; KLÖR, HANS-ULRICH[1]; STEGMAIER, CHRISTA[2]; BRENNER, HERMANN
haug@dzfa.uni-heidelberg.de
[1]*Medical Clinic III, University of Giessen;* [2]*Saarland Cancer Registry, Saarbrücken*

New stool tests might offer promising approaches for non-invasive colorectal cancer (CRC) screening, but data from large-scale epidemiologic studies are scarce. The aim of this study was to investigate the potential of a new test for faecal tumour M2-PK, an isoform of the glycolytic enzyme pyruvate kinase which characterises the metabolism of tumour cells, to discriminate patients with CRC from an unselected average-risk population. Faecal tumour M2-PK concentrations were examined among 917 unselected average risk people aged 50–75 years and among 68 CRC patients by means of the ScheBo® Tumour M2-PK Test, a sandwich enzyme-linked immunosorbent assay (ELISA). The test allows quantitative measurement of tumour M2-PK in 20 mg of native stool with a lower detection limit of 2 U/ml. Sensitivity and specificity of the test were calculated at different cut-off-values, and receiver-operating characteristics curves (ROC) were constructed to visualise the discriminatory power of the test. The median (interquartile range) faecal tumour M2-PK concentration was <2 U/ml (<2–3.2) among the population sample and 15.8 U/ml (5.1–65.1) among CRC patients ($p < 0.0001$). At a cut-off-value of 5 U/ml sensitivity and specificity were 78% and 83%, respectively. Sensitivity was slightly higher for colon than for rectum cancer. The ROC analysis yielded an area under the curve of 0.735. Despite the need of further investigations to assess the stage-dependence of this marker and the potential to detect adenomas, its performance characteristics regarding cancerous lesions as well as its practicability and simple analysis suggest that the tumour M2-PK stool test may be a promising tool for CRC screening in a population setting.

VISUAL CAPACITY, OUTDOOR ACTIVITIES AND LIFE SATISFACTION OF OLDER ADULTS

HEYL, VERA; WAHL, HANS-WERNER; MOLLENKOPF, HEIDRUN
heyl@dzfa.uni-heidelberg.de

This study examined the role of vision in connection with other predictors of out-of-home everyday functioning and emotional well-being among older adults in different contexts. The results are based on a sample of 1519 elderly (55–98 years) from Germany, and comparative samples from Finland ($n = 610$) and Italy ($n = 600$). Although all of the participants were living in private households, half resided in urban areas, while the other half resided in rural regions. Structural equation models supported the hypothesis of cross-culturally invariant basic relations among age, vision, intellectual functioning, out-of-home everyday functioning and emotional well-being. In detail, vision mediated the effect of age on out-of-home ADL/IADL (Activities of Daily Living/Instrumental Activities of Daily Living) and out-of-home leisure activities, intellectual functioning mediated the effect of vision on out-of-home leisure activities, and all effects on emotional well-being were mediated by out-of-home leisure activities. Besides these basic mechanisms, the results also indicate contextual variations: First, social resources contributed less while outdoor motivation contributed more to out-of-home leisure activities in the German urban than in the German rural sample. Second, outdoor motivation was significantly related to social resources in the German urban, but not in the German rural sample. Third, income-per-head contributed modestly but significantly to out-of-home leisure activities in the East German, but not in the West German urban and rural samples. On a more general level, it is concluded that in different regional contexts, different contextual resources are crucial for maintaining everyday competence and that visual capacity plays an important role in this network of resources.

AGEING AND PERSON-ENVIRONMENT FIT IN DIFFERENT URBAN NEIGHBOURHOODS

HIEBER, ANNETTE; OSWALD, FRANK; WAHL, HANS-WERNER; MOLLENKOPF, HEIDRUN
hieber@dzfa.uni-heidelberg.de

Person–environment relations in old age can be regarded from the perspective of individual environmental needs (P), from the perspective of existing environmental amenities at home and in the neighbourhood (E) or from the perspective of fit between environmental needs and residential conditions related to social and physical environmental features (P $\times$ E). The first aim of this study is to establish a set of person–environment fit indices, according to basic, comfort-oriented, as well as social needs and to describe stability and change over time in these fit domains. The second aim is to explain outdoor place attachment—which can be regarded as a major indicator of a "good life" in the community—using a set of person- and environment-related predictors. Data from a randomised mail-questionnaire study with $N = 217$ elders at T1 and T2 (3 years after T1) serve as the empirical basis of the study. The sample is stratified by age group (51–60, 61–70, 71–80), gender (51% women) and three different urban neighbourhood types. The results concerning the basic physical amenities fit index shows different changes for districts and age groups over time. The comfort-oriented fit index was quite stable averaged across all districts, but, as additional analyses revealed, decreased for those residing in the most pleasant district. The social fit index increased in the district with best access to public transportation and decreased in the most pleasant districts. Regression analyses run separately for the three districts revealed the impact of person–environment fit indices as predictors for outdoor place attachment.

PERCEPTION OF RESOURCES AND THEIR AGE-DIFFERENTIAL RELATIONSHIP TO SUBJECTIVE WELL-BEING

JOPP, DANIELA; LEIPOLD, BERNHARD[1]
jopp@dzfa.uni-heidelberg.de
[1] *Free University of Berlin*

Personal resources represent the basic prerequisite for successful development and ageing. In order to invest one's resources in optimal ways leading to positive outcomes such as high subjective well-being, the individual's perception of these resources is crucial. Moreover, resource loss is considered as a specific developmental trigger. Several studies involving young and middle-aged persons have shown that resource loss is accompanied by depression and low well-being. Whether this effect holds also for older individuals is an open question. Given that old and very old age is characterised by a decline in multiple domains of functioning, it may be supposed that older individuals learn to deal with these negative changes and thus feel less influenced. The relationship between resource perception and well-being was examined investigating a sample of 40 young (20–40 years) and a subsample of 42 old persons (70–90 years) of the ALLEE-Study (Altern und Lebenserfahrung). Age groups did not differ in their perception of resource status and importance, but in resource change. Young individuals experienced more gains, old individuals more losses. Regarding the relationship between resources and well-being, resource status was the most powerful predictor of well-being in both groups. As had been hypothesised age differences emerged with respect to resource changes: Resource loss was negatively associated with well-being in the young, but not in the old age group. Thus, results indicate that the importance of resource loss changes over the life-span, calling for further research into the mechanism responsible for this effect.

TECHNOLOGY AS A SUPPORT AND CHALLENGE FOR AUTONOMOUS LIVING IN OLD AGE

KASPAR, ROMAN; MOLLENKOPF, HEIDRUN; BECKER, STEFANIE
kaspar@dzfa.uni-heidelberg.de

In light of a technological landscape that is changing at an ever faster rate, the ability to use complex technology has become a key competence for independent living and successful participation in society. Elderly people, it is often assumed, might lose out in this trend towards modernisation. Especially in old age, when access to and instruction in using modern technology is no longer provided by educational or occupational institutions, the maintenance of technology-related competence may increasingly depend on individual interests and possibilities. This study attempts to delineate the vital role of personal interests and individual biography as predispositions for current use and appraisal of technology. Data stem from a national representative survey conducted in 1999 with a total of 1,417 community dwelling individuals aged 55–98 (mean age 69.7 years; 701 men, 716 women). On the basis of both biographical information concerning experiences with technology and subjective evaluation of technology in general, five prototypical technology-related lifestyles—each differing substantively in their commitment to technology—were identified. Apart from being associated with specific socio-demographic characteristics, the five extracted profiles differed with respect to underlying motives (i.e. subjective importance of different life domains) as well as possession and use of technology. Even if older individuals differ greatly with respect to technological experience and acceptance, our analyses revealed subgroups with characteristic communalities. To address these specific technological backgrounds, identifying the needs and attitudes of the older user would help to make future technology more appealing for the elderly.

STRESSFUL LIFE-EVENTS IN MIDDLE ADULTHOOD: INFLUENCE ON MENTAL HEALTH?

MALLAU, ANNA; SCHMITT, MARINA; VOSS, ELKE
mallau@dzfa.uni-heidelberg.de

A wide range of research studies document the relation between stressful life-events and mental disorders. Nevertheless, most of these studies are subject to restrictions concerning cross-sectional design and the use of clinical samples or neglect age-specific approaches concentrating on middle-adulthood. Therefore, the purpose of this study was to examine (a) the amount and kind of critical life-events in middle adulthood, (b) the existence of a cumulative effect of critical life-events on mental disorders and (c) the prediction of mental disorders by specific stressful events. Data are drawn from $N = 448$ individuals (mean age at T1: 44.2 years) participating at both measurement points (T1–T2: 4.1 years) of the Interdisciplinary Longitudinal Study of Adult Development (ILSE). Point prevalence rates of mental disorders were calculated with the help of data from a structured clinical interview based on DSM-III-R (Diagnostic and Statistical Manual of Mental Disorders). Using content analysis, recent stressful life-events reported in a semi-structured interview were classified into 34 categories. Results show a high amount of stressful life-events in middle adulthood. Most of the stressful life-events occurred in the social, health and occupational domains. Besides, a cumulative effect of critical life-events on the prevalence of mental disorders, some significant relations between the incidence of mental disorders and specific life-events (e.g. unemployment, problems in social relationships) occurred. The consequences of these results on mid-life and late-life development and on the implementation of prevention strategies are currently discussed. Further research should examine the role of resources as possible mediators of the relations between stressful life-events and mental health.

SOCIAL PARTICIPATION IN VERY OLD AGE

NAUMANN, DÖRTE; HIMMELSBACH, INES; OSWALD, FRANK
naumann@dzfa.uni-heidelberg.de

Social participation is an important indicator of quality of life. However, little is known about how social participation is negotiated in the everyday lives of very old people. Age-related research on social ecology suggests that societal participation may evolve over the life course due to aspects of ageing and social change. Thus, one can assume that the structure and meaning of societal participation differs in the third and fourth age. In this work, preliminary qualitative and quantitative findings on the structure and meaning of societal participation among community-dwelling older adults who live alone (aged between 75–89 years) are presented. Data are drawn from the European project ENABLE-AGE, consisting of a longitudinal survey ($N = 1918$) and an in-depth study ($N = 200$) in urban single households in Germany, the UK, Sweden, Hungary and Latvia. The project focused on the relationship between the home environment and healthy ageing with a broad understanding of the latter in terms of independence, well-being and social participation. One focus of the qualitative in-depth study, framed in a Grounded Theory approach, is to deepen the understanding of the structure and meaning of social participation in relation to the home environment in very old age. Findings suggest that both active and passive patterns of participation are important for well-being and that participation depends on the psycho-social and physical relationship between the person and the environment. All in all, results support the need to ensure barrier-free environments to enable very old persons to make a valued contribution to society.

HELICOBACTER PYLORI AND HEPATITIS A VIRUS INFECTIONS AND THE CARDIOVASCULAR RISK PROFILE IN PATIENTS WITH DIABETES MELLITUS: RESULTS OF A POPULATION BASED STUDY

ONGEY, MERCY; BRENNER, HERMANN; THEFELD, WOLFGANG[1]; ROTHENBACHER, DIETRICH
ongey@dzfa.uni-heidelberg.de
[1] *Robert Koch Institute, Berlin, Germany*

The objective of this study was to investigate the associations of sero-positivity for *Helicobacter pylori* (HP) and Hepatitis A virus (HAV) infection with prevalence of cardiovascular diseases (CVD) and CVD-risk markers in a large population-based sample of patients with diabetes mellitus (DM), who are at high risk of developing CVD. Several studies have suggested that chronic infections are associated with the development of atherosclerosis and coronary heart diseases (CHD). This analysis is based on the German National Health Interview and Examination Survey which was conducted in 1998. We identified all subjects with prevalent DM aged 40–79 years. HP and HAV status were measured by serum immunoglobulin G antibodies. Prevalence of several CVD events (myocardial infarction, stroke and CHD) was recorded. In addition, serum levels of total triglycerides, total cholesterol, HDL cholesterol, LDL cholesterol and lipoprotein (a) were measured. Among the 4,285 participants of the German Health Survey aged 40–79 years, we identified 365 patients with DM. 32.1% of these had at least one CVD and there was a clear increase of CVD with age. Sero-prevalence of HP or HAV was neither associated with the prevalence of CVD nor with mean levels of blood lipids after multivariate adjustment for covariates. In this large group of 365 patients with DM no association of HP and HAV sero-prevalence with presence of CVDs or the level of serum lipids was established. Therefore it seems unlikely that HP and HAV sero-prevalence influence CVD progression in patients with diabetes.

MARKERS OF SYSTEMIC INFLAMMATION AND PAIN IN CHRONIC MUSCULOSKELETAL DISEASES

RAUM, ELKE; STÜRMER, TIL[1]; BRENNER, HERMANN
raum@dzfa.uni-heidelberg.de
[1]*Division of Pharmacoepidemiology, Brigham and Women's Hospital, Boston, USA*

Although osteoarthritis (OA) and other chronic musculoskeletal diseases lack the large-scale systemic inflammatory response of rheumatoid arthritis, there is increasing interest in a potential role of subclinical inflammatory processes even for these diseases. We therefore assessed the association between high-sensitivity C-reactive protein (hsCRP) and pain in patients with OA and chronic lower back pain (cLBP). HsCRP was measured once among 770 patients with advanced OA of the hip or the knee. There were 335 hsCRP-measurements from 41 patients with cLBP. Intensity of pain was measured using visual analogue scales (VAS, 0–100). The association between pain and hsCRP was analysed with multivariable regression models. For patients with cLBP statistical methods for repeated measurements (GEE) were used. The median level of pain indicated on the VAS was 73 and 30 in patients with OA and cLBP, respectively. The (geometric) mean hsCRP was 2.5 mg/l among patients with OA and 1.31 mg/l for all measurements of patients with cLBP. For patients with OA, every increase of 10 mm on the VAS was associated with a 5.7% increase in mean hsCRP (95% confidence interval: 1.1–10.4) controlling for known or suspected predictors of hsCRP. For patients with cLBP no significant association between pain and hsCRP was found in the multivariable model. Severity of pain was associated with hsCRP in patients with

OA, but not in patients with cLBP. These results might reflect a differential role of a systemic inflammatory response for these two entities of chronic musculoskeletal diseases.

MODELLING STABILITY OF LIFE SATISFACTION IN OLDER AGE

SCHILLING, OLIVER
schilling@dzfa.uni-heidelberg.de

Empirical evidence fails to show age related decline in life satisfaction (LS) in old age. Given the frequent declines in objective quality of elders' lives, this finding has been labelled a "stability despite loss paradox" in gerontological discussions. However, evidence of this nature has been mainly derived from cross-sectional age group comparisons, and longitudinal analyses are the method of choice for analysing intra-individual change. Using data from the German Socio-Economic Panel, development of LS in old age was analysed longitudinally. To model true-score stability of single item measures of LS over 16 annual panel waves (1984–1999), autoregressive (quasi-Markov) structural equation models were specified. Nested model comparison strategies were applied to test hypothetical developments of LS in old age. Results indicated high "monotonic" true score stability in LS, which was not specific to old age but could be found across the whole adult life span. Neither true-score stability, nor variances increased substantially in later life. Notably, a decline in mean satisfaction scores was found, in contrast to the frequently observed findings of cross-sectional mean level stability across old age.

GENDER AS A PREDICTOR OF PARTICIPATION IN GERIATRIC REHABILITATION

SCHÖNEMANN-GIECK, PETRA; COFIE-NUNOO, DEREK; EHLERT, CLAUDIA
schoenemann@dzfa.uni-heidelberg.de

Only recently, are gender-specific differences in health care increasingly taken notice of. Though the results are ambivalent, there is evidence for a lower participation rate of female patients. From a medical perspective, this gender-specific difference is not well founded, because women benefit from interventions to the same degree as men do. In addition, there are almost no studies referring to gender-specific differences in geriatric rehabilitation. Thus, the aims of the study were (a) to investigate gender-specific differences in participation rates of geriatric rehabilitation, (b) to evaluate the success of geriatric rehabilitation with respect to gender and (c) to investigate the role of additional subjective and objective characteristics for geriatric rehabilitation. Within the "Wiesbaden Network of Geriatric Rehabilitation" 106 geriatric at-risk persons who lived at home were identified over a period of 18 months by administering a standardised screening instrument. Eighty-one of them (76%) agreed to participate in this study and provided data relevant for geriatric rehabilitation. Forty-two individuals were sent to rehabilitation by their family doctor. A selectivity analysis reveals that the female participation rate in geriatric rehabilitation is indeed lower than that of male patients. Logistic regression confirmed that participation is more likely for men, but additionally demonstrated that persons needing help to dress and undress and younger patients have a better chance to receive geriatric rehabilitation while subjective health and motivation had no impact. No gender differences in rehabilitation success were obtained. More attention should be paid to who gets the opportunity for geriatric rehabilitation.

LONG-TERM EFFECTS OF RISK FACTOR MODIFICATION IN CARDIOVASCULAR REHABILITATION

TWARDELLA, DOROTHEE; KUEPPER-NYBELEN, JUTTA; ROTHENBACHER, DIETRICH; HAHMANN, HARRY[1]; WÜSTEN, BERND[2]; BRENNER, HERMANN
twardella@dzfa.uni-heidelberg.de
[1]*Klinik Schwabenland, Isny-Neutrauchburg;* [2]*Klinik am Südpark, Bad Nauheim*

To evaluate systematically the key determinants of long-term prognosis among coronary heart disease (CHD) patients undergoing rehabilitation (rehab), a prospective cohort study (KAROLA) was started in January 1999 at two cooperating clinics. Over a period of 17 months 1,206 consecutive patients between 30 and 70 years of age who underwent in-patient rehabilitation due to CHD were recruited. Baseline data were collected via patient and medical questionnaires, and a blood sample was drawn at discharge from rehab. Active follow-up examinations were conducted 1 and 3 and years after discharge, and a 4.5 year follow-up is currently implemented. Data regarding risk factors, treatment and various health outcomes including secondary cardiovascular disease events are collected in each case via a patient questionnaire as well as a questionnaire from the patient's general practitioner (GP). Furthermore, blood samples are drawn by the GP, and the vital status and, if deceased, cause of death are obtained from patients not responding to the follow-up questionnaires. Selected research findings of KAROLA are presented: Analysis of cardiovascular risk factors showed that during in-patient rehab levels improve significantly. However, during the year following rehab these improvements are only partly sustained, highlighting the need for more effective maintenance of risk factor modification in subsequent outpatient care. Where risk factor modifications are maintained, they may have a large impact on prognosis. This is illustrated for smoking cessation, which leads to a major reduction of the risk of secondary cardiovascular disease events already within the first year after rehab.

CHRONIC INFECTION WITH *HELICOBACTER PYLORI* AND SYSTEMIC INFLAMMATORY RESPONSE UNDER CONSIDERATION OF THE INTERLEUKIN-1 RECEPTOR ANTAGONIST GENE POLYMORPHISM IN HEALTHY ADULTS

ZUMKELLER, NATALIA; KOENIG, WOLFGANG[1] HOFFMANN, MICHAEL H.[2]; KOLB, HUBERT[3]; BRENNER, HERMANN; ROTHENBACHER, DIETRICH
zumkeller@dzfa.uni-heidelberg.de
[1]*Department of Internal Medicine II-Cardiology, University of Ulm Medical Center, Ulm;* [2]*Department of Clinical Chemistry, University of Freiburg;* [3]*German Diabetic Clinic, Research Institute at the University of Düsseldorf*

Helicobacter pylori infection persists life long and in most cases causes chronic gastritis. Clinical sequels are peptic ulceration and gastric adenocarcinoma. It has been suggested that both, virulence factors of *H. pylori* and host polymorphisms determine the clinical outcome. We evaluated the combined effects of the interleukin-1 receptor antagonist (IL-1RA) gene polymorphism and *H. pylori* infection on markers of a systemic inflammatory response taking into account virulence markers of infection. 479 occasional blood donors of the University of Ulm blood donor centre, aged 40–68 years, were recruited in the context of a case-control study, conducted between October 1996 and November 1997. A linear regression method was employed to estimate the association of the seroprevalence of antibodies against *H. pylori*, its virulence factors (CagA, VacA) and IL-1RA gene polymorphism with serum concentrations of Interleukin (IL)-6, IL-8 and tumour-necrosis factors (TNF)-α (homozygosity for allele 2 (IL-1RN*2) vs. others). Serum concentrations of IL-6, IL-8 and TNF-α were not statistically significantly higher in subjects having antibodies against *H. pylori*, or more specifically against CagA and VacA, and being homozygous for the pro-inflammatory IL-1RN*2 allele compared to others after adjustment for covariates. Our results are consistent with previous indications that the pro-inflammatory effect of *H. pylori* infection may be restricted to the mucosal level only and extend these findings in that they indicate the absence of a systemic inflammatory response even in the presence of homozygosity for the pro-inflammatory IL-1RN*2 allele.